Treating Disordered Speech Motor Control

FOR CLINICIANS BY CLINICIANS
Deanie Vogel and Michael P. Cannito, Series Editors

This book, *Treating Disordered Speech Motor Control*, is the 12th book in the For Clinicians by Clinicians series of texts on the diagnosis and clinical management of speech, language, and voice disorders. Each text provides a contemporary perspective on one major disorder or clinical area and is designed for use in clinical methodology courses and continuing education programs. Authors have been selected who represent a broad spectrum of clinical interests and theoretical positions and who hold the common belief that their viewpoints, experiences, and successes should be shared in order to provide a forum for clinicians by clinicians.

The idea for this series came from Dr. Harris Winitz, who served as editor of the series until 1997. During Winitz's tenure as series editor, many important titles were added to the series, including the following volumes: *Treating Language Disorders, Treating Articulation Disorders, Case Studies in Aphasia Rehabilitation, Treating Cerebral Palsy, Alaryngeal Speech Rehabilitation, Treating Disordered Speech Motor Control, Cleft Palate,* and *Language Intervention: Beyond the Primary Grades.*

The last four additions to the series, *Aging and Communication, Alaryngeal Speech Rehabilitation, Evaluation of Dysphagia in Adults,* and this revision of *Treating Disordered Speech Motor Control,* have been guided by the new series co-editors, Deanie Vogel and Michael P. Cannito. Their intent is to continue the rich tradition of this important series that was established many years ago by Dr. Winitz.

Treating Disordered Speech Motor Control

For Clinicians by Clinicians

Second Edition

Edited by
Deanie Vogel
and
Michael P. Cannito

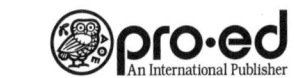

8700 Shoal Creek Boulevard
Austin, Texas 78757-6897
800/897-3202   Fax 800/397-7633
www.proedinc.com

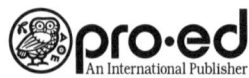
An International Publisher

© 2001, 1991 by PRO-ED, Inc.
8700 Shoal Creek Boulevard
Austin, Texas 78757-6897
800/897-3202   Fax 800/397-7633
www.proedinc.com

All rights reserved. No part of the material protected by this copyright notice may be reproduced or used in any form or by any means, electronic or mechanical, including photocopying, recording, or by any information storage and retrieval system, without prior written permission of the copyright owner.

Library of Congress Cataloging-in-Publication Data

Treating disordered speech motor control / edited by Deanie Vogel, Michael P. Cannito.—2nd ed.
    p.   cm.—(For clinicians by clinicians)
    Includes bibliographical references and index.
    ISBN 0-89079-869-9 (alk. paper)
    1. Language disorders. 2. Motor cortex. I. Vogel, Deanie. II. Cannito, Michael P. III. Series.
    [DNLM: 1. Speech Disorders—therapy. 2. Apraxia, Ideomotor—physiopathology. 3. Apraxia, Ideomotor—therapy. 4. Speech Disorders—physiopathology. WL 340.2 T784d 2001]
RC423.T72 2001
616.85'5—dc21
                                                            00-045874
                                                                     CIP

This book is designed in Palatino and Eras.

Printed in the United States of America

1 2 3 4 5 6 7 8 9 10   05 04 03 02 01

To Robin, for your courage and ability to love life in spite
of overwhelming circumstances,
and to Arnie

—DV

To my daughters, Caitlin and Tess, just for being you

—MPC

Contents

Contributors ▪ **ix**

Preface ▪ **xi**

1 Comanagement of Disordered Speech Motor Control: The Roles of the Neurologist and the Speech–Language Pathologist ▪ **1**
Robert Lozano

2 Pharmacologic Approaches to Speech Motor Disorders ▪ **27**
David B. Rosenfield

3 Dysarthria Evaluation and Treatment: The Basics ▪ **79**
Vicki L. Hammen

4 A Top-Down Approach to Treatment of Dysarthric Speech ▪ **119**
Deanie Vogel, Lynda Miller, and Jane Mertz Garcia

5 Dysarthria: A Breakdown in Interpersonal Communication ▪ **157**
Rosemary Lubinski

6 Phonological Encoding and Speech Programming: The Disorders of Paraphasias and Apraxia of Speech ▪ **195**
Robert S. Pierce

7 Nature and Management of Acquired Neurogenic Dysfluency ▪ **239**
Michael P. Cannito, Jon Deal, and Anthony DiLollo

8 Neurogenic Disorders of Prosody ▪ **277**
Samuel Amebu Seddoh and Donald A. Robin

9 Neurological Aspects of Spasmodic Dysphonia ▪ **321**
Michael P. Cannito

10 Noninvasive Instrumentation in the Treatment of Stuttering ▪ **377**
Ben C. Watson and Peter J. Alfonso

11 Developmental Apraxia of Speech: Advances in Theory and Practice ▪ **413**
Thomas P. Marquardt, Harvey M. Sussman, and Barbara L. Davis

Author Index ▪ **475**

Subject Index ▪ **485**

Contributors

Peter J. Alfonso, PhD
Haskins Laboratories
New Haven, CT 06501

Michael P. Cannito, PhD
School of Audiology and Speech–
 Language Pathology
University of Memphis
Memphis, TN 38105

Barbara Davis, PhD
Department of Communication
 Sciences and Disorders
University of Texas at Austin
Austin, TX 78712

Jon Deal, PhD
Audiology and Speech Pathology
 Service
Department of Veterans Affairs
 Medical Center
Columbia, MO 65201

Anthony DiLollo, MS
School of Audiology and Speech
 Pathology
University of Memphis
Memphis, TN 38105

Jane Mertz Garcia, PhD
Communication Sciences and
 Disorders, Family Studies &
 Human Services
Kansas State University
Manhattan, KS 66506-1403

Vicki Hammen, PhD
Arnette Clinic
Lafayette, IN 47904

Robert Lozano, MD, PhD
Private Practice
Brownsville, TX 78520

Rosemary Lubinski, PhD
Department of Communication
 Disorders and Sciences
University of Buffalo
Buffalo, NY 14214-3005

Thomas P. Marquardt, PhD
Department of Communication
 Sciences and Disorders
University of Texas at Austin
Austin, TX 78712

Lynda Miller, PhD
Smart Alternatives
Austin, TX 78704

Robert S. Pierce, PhD
School of Speech Pathology
 and Audiology
Kent State University
Kent, OH 44242

Donald A. Robin, PhD
Department of Communication
 Disorders
San Diego State University
San Diego, CA 92182

David B. Rosenfield, MD
Stuttering Center and Speech Motor
    Control Laboratory
Department of Neurology
Baylor College of Medicine
Houston, TX 77030

Samuel Amebu Seddoh, PhD
Department of Speech Pathology
    and Audiology
Southern University
Baton Rouge, LA 70813

Harvey M. Sussman, PhD
Department of Linguistics
Department of Communication
    Sciences and Disorders
University of Texas at Austin
Austin, TX 78712

Deanie Vogel, PhD
Communication Disorders Program,
    Our Lady of the Lake University
Department of Medicine, Division
    of Neurology
The University of Texas Health
    Science Center
San Antonio, TX 78207

Ben C. Watson, PhD
Department of Otolaryngology,
    Division of Research
New York Medical College
Vahalla, NY 10595

Preface

This book about neuromotor disturbances of speech production is the second edition of the volume published in 1991. The book's purposes are (a) to look at the phenomena in question somewhat more broadly than is typical for books about motor speech disorders, (b) to provide an update of some issues in disordered speech motor control, and (c) to integrate recent clinical information from various disciplines, particularly speech–language pathology and neurology. It is not our intent to provide a comprehensive textbook on normal and disordered speech neurophysiology. This book is aimed primarily at the practicing professional readership; thus much of the material contained herein is technical and specialized. It should also be quite useful, however, to advanced graduate students in the area of neuropathologies of communication, perhaps as supplemental reading material to a more basic text.

The term *speech motor control* in the title of this book is used to refer to a quite broad process that includes premovement organization as well as motoric execution and modulation; in our view, without organization there can be no control. As a consequence of this orientation, we have included substantial content not only from the phonological domain of language, but from the affective and pragmatic arenas as well.

A number of content themes underlie and link the various chapters in this volume. For example, in Chapter 2, in addition to discussing the underlying causes of specific disorders of speech motor control and the effects of pharmacology on speech disorders, Rosenfield reviews neuroanatomy and neurophysiology. Cannito expands on this review in Chapter 9, in his description of spasmodic dysphonia.

An additional theme, *assessment*, is addressed by Hammen in Chapter 3—a new chapter in this second edition. Hammen discusses assessment of dysarthria using a variety of clinical measures. Other assessment procedures are introduced in Chapter 1 by Lozano and in Chapter 6 by Pierce. Lozano, a speech–language pathologist and a neurologist, describes assessment of the patient with disordered speech motor control from the viewpoint of both professions. Pierce, from a psycholinguist perspective, writes of assessment procedures that can be used to differentiate apraxia of speech from phonemic paraphasias. In Chapter 10, Watson and Alfonso describe their work in assessment by means of instrumentation.

Therapeutics is another frequently occurring content theme in this text. In Chapters 3–8, 10, and 11, contributors offer treatment suggestions. Hammen presents basic treatments for dysarthria, and Vogel, Miller, and Garcia describe a "top-down," communication-oriented approach to the treatment of dysarthric speech. Lubinski writes of the roles that the dysarthric patient, the family, and the speech–language pathologist play in the therapeutic process. Pierce offers descriptions of treatment programs designed to remediate apraxia of speech or to decrease or eliminate phonemic paraphasia. Cannito, Deal, and DiLollo outline general schema within which to approach treatment of neurogenic dysfluency. Seddoh and Robin focus on treatment of disordered prosody; Marquardt, Sussman, and Davis suggest methods for treating developmental apraxia of speech. Each of these chapters is supported with literature reviews and extensive case study material.

Two additional content themes in this volume are *neuromotor dysfunction* and *communication*. In Chapter 2, Rosenfield discusses neuromotor disorders in general, while in Chapter 9, Cannito writes of neuromotor dysfunction in spasmodic dysphonia. Watson and Alfonso, in Chapter 10, discuss the use of instrumentation in cases of neuromotor dysfunction. In Chapter 7, Deal, Cannito, and DiLollo concentrate on neuromotor dysfunction in neurogenic dysfluency. Focusing on the communication process in Chapter 4, Vogel, Miller, and Garcia offer an approach to improve the dysarthric patient's overall communicative ability, and Lubinski, in Chapter 5, suggests how families can improve their communication with the dysarthric patient. In Chapter 1, Lozano presents his views on communication from a slightly different perspective by offering suggestions for clearer communication between speech–language pathologists and physicians.

The editors wish to acknowledge the contributions of James Patton and other members of the staff at PRO-ED. Their wise suggestions and their cooperation in producing this second edition in particular, and the entire For Clinicians by Clinicians series in general, are much appreciated.

Chapter 1

Comanagement of Disordered Speech Motor Control: The Roles of the Neurologist and the Speech–Language Pathologist

Robert Lozano

Lozano, a speech–language pathologist who became a neurologist, discusses patient management from the point of view of each discipline and outlines assessment and treatment procedures conducted by the professionals from both areas. Finally, he underscores the need for cooperation between professionals from each discipline in order to provide the best care available for the communicatively impaired patient.

1. What is the most important part of the neurologic examination?
2. How does the speech–language pathologist's approach differ from the neurologist's approach to patient management?
3. Which skills did Lozano find easy to transfer from speech–language pathology to medical practice?

※　※　※

As I rounded the corner to enter the hospital room, I could hear my next patient before I could see him. He was complaining to his roommate that he wished he had never mentioned "it" because now more doctors would be coming to see him and probably they would "do more tests." "It" was a momentary visual blurring that occurred as he was walking and turning around, and "it" was the reason I was consulted. I had not seen the patient yet, but already I knew from hearing him speak that his neurologic examination would be abnormal. His speech was marked by prominent ataxic dysarthria with monopitch, an occasional pitch break, and an explosive quality. I could hear the dysmetria in his articulation; I had learned to recognize it when I was a speech–language pathologist.

It was extremely flattering to be asked to write a chapter for this book. "We want you to contribute because of your unique perspective," I was told. I suppose the foundation of my "uniqueness" was laid when I completed my master's degree in speech pathology, entered the doctoral program at Wayne State University, and was awarded a traineeship in speech pathology at the Allen Park, Michigan, Veterans Administration Medical Center. There I developed an interest in the acquired speech and language disorders of neurologically impaired adults. Later, I received my Certificate of Clinical Competence in Speech Pathology from the American Speech-Language-Hearing Association (ASHA).

Still later, I completed my PhD degree in speech pathology and became the director of speech and language pathology at the Rehabilitation Institute in Detroit, Michigan. For a while, things were going pretty well. Then, for various reasons, I left the Institute and went to medical school. I received my medical degree from Michigan State University and completed a year of residency in internal medicine. Then I finished a 3-year residency in neurology at the University of Texas Health Science Center in San Antonio and started private practice in Texas.

If I am unique, I suppose it is because of my experience on both sides of the street. I was a clinical speech–language pathologist working with communication disorders of neurologically impaired adults, and then I became a physician diagnosing and treating neurologic illnesses of which aphasia or dysarthria may be a symptom or a sign.

When I made the transition from speech–language pathology to medicine, one speech–language pathologist friend of mine dubbed me a "defector." What gave that endearing nickname meaning was the sense of friendly rivalry and competition that may exist between speech–language pathology and neurology. I had gone over to the other side. But rather than experiencing defection, I feel more like a person who has undergone a personal evolution, one that began in speech–language pathology and continued to grow in neurology. For me, the two professions represent different points on the same continuum. Caring for the patient is the desire of both professions. Of course there are differences as well as similarities in the two professions, and I will discuss a number of them in this chapter.

Preparation

Academic Preparation

The academic preparation for speech–language pathology is slightly different from the academic background needed for medicine. In speech–language pathology, there is an undergraduate core curriculum designed to prepare the student for the graduate courses necessary to obtain the master's degree, certification by ASHA, and state licensure. Academic courses are required in areas such as anatomy of the speech and hearing mechanism, neuroanatomy, speech physiology, acoustics, phonetics, linguistics, psychology, and psycholinguistics. In some states in the United States, persons with an undergraduate degree in speech–language pathology can provide services as assistants under the supervision of a licensed speech–language pathologist who has completed a master's degree. At this time, the bulk of services provided in this way is in the schools.

The doctorate in speech–language pathology is, basically, a science degree. At the present time there is no clinical doctorate. To pursue the doctorate is a personal decision; the doctoral degree is not a requirement for certification or state licensure.

The traditional undergraduate preparation for medicine includes courses in biology, general chemistry, organic chemistry, physics, physiology, and biochemistry. In part, some medical schools want a measure of how well an individual is able to handle several science classes simultaneously. Medical schools accept students with a variety of undergraduate majors so long as the student has completed the prerequisite science classes satisfactorily and so long as the school feels that the candidate will make a valuable contribution as part of that particular medical school's class. It seems, however, that students with a major in science are preferred by committees selecting candidates for medical school.

Clinical Preparation

Clinical training in speech–language pathology may begin at the undergraduate level, and it is an integral part of the graduate curriculum. Supervised clinical practica in a range of speech, language, voice, and hearing disorders are required. In most medical schools, the medical student enters the clinical practicum years after spending 2 years studying basic science (e.g., microbiology, pharmacology, pathology, physiology). During the third and fourth years of medical school, the student enrolls in courses in internal medicine, pediatrics, psychiatry, obstetrics–gynecology, and surgery. Here the abstract of classroom science merges with the reality of the sickness, disease, and pestilence found in the clinic–hospital setting.

In almost every state in the United States, a physician must undergo at least one year of postgraduate training before becoming licensed. The trend in American medicine has been for the recent medical graduate to select a multiyear training program in a specific area of medicine, for example, in internal medicine, obstetrics–gynecology, family medicine, or pediatrics. At least a year of internal medicine or its equivalent must be completed prior to entering a 3-year neurology residency. Postgraduate medical training is vigorous and includes long periods of being on call, during which the resident may have a continuous work period of 30 hours or more.

In speech–language pathology, after completing a graduate program, the student must undergo a supervised work experience during the clinical fellowship year (CFY). The specialization that occurs in speech–language pathology depends not only on the student's academic training program but also depends heavily on the type of workplace the student selects to complete the CFY. School-based speech–language pathologists develop more experience and expertise in articulation disorders and language delay, whereas those who are medically based learn more about neurogenic communication disorders such as aphasia and dysarthria as well as swallowing disorders. Speech–language pathology specialization then is driven by the experiences of the individual clinician.

I think speech–language pathologists know more about what neurologists do than vice versa. Usually, the speech–language pathologist must educate the physician regarding the benefits of speech and language therapy for the patient with a communication disorder. This is necessary so that physicians will make the appropriate patient referrals. Speech–language pathologists should remember that they offer important and beneficial services to patients and that they need to communicate this fact to physicians. Speech–language pathologists should also be aware that physicians also do their share of educating. For example, a physician arriving at a hospital for the first time must make the existing medical staff aware of what the physician can do for the patients at that facility.

I believe my experiences in speech–language pathology have been extremely valuable to me as a physician. There are a number of skills that I learned as a speech–language pathologist that I continue to use as a neurologist. For example, the interviewing skills I used as a speech–language pathologist transferred easily to my medical practice. And listening skills are crucial in both speech–language pathology and medicine. Listening to the patient and caring about those things that are important to the patient are the most valuable skills any health care provider can possess. The ability to observe patient behavior critically is a skill learned by speech–language pathologists and used extensively by neurologists. I learned to appreciate how an illness or disability affects the patient and the patient's position in the family and in society during the years I was a speech–language pathologist. From the perspective of seeing patients as people, compassion for others may grow. As a speech–language pathologist, I learned to set aside the goals of a treatment session to comfort a distraught patient.

The Neurologist's Approach to Patient Management

For the neurologist, the knowledge of the anatomy, physiology, and pathophysiology of the nervous system provides the conceptual framework for problem solving. Each patient presents a unique set of circumstances and complaints that is dissected by careful history taking. The neurologist's goals are to provide answers to the questions, Where is the lesion? and What is the nature of the lesion? After the diagnosis is made, appropriate treatment can begin or the appropriate referral can be made.

The History

The history is the most important part of the neurologic evaluation. While the history is taken, the neurologist forms a set of hypothetical diagnoses. With selected follow-up questions, each hypothetical diagnosis is tested and ranked according to the likelihood of its occurrence. This has been referred to as "hypothesis-driven" history taking. Information is gathered on essential basic factors, including the age and sex of the patient, onset of the problem, progression of symptoms, duration and course of the problem, and predisposing conditions. This information is used by the neurologist to decide the level of the nervous system at which the lesion is located and the disease process most likely involved.

Neurologic Examination

The *neurologic examination* provides a detailed evaluation of the integrity of the nervous system. Generally, the complete neurologic examination consists of an evaluation of the patient's mental status, cranial nerves, motor system, sensory system, and gait. The *mental status examination* tests alertness, orientation, attention, memory, and speech and language functions. This examination may include determining if the patient is aware of the time, date, and place of the examination and asking the patient to do mathematical calculations, interpret proverbs, and solve hypothetical problems such as, What would you do if you smelled smoke in a crowded theater? The *cranial nerve examination* involves evaluation of the function of nerves with nuclei located above the spinal cord. The cranial nerves important to speech motor control, their functions, and methods for testing them are listed in Table 1.1.

An *evaluation of the motor system* includes noting appearance of the muscles and an examination of muscle tone and strength. Some neurologists include coordination and deep tendon reflex testing in their evaluation of the motor system. Passive movements are evaluated while moving the patient's limb as the patient maintains the limb in a state of relaxation. Active movements are evaluated as the patient carries out movements described by the examiner.

Sensory system testing involves assessing temperature, pain, light touch, vibration, and proprioception throughout the body. The examiner may pinch the patient's muscles or press on structures that are

Table 1.1
Cranial Nerves Involved in Speech Motor Control

Cranial Nerve	Function	Method of Evaluating
V. Trigeminal	Sensation from masseters, palate, and pharynx	With a pin, examiner pricks patient's face first on one side, then the other. Examiner asks patient to identify location of pinprick.
	Motor to mandibular muscles	Patient asked to simulate a bite while examiner attempts to pry patient's jaw apart. Examiner checks for jaw weakness.
		Patient relaxes and opens jaw slightly. Examiner taps on patient's jaw to test for jaw-jerk.
VII. Facial	Sensation from anterior tongue; motor to face	Examiner observes patient's face for movement, tics, tremors. Asks patient to wrinkle forehead and look upward. Patient puffs out cheeks. Examiner squeezes cheeks in to force expulsion of air.
IX. Glosso-pharyngeal	Sensation from posterior tongue	While patient phonates, examiner observes elevation of palate and contraction of pharyngeal wall.
X. Vagus	Motor to larynx, pharynx, and soft palate	Examiner assesses phonatory capabilities while patient phonates.
XII. Hypoglossal	Motor to tongue	Patient presses tongue to inside of right, then left cheek while examiner palpates from outside.
		Patient protrudes and retracts tongue as rapidly as possible. Examiner checks for alternate motion rate.
		Patient moves tongue from side to side as rapidly as possible. Examiner checks for lateralization and rate.

sensitive to pressure, for example, the larynx. Or, the examiner may test the ability to identify light touch as the patient's skin is stroked or touched with a light pinprick. Gait and station are also tested as the patient performs a number of standing and walking exercises.

There are several branching steps that can be included in the neurological examination. These steps are used to evaluate a possible abnormality further or to define better the level in the nervous system at which a dysfunction may be present. Specific maneuvers are used to elicit pathologic signs, many of which have been named for dead neurologists. For example, when stroking the lateral aspect of the sole of the patient's foot, the examining neurologist is attempting to observe whether the patient's big toe moves up or down. An upward moving toe (*dorsoflexion*) is a pathologic sign of an upper motor neuron lesion affecting that extremity and is referred to as the *Babinski reflex*. Because a further description of the clinical neurological examination is beyond the scope of this volume, the interested reader is encouraged to consult Brookshire (1997) or Duffy (1995) for more information on this topic.

As a speech–language pathologist, I was never favorably impressed with the speech and language evaluations conducted by a neurologist. I found these evaluations to be too brief and lacking in depth and detail. Please spare me, "Say Methodist–Episcopal"! Yet as a neurologist, I found myself thinking how long, detailed, and burdensome are the evaluations conducted by the speech–language pathologist. Please spare me, "Say pa/ta/ka"! The point here is that the speech evaluation serves a different function for each discipline. The neurologist is conducting a screening of speech functions, looking for errors that will confirm the suspicion of a lesion. Speech and language screening is just a portion of a complete neurologic examination. The speech–language pathologist's evaluation, on the other hand, involves taking an inventory of communication skills, analyzing errors, and forming a basis for diagnosing and treating the patient's communication disorder. Of course, within the current climate of health care and with demands from third-party payers, speech–language pathologists are compelled to conduct their evaluations in much less time than before.

In general, there should be no real surprises during the neurologic exam. Examination results should confirm the verbal hypotheses formed during the history taking. If the examination results do not fit the hypotheses formed from the existing history, further information must be obtained.

Neurologic Diagnosis

The neurologist who conceptually applies the neuroanatomical grid to the results of the patient's history and neurological examination is attempting to answer the question, What is the lesion? To answer the question, Where is the lesion? the neurologist references the probable location of the lesion against those neuropathologic processes that can occur at that site. The possible etiologies arising from this cross-referencing are the differential diagnoses of the patient's problem.

Neurologists relish differential diagnoses. A *differential* is a list of the possible diagnoses that may account for the patient's neurologic condition. The spectrum of etiologies of a particular condition are held up for scrutiny. For example, the neurologist considers the question, Is the patient's neurologic deficit compatible with dysfunction caused by tumor, ischemia, degenerative processes, infection, or metabolic dysfunction? In a sense, the neurologist approaches the patient's problem as a marvelous intellectual puzzle that can be solved with information from the history; knowledge of neuroanatomy, neurophysiology, and neuropathology; logic; and confirmation from the results of the neurologic examination. Typically the level of the lesion is determined first, and then the neurologist speculates about which disease processes are present at that location. In neurology circles, great accolades are given to those neurologists who can produce a range of possible diagnoses. Although the list should be complete and include uncommon diseases, emphasis should be placed on typical presentations of common diseases. There is a saying among neurologists in South Texas that goes, "When you're out on the ranch and you hear hoofbeats, the first thing you think of should not be zebras." Some neurologic causes of and, therefore, diagnoses that may be considered in conditions producing disordered speech motor control are listed in Table 1.2.

Laboratory Tests

Once the differential diagnoses have been determined, additional laboratory tests may be ordered. Needed information may come from blood analysis, examination of the cerebrospinal fluid, neurologic electrophysiology evaluations, and special imaging procedures. The

Table 1.2
Common Underlying Neurologic Causes
of Disordered Speech Motor Control

Myasthenia gravis

Eaton-Lambert syndrome

Parkinson's disease

Progressive supranuclear palsy

Olivopontocerebellar degeneration

Alzheimer's disease

Multiple sclerosis

Encephalopathies—toxic-metabolic, progressive multifocal leukoencephalopathy

Cerebellar degeneration—idiopathic, toxic

Amyotrophic lateral sclerosis

Wilson's disease

Huntington's disease

Tourette's syndrome

Thyroid disease

Parathyroid disease

Ischemia

Stroke

Tumors—carcinoma (primary, metastatic)

Encephalitis

Meningitis

Lues

Jacob-Creutzfeldt disease

Trauma—traumatic brain injury

Toxins—alcohol, lead, mercury, drugs

Cerebral palsy

Metabolic derangements—hyponatremia, hypokalemia, hypoglycemia, vitamin deficiencies

---

added information is obtained in order to exclude some diagnoses and to support the most likely one. The choice of laboratory tests selected is based on information regarding the suspected disease and the pathologic findings.

Many tests are performed so frequently that they are considered routine; the *complete blood count* (CBC) is an example. The CBC provides the physician with a quantitative and qualitative analysis of the patient's blood. The number of *leukocytes*, or *white blood cells* (WBCs), will increase with infection and stress. The differentiation of WBCs into types is also helpful in diagnosis. The number of *red blood cells* (RBCs) provides a measure of the body's ability to produce blood cells and also is used to identify the presence of anemia. Further hematologic measures can provide information regarding the amount of *hemoglobin* (the oxygen-carrying component in the RBCs) and the *hematocrit* (the percentage of RBC mass compared to the blood volume). The average size of the RBCs is referred to as the *mean corpuscular volume* (MCV). Increased MCVs are detected in certain disease states.

The CBC can yield important information. For example, a patient who had undergone stomach surgery several years previously developed difficulty walking and dysarthric speech. A CBC revealed a normal WBC and decreased numbers of RBCs with decreased hemoglobin and hematocrit; MCV was enlarged. Based on the results of the CBC, together with the patient's history of stomach surgery, the physician decided to check the patient's vitamin B12 level and review the patient's history of alcohol intake, which could affect B12 levels. The physician reasoned that the previous surgery had resulted in impaired vitamin B12 absorption, and that the patient was suffering neuronal damage secondary to vitamin B12 deficiency. That was a possible cause of the patient's walking and speech difficulties.

Metabolic screening is another frequently ordered laboratory test. This procedure varies from community to community and is based on the capability of the laboratory equipment available in a particular locale. The following example illustrates how the metabolic screen was helpful in treating an elderly person who was taking oral hypoglycemic medication for diabetes. The patient was brought into the emergency room of a local hospital after developing slurred speech and confusion. As part of a metabolic screen, the patient's serum glucose was checked and was found to be abnormally low. After adjustment of the glucose level, the patient's speech and mental functioning returned to normal.

There are patients for whom special blood studies may be indicated. For example, *Wilson's disease* is a familial metabolic disorder with abnormal copper metabolism that produces deposits of copper and consequent degeneration of the liver and basal ganglia. Dysarthria is a common consequence of Wilson's disease. It is important to check serum ceruloplasmin (a transport protein for copper) and serum copper levels in a patient for whom Wilson's disease is suspected.

Examination of the *cerebrospinal fluid* (CSF) may be necessary in some cases. Essential examination of CSF must include cell count and differential glucose and protein. The cells are identified and quantified. The specific findings in the CSF may be very important for the confirmation of the proposed diagnosis. Increased WBCs in the CSF may signal infection. An excessive number of RBCs in the CSF may indicate the presence of a subarachnoid hemorrhage. Glucose is actively transported in the CSF. An abnormally low CSF glucose level often is indicative of inflamed meninges. In classic tuberculosis meningitis, the CSF glucose is extremely low, and central nervous system syphilis is often revealed by hundreds of WBCs in the CSF with a predominance of lymphocytes. So it becomes obvious that the specific findings in the CSF may be very important for the confirmation of the proposed diagnosis.

Depending on the anticipated diagnosis, additional special tests on the CSF may be needed. For example, in suspected multiple sclerosis, most neurologists would request the determination of gamma immunoglobins (IgG) for evidence of increased levels. In such patients, examination of the CSF with electrophoresis may reveal the presence of oligoclonal bands that tend to support the diagnosis of multiple sclerosis.

Special imaging techniques are very useful for diagnosis. In multiple sclerosis, *magnetic resonance imaging* (MRI) has been extremely useful in detecting white matter plaques. MRI also has been helpful in demonstrating the presence of occult tumors. *Computerized tomography* (CT) has contributed to the confirmation of the diagnosis of stroke, hemorrhage, and tumor. Examples of MRI and CT scans of patients who exhibited disordered speech motor control are shown in Figures 1.1 and 1.2.

Specific electrophysiologic studies may be required for patients with neuromuscular disorders. *Nerve conduction velocities* (NCV) and *electromyography* (EMG) may be used in diagnosis. The recording of

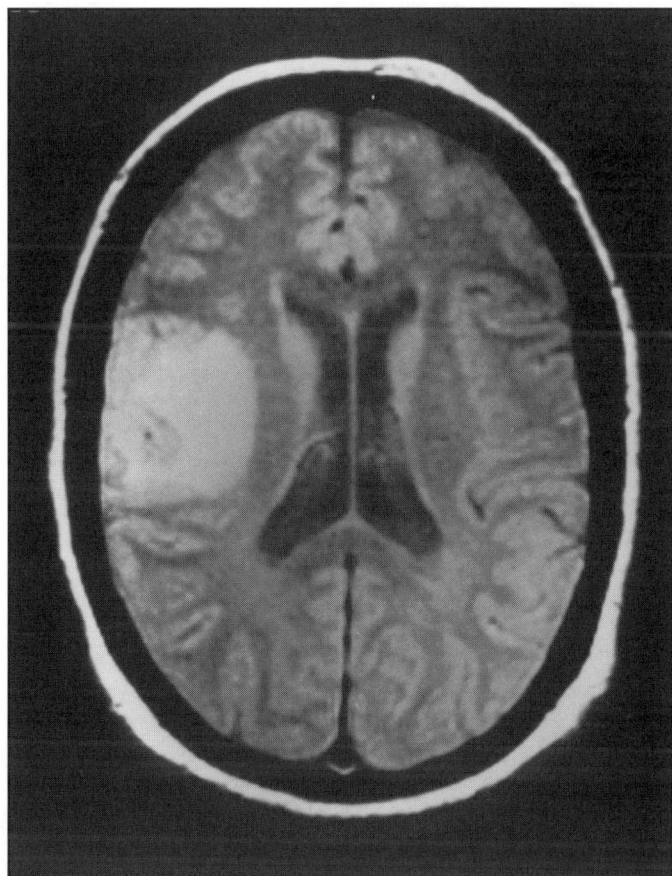

Figure 1.1. Head MRI, T1 image. A 53-year-old female with a history of breast cancer presented with seizure, mild left facial palsy, and mild dysarthria. Diagnosis: Single metastatic tumor in right hemisphere.

muscle fasciculations and denervation potentials may substantiate denervation changes found in amyotrophic lateral sclerosis (ALS). A biopsy of muscles may be needed to determine correct neuromuscular diagnosis.

Treatment

For the neurologist, arriving at a diagnosis may be easier than selecting the most effective treatment. There can be a wide range of acceptable

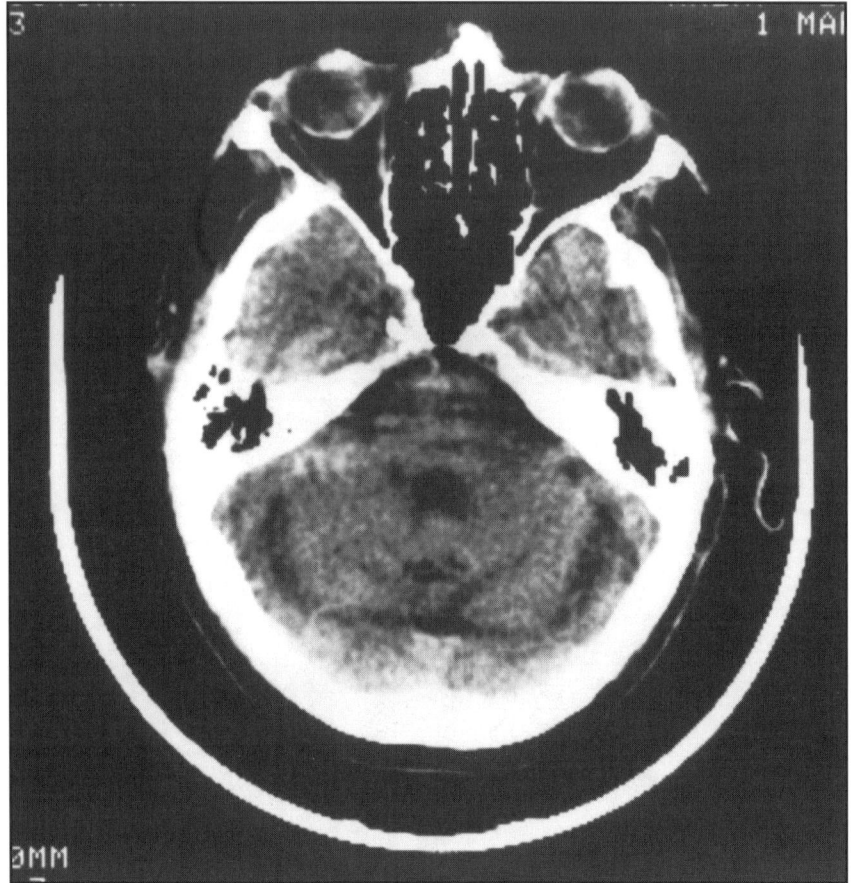

Figure 1.2. CT-scan image. A 65-year-old male with long-standing gait ataxia, extremity dysmetria, and ataxic dysarthria. Diagnosis: Marked cerebellar atrophy, possible cerebellar stroke.

medical therapies for some disorders, due in part to the seemingly continuous introduction of new therapeutics. This is highly praised by some as medical progress. Sometimes, when a new medication or surgery is found to be efficacious for treating a certain disease, the news appears in the popular press and public interest is aroused. If the new cure is not available in the United States due to restrictions set by the Food and Drug Administration (FDA), for example, some patients will travel to countries outside the United States where they can obtain the cure. In reality, these new cures may not be any more effective than the existing "tried and true" therapies that, because of their easy availability, may also be less expensive. As a rule, the experimental trials comparing one therapy with another lag long behind the excitement generated by the popular press. To be sure, new instrumentation and treatment programs become available in speech–language pathology that improve the quality of a patient's life. In medicine, new treatment programs—if effective—can extend that life.

Typically, the physician begins the patient on a therapeutic trial of medication or refers the patient for another type of therapy or for surgery. The neurologist makes adjustments to the treatment regime pragmatically, based on the success or failure of the current treatment. Usually a neurologist who refers a patient to a speech–language pathologist has identified the patient's neurologic problem and the referral is part of an overall treatment plan. Most neurologists categorize the speech–language pathologist as an allied health professional just as they would categorize the physical or occupational therapist. These professionals are considered by the physician to be members of the rehabilitation team.

Referral to a Speech–Language Pathologist

A consultation request from the neurologist to the speech–language pathologist may read: "Patient had stroke, has slurred speech; please evaluate and treat." Now the patient has been placed in the care of the speech–language pathologist for the remediation of the communication disorder. The speech–language pathologist has been trained to take the history of the patient's communication impairment, to select the appropriate diagnostic measures, and to design and carry out the plan for the treatment of the disorder. I have found that many neurologists have no idea that speech–language pathologists have a master's level education, that there exists a national organization with criteria for certification of speech–language pathologists, and that in most states speech–language pathologists must be licensed to practice. A neurologist who has a patient with a communication disorder for which there is no effective medical therapy hopes that the speech–language pathologist can improve the patient's ability to communicate and, therefore, improve the quality of the patient's life.

The efficacy of speech–language therapy has been questioned by some physicians. As a speech–language pathologist, at times I felt there were hordes of demonic physicians roaming the countryside chanting, "Why bother with speech therapy? It doesn't work!" Despite evidence that speech therapy for neurogenic communication disorders *does* work (Aftonomos, Appelbaum, & Steel, 1999; Albert, 1998; Dworkin, Abkarian, & Johns, 1988; Elman & Bernstein-Ellis, 1998; Ramig, 1998; Robey, 1998; Vogel, Cannito, Salvatore, & Marquardt, 1998; Wertz et al., 1981, 1986) even at this time, some neurologists question its efficacy. This "no benefit" attitude also has been helped to be dispelled by the fact that third-party payers have recognized the benefit of speech–language therapy and have offered reimbursement for the services of a speech–language pathologist.

It is my hunch that the assumption that speech or language therapy does not work is based in part on the speech and language examination conducted by the neurologist. The typical neurologist—that is, one who does not have a special interest in higher cortical functioning in general or in speech and language in particular—evaluates the patient's speech and language only for the purpose of determining the presence of aphasia versus dementia or confused mental state. The neurologist usually makes a modest effort to classify the type of aphasia for anatomic correlation, then refers the patient to a speech–language pathologist for a thorough evaluation and subsequent treatment for the communication disorder. Eventually the patient returns to the neurologist, who reevaluates the communication disorder and determines whether residual speech or language impairment is present. Usually it is. Although the patient's speech intelligibility and language skills may have improved with therapy, residual speech or language impairment may persist. The presence of this residual deficit may account for the neurologist's skepticism.

I believe that almost all patients who have a speech or language problem secondary to neurologic impairment should be evaluated by a speech–language pathologist. I also believe that a competent speech–language pathologist can decide who may and who may not benefit from a trial of treatment; furthermore, not all patients need speech–language therapy. There are some who will achieve good recovery without intervention, and there are some who will never be capable of effective communication. It is also important to recognize that not all patients want speech–language services. Time is most effectively spent with patients who are motivated. Rather than treatment, a reevaluation at a later time is appropriate for some patients. Just as physicians are skeptical of referring patients to surgeons who always recommend a specific operation, they tend to be somewhat wary of referring a patient to a speech–language pathologist who recommends therapy for all patients regardless of how dismal the prospects for a successful outcome may be. Certainly, recent changes in health care reimbursement have affected this decision.

The Speech–Language Pathologist's Approach to Patient Management

Diagnosis and Treatment

Although I believe this is happening much less frequently now than previously, some patients who arrive for a speech and language evaluation do not know just why they are there. Often a patient will express great relief upon meeting a professional whose purpose is to focus on remediation of the communication disorder. During the initial interview, when obtaining information about the patient's background, the speech–language pathologist also gathers a spontaneous speech and language sample and estimates the patient's mental status and ability to comprehend verbal messages. The speech–language pathologist is concerned with answers to the questions, Does the patient have a communication disorder? What are the patient's residual capabilities? and How can I facilitate the improvement of the patient's communication skills? To answer these questions, the speech–language pathologist conducts a diagnostic assessment.

The speech–language pathologist selects diagnostic instruments to establish and record the patient's communicative abilities. In the formal evaluation, standardized procedures are employed for obtaining samples of the patient's speech and for scoring those samples. The formal speech and language evaluation administered by the speech–language pathologist is more detailed and quantifiable than the speech and language screening examination administered by the neurologist.

After the assessment, the communication disorder is classified. It is interesting that there appear to be "lumpers" and "splitters" among both neurologists and speech–language pathologists. Many neurologists tend to split language disorders—that is, *aphasia*—into groups by type while lumping speech disorders—that is, *dysarthria*—together. Speech–language pathologists, on the other hand, may lump aphasia while splitting dysarthria into groups by patterns of characteristics. Tables 1.3 and 1.4 list dysarthria types and aphasia syndromes.

Once the level of residual function has been determined, the speech–language pathologist can design a treatment program to facil-

Table 1.3
Dysarthria Types and Their Highest Ranked Symptoms

Dysarthria Type	Highest Ranked Symptoms
Flaccid	Hypernasality Imprecise consonants Breathiness
Spastic	Imprecise consonants Monopitch Reduced stress
Ataxic	Imprecise consonants Excess and equal stress Irregular articulatory breakdown
Hypokinetic	Monopitch Reduced stress Monoloudness
Hyperkinetic (Chorea)	Imprecise consonants Prolonged intervals Variable rate
Hyperkinetic (Dystonia)	Imprecise consonants Distorted vowels Harsh voice quality
Mixed (ALS)	Imprecise consonants Hypernasality Harsh voice quality
Mixed (MS)	Impaired loudness control Harsh voice quality Defective articulation
Mixed (Wilson's disease)	Monopitch Monoloudness Reduced stress

Note. Adapted from *Motor-Speech Disorders*, by F. L. Darley, A. E. Aronson, and J. R. Brown, 1975, Philadelphia: Saunders. Copyright 1975 by W. B. Saunders Company. Adapted with permission.

Table 1.4
Classifications of Aphasia Syndromes

Type	Task	Symptoms
Broca's	Spoken discourse Auditory language comprehension Sentence repetition	Nonfluent speech Relatively normal Abnormal
Global	Spoken discourse Auditory language comprehension Sentence repetition	Nonfluent speech Poor Poor
Transcortical Motor	Spoken discourse Auditory language comprehension Sentence repetition	Nonfluent speech Relatively normal Relatively normal
Mixed Transcortical	Spoken discourse Auditory language comprehension Sentence repetition	Nonfluent speech Abnormal Relatively normal
Wernicke's	Spoken discourse Auditory language comprehension Sentence repetition	Fluent speech* Poor Poor
Conduction	Spoken discourse Auditory language comprehension Sentence repetition	Fluent speech* Relatively normal Poor
Transcortical Sensory	Spoken discourse Auditory language comprehension Sentence repetition	Fluent speech* Poor Relatively normal
Anomic	Spoken discourse Auditory language comprehension Sentence repetition	Fluent speech Relatively normal Relatively normal

*Although output is fluent, it is paraphasic and may contain low information content.

itate improvement of communication. Most therapy for neurologically based speech disorders involves providing stimulation and teaching compensatory strategies. The patient's residual communicative strengths can be used to improve impaired communication skills. The structuring of individualized treatment is not a trivial task. The best speech–language clinicians are those who are resourceful and imaginative in designing treatment programs.

In summary, neurologists have a "disease-state" orientation to patient management. They obtain a history and conduct an examination to discover features of dysfunction as evidence of lesions in the patient's nervous system. They then attempt to localize and determine the etiology of the lesion, and this information aids them in making decisions regarding which treatment to recommend.

The speech–language pathologist's approach to management of the patient with a neurogenic motor speech disorder is a functional one. The clinician must determine not only what the patient cannot do but also what the patient can do. After determining a patient's communicative strengths and weaknesses, speech–language pathologists design treatment programs using the strengths to improve the weaknesses. The goal is to restore speech intelligibility to a level as near to premorbid ability as is possible. If effective verbal communication cannot be restored, the patient must be instructed in how to use augmentative and alternative methods of communication.

Case Studies

In this section, two patients with neurologically based speech disorders will be described. In the first case, the speech–language pathologist was an integral part of the patient's management plan.

 CASE 1

One night while at a party, I was approached by the wife of an attorney who knew I was both a physician and a speech–language pathologist. This lady wanted me to meet her husband, a 28-year-old attorney who had no significant past medical history but who recently had been experiencing some speech difficulties. When I met him, I noted that his speech was slow and labored. He told me that people were beginning to notice that he "sounded different" and that often he was asked if he had a cold. He was especially concerned because his profession demanded good communication skills.

The attorney told me that he had been feeling weak and that, lately, both of his hands had become clumsy. In addition, he reported that occasionally he felt as if fluid was beginning to regurgitate through his nose. As I listened to him, I noted that his speech was slow and deliberate with a suggestion of mild hypernasality and mild imprecise articulation. I recommended that he consult a neurologist and a speech–language pathologist.

Results of the neurological evaluation revealed weakness and fasciculations in his extremities and the presence of mild spasticity and hyperreflexia (exaggeration of the deep tendon reflexes). Sensation was intact.

The patient exhibited no higher cortical dysfunction, but he did have inadequate velopharyngeal closure and slowed tongue movements, which are evidence of cranial nerve motor impairments. His mild spasticity and increased deep tendon reflexes were signs of upper motor neuron dysfunction, whereas the fasciculations that were evident were indicative of lower motor neuron disease. There were signs of mixed upper and lower motor neuron lesions at the level of and below the medulla.

When a neurologist is confronted with this constellation of symptoms and signs, he must include motor neuron disease in the differential diagnosis. Treatable causes of motor system dysfunction, such as thyroid disease and heavy metal poisoning, must be considered and ruled out. Other possible causes of similar dysfunction include bulbar-cervical spinal cord diseases such as bulbomyelia. Tumor and multiple sclerosis must be considered, as well.

Laboratory tests and neuroimaging were ordered. Electromyography supported the clinical suspicion of denervation changes. Blood chemistry and special tests were not diagnostic. Imaging did not reveal a tumor or changes consistent with structural pathology. A presumptive diagnosis of amyotrophic lateral sclerosis (ALS), a progressive, devastating and, to date, incurable disease was made.

Results of the speech evaluation revealed a severe dysarthria. Initially, treatment for the speech impairment focused on tongue strengthening exercises, but, as the patient's condition gradually worsened, the focus of therapy was changed to control of speech rate. Eventually, despite the patient's efforts to talk, he could no longer use verbal communication effectively and an electronic communication board with a printer was introduced. Unfortunately, his communication remained severely impaired.

The patient experienced progressive deterioration of strength throughout his body. He lost his job. He became wheelchair bound. Swallowing became increasingly difficult for him. After several years of debilitation and emotional distress, the patient died.

The neurologist's role in the management of this patient was to establish the correct diagnosis with special emphasis on ruling out treatable causes of denervation and motor dysfunction and to consider medical management to treat the symptoms such as spasticity. The speech–language pathologist's role was to diagnose the speech problem, attempt to preserve communication, introduce compensatory techniques, and ultimately facilitate the use of methods of communication that augmented or were alternatives to speech. In other words, the speech–language pathologist's responsibility was to help the patient achieve optimum communication despite his debilitating neurologic condition. In addition, the speech–language pathologist managed the patient's dysphagia, recommending the most effective and efficient methods for facilitating safe swallowing.

When faced with a patient with an incurable disease, the physician may feel powerless to help the patient and so may resort to therapies that have questionable effectiveness or that have been reported successful by anecdote rather than by results of controlled treatment studies. The physician may think, *What harm can it do?* and encourage the patient to try an unproven therapy. Unfortunately, the patient's hopes of being cured are raised, then crushed, with each unsuccessful therapeutic trial. It is my opinion that honest communication between the patient and physician should guide the treatment. Supportive care is essential. The plight of patients with ALS is this: Their bodies are wasted; they have no strength to perform basic self-care; it is likely that they are unable to speak so that they can be understood; and they may have significant swallowing and feeding difficulties. At the same time, they have retained sensation so that they may have physical pain, yet are unable to move; and they have retained their mental functions so that they are aware of all that is happening to them.

In this case, the speech–language pathologist's task was a formidable one. The treatment goals had to be altered as the patient's medical condition and communication deteriorated, until ultimately he was forced to abandon verbal communication. Alternate methods of communication were attempted, and methods were selected that were the most effective for allowing the patient to express his needs. How can anyone overestimate the value of being introduced to a communication system that is the debilitated, dependent patient's only way to express himself, to communicate with others? I believe that all such patients should be referred to a speech–language pathologist.

 CASE 2

In this case, I did not refer the patient to a speech–language pathologist. He was a 67-year-old, right-handed man who had been admitted to the hospital for further evaluation of a pleural effusion and possible open lung biopsy. About 12 years previously, he had developed a sudden unsteadiness and weakness in his left leg. This eventually improved; however, over the years his ability to walk in a steady manner had gradually declined so that when I first saw him, he was using a walker for assistance. His speech was affected; I recognized the characteristics of ataxic dysarthria. His handwriting had deteriorated, and he had difficulty coordinating his hands and fingers to do fine motor tasks. As he spoke, I noticed that his grammar and syntax were appropriate and that he had no word retrieval difficulties. He denied memory loss. He had experienced an episode of blurred vision while using his walker when he had attempted to turn around; this episode had lasted approximately 1–2 seconds. He denied tinnitus, vertigo, diplopia (double vision), amaurosis fugax (transient monocular blindness), weakness, or sensory loss.

At this point, my hypothesis was a lesion in the cerebellum, and I asked some follow-up questions to probe for a possible etiology. Although this man was a smoker, he had no history of cancer, but he did have a pleural effusion from undiagnosed disease. He had used alcohol excessively 12 years before, at the time when he had noticed his first symptoms, but he had quit drinking and had abstained for several years. There was no family history of neurological disturbances similar to those he reported, nor of metabolic disease.

The pertinent findings of his neurologic examination were the following: nystagmus on lateral gaze and preserved strength throughout. Appendicular dysmetria (inability to gauge the distance, speed, and power of a movement) and dysdiadochokinesis (inability to perform and sustain rapid alternating movements) were present bilaterally. He could not stand with his feet together and his gait was wide-based. He had difficulty when he attempted to turn, and he nearly fell each time he tried to do so.

Laboratory examination revealed normal metabolic parameters including thyroid functions. CT scan of the head showed marked diffuse cerebellar atrophy. No tumor or infarction was seen. The most likely diagnosis was a form of idiopathic or nonfamilial cerebellar degeneration. Alcoholic cerebellar disease and a form of cerebellar paraneoplastic syndrome (tumor) were possibilities. As I considered referring him to a speech–language pathologist, I asked him how he felt about his speech. Although he recognized his speech was "not like it used to be," he told me that he was not especially disturbed by it and felt that by speaking slowly he could be understood. However, he was very stressed by his decreased ability to walk. I referred this patient to a physical therapist but did not refer him to a speech–language pathologist. At that point, I wondered if the "defector" was also a "traitor."

Later this patient underwent open lung biopsy, which diagnosed carcinoma. At that time, further staging procedures were being considered.

Summary

In summary, the best care for the patient with a communication disorder is achieved when the neurologist and the speech–language pathologist realize that each offers different, yet competent, services that benefit the patient and when they agree to cooperate in patient management. Successful comanagement of the patient is accomplished more efficiently when the speech–language pathologist and the neurologist realize that there are strengths and shortcomings in both professions.

The speech and language disorders of neurologically impaired adults sparked my interest in medicine and neurology. I have cared for patients both as a speech–language pathologist and as a neurologist. As a member of both professions, I have learned this: Listen to your patients, attend to their concerns, maintain open communication with them, give them your best and most honest effort, and you will help them.

References

Aftonomos, L. B., Appelbaum, J. S., & Steele, R. D. (1999). Improving outcomes for persons with aphasia in advanced community-based programs. *Stroke, 30*, 1370–1379.

Albert, M. L. (1998). Treatment of aphasia. *Archives of Neurology, 55*, 1417–1419.

Brookshire, R. H. (1997). *Introduction to neurogenic communication disorders* (5th ed.). St. Louis: Mosby.

Darley, F. L., Aronson, A. G., & Brown, J. R. (1975). *Motor-speech disorders*. Philadelphia: Saunders.

Duffy, J. R. (1995). *Motor speech disorders: Substrates, differential diagnosis, and management*. St. Louis: Mosby.

Dworkin, J. P., Abkarian, G. G., & Johns, D. F. (1988). Apraxia of speech: The effectiveness of a treatment regimen. *Journal of Speech and Hearing Disorders, 53*(3), 280–293.

Elman, R. J., & Bernstein-Ellis, E. (1998). The efficacy of group communication treatment in adults with chronic aphasia. *Journal of Speech-Language-Hearing Research, 42*, 411–419.

Ramig, L. O. (1998). Treatment of speech and voice problems associated with Parkinson's disease. *Topics in Geriatric Rehabilitation, 14*(2), 28–43.

Robey, R. R. (1998). A meta-analysis of clinical outcomes in the treatment of aphasia. *Journal of Speech-Language-Hearing Research, 41*, 172–187.

Vogel, D., Cannito, M. P., Salvatore, A., & Marquardt, T. (1998, February). *Effects of treatment on affect production in Parkinson's disease*. Paper presented to the Conference on Motor Speech, Tucson, AZ.

Wertz, R. T., Collins, M., Weiss, D., Kurtzke, J., Friden, T., Brookshire, R., Piercew, J., Holtzapple, P., Hubbard, D., Porch, B., West, J., Davis, L., Matovitch, V., Morley, G., & Resurrection, E. (1981). Veterans Administration cooperative study on aphasia: A comparison of individual and group treatment. *Journal of Speech and Hearing Research, 24*, 580–594.

Wertz, R. T., Weiss., D., Aten, J. L., Brookshire, R. H., Garcia-Bunuel, L., Greenbaum, H. J., Marshall, R. C., Vogel, D., Carter, J. E., Barnes, N. S., & Goodman, R. (1986). Comparison of clinic, home, and deferred language treatment for aphasia: A Veterans Administration cooperative study. *Archives of Neurology, 43*, 653–658.

Chapter 2

Pharmacologic Approaches to Speech Motor Disorders

David B. Rosenfield

Rosenfield discusses principles of pharmacologic therapeutics, basic aspects of pharmacology, and particular neurologic diseases that can compromise speech. He discusses various medications used to treat these disturbances, as well as their possible side effects.

1. *List the major movement disorders discussed by Rosenfield and the drugs that can be used to treat these disorders. Name the side effects of each of these drugs. If some symptoms are reduced with the administration of a particular drug but other symptoms increase, what factors are important in deciding whether or not that medication should be continued?*

2. *Is it probable that a drug will be discovered that will cure stuttering? Discuss the different parts of the brain involved in speech production that might be involved in stuttering. Is the etiology of stuttering different for different people?*

3. *What are some of the diseases associated with spasmodic dysphonia? What pharmacologic therapies are efficacious for treatment of this disorder?*

✵ ✵ ✵

One should not undertake a discussion of the pharmacologic therapies of speech motor disturbances without first dispelling some misconceptions about this subject. First, there is the assumption that because these therapies exist, cures are available. Also, there is the idea that speech motor disturbances have an underlying locus of breakdown that can be medicinally "fixed." Finally, there is the supposition that disturbances of nervous system motor output can themselves be fixed. None of these assumptions is true.

It is this conundrum of implausibilities that underlies this chapter. Add to this an awareness that speech–language pathologists do not prescribe medicine and that most graduate programs in speech–language pathology do not require students to learn pharmacology and the question becomes, Why include a chapter on neuropharmacology in a book for the speech–language clinician? There are several answers.

First, many patients with movement disorders affecting speech are treated routinely with pharmacologic agents. Understanding the effects of such medications should enhance the speech–language pathologist's interaction with both patient and neurologist. Second, the fact that patients tend to see their speech–language pathologists more often than they see their physicians suggests that the informed clinician may participate more effectively in the monitoring of symptomatic changes or side effects that may be related to a particular pharmacologic regimen. Finally, there is growing interest in experimentation with pharmacologic trials for patients with "idiopathic" speech disorders, such as spasmodic dysphonia or stuttering. Typically such patients are seen by speech–language pathologists but might not routinely be referred to a neurologist. It seems prudent to suggest that the practicing speech clinicians have a realistic appreciation of the current status of pharmacotherapies for these disorders and their limitations.

The employment of medication in treating a particular symptom is not simple. Different drugs can have different effects in different patients. Too often a patient may have a symptom that worsens with time. The physician may not know whether the symptom is worsening from the disease or from side effects of the drug that is being employed to treat the underlying ailment.

It is my personal experience that attentive speech–language pathologists can be of considerable assistance in providing health care. Doctors welcome personnel with the types of skills that the speech–language pathologist has. These skills come from experience, from being attuned to a particular presentation of symptoms, from knowledge pertaining to medications, and from a knowledge of pharmacology. The remainder of this chapter provides information in three broad categories. The first is a survey of fundamental concepts pertinent to an understanding of pharmacology in general. These concepts include principles of therapeutics, sources of drug information, and information regarding neurotransmitters. Second, the disorders of movement are treated somewhat extensively, including discussions of etiology, symptomatology, and the positive and negative effects of medication. These disorders characteristically involve neurochemical systems and frequently are managed by pharmacologic means. Collectively, movement-disordered patients comprise the largest population for whom pharmacologic approaches to speech motor control may be of interest. The final topic area involves pharmacologic issues relevant to other speech disturbances and includes discussions of normal speech motor control, stuttering, and spasmodic dysphonia. Throughout this chapter, frequent reference will be made to a variety of neuroanatomical structures.

Fundamental Concepts

Principles of Therapeutics

Well-designed and well-executed clinical trials exemplify the application of the scientific method to clinical decision making. Clinical trials form the basis for physicians' therapeutic decisions. In excellent summaries of the scientific requirements for clinical trials (Hill, 1960, 1962), it is agreed that the sine qua non of any clinical trial is its controls. There are many different types of controls, and one should understand that a controlled trial is not the same as a randomized double-blind trial. Although the randomized double-blind controlled trial is the most effective design for distributing variables between treatment and control groups, it is not always optimal or ethical. It is not always possible to employ this design to study disorders that are rare; study populations of patients that cannot, due to regulation or ethics or both, be studied; or study treatment of patients with a uniformly fatal disorder (Hill, 1960, 1962).

Results of clinical trials of therapeutic agents may not generalize to use with all patients. This is because often patients selected for experimental drug trials do not have coexisting diseases, and usually such trials assess the efficacy of only one or two drugs rather than the many drugs that may be taken by a patient who is not in the study. Clinical trials usually are conducted over small periods of time and usually involve small numbers of patients. Compliance may be better controlled for patients participating in experimental trials than for those who are not. These factors lead to the following conclusions.

1. Even if the findings of a well-executed clinical trial of a drug are understood, a physician only can hypothesize about what effects that drug will have on a particular patient. One cannot assume that what occurred in patients participating in the drug trial will also occur in other patients; thus, a physician uses the results of earlier clinical trials to establish an experiment for each patient. The physician must detect side effects and also must determine whether these effects truly are a result of the drug administered. Approximately one half or more of both the useful and adverse effects of drugs that have not been recognized in initial formal trials are subsequently discovered and reported by practicing physicians (Ingelfinger, Mosteller, Thibodeau, & Ware, 1983).

2. If a drug does not produce its anticipated effect in one patient, it cannot be assumed that the effect cannot occur in that patient or in another patient. Many factors may contribute to a drug's lack of efficacy in an individual patient. Some of these factors are misdiagnosis, poor compliance by the patient with the regimen, improper dosage or dosage intervals, simultaneous development of another disease, use of other agents that interact with the primary drug to nullify or to alter its effects, undetected genetic or environmental variables that modify the disease or the pharmacological actions of the drug, and unknown therapy by another physician who is caring for the same patient. Even if the medication appears to be efficacious and without harm, a physician must not attribute uncritically all improvement to the therapeutic regimen chosen. Nor can a physician assume that a deteriorating condition reflects only the natural course of the disease.

3. Rational drug therapies are based upon critical observations. A physician, in effect, employs as scientific an approach in treating each individual patient as do researchers when formally investigating drugs.

Therapy itself is a science. All treatments of all patients should focus upon each patient as an individual. Individual patients can demonstrate wide variability of response to the same drug. The basic concepts that underlie these sources of variability include the prescribed dose, the administered dose, and the concentration of the medication at the locus of action. These three factors alter the intensity of the effect (Koch-Weser, 1972).

Patient noncompliance, as well as possible medication errors, can result in the prescribed dose differing from the actual dose taken by the patient. The administered dose will have varying effect upon the concentration of the medication at the intended locus of action. The amount of medication delivered to this locus of action depends upon the rate and degree of the drug's absorption, the patient's body size and composition, the distribution of the medicine in body fluids, the degree of chemical binding of the drug in plasma and tissues, and the rate of elimination from the body. The relationship between the concentration of the medicine at the locus of action to its intensity of effect upon the patient is altered by drug-receptor interactions, the overall functional state of the patient, and any placebo effects.

The relationship between the administered dose and the concentration of medication at the locus of action, as well as the relationship between the concentration of the medication at the locus of action to the intensity of the effect, is further acted upon by physiological variables, pathological factors, genetic factors, interaction with other drugs, and development of drug tolerance by the patient. Nothing mandates that any particular patient will have any particular response to any particular drug. There are multiple variables within each individual patient (Nies & Spielberg, 1996).

Sources of Drug Information

Textbooks on pharmacology and therapeutics, leading medical journals, drug compendia, professional seminars, meetings, and advertisements are all sources of drug information. *Goodman and Gillman's "The Pharmacological Basis of Therapeutics"* (Hardman & Limbird, 1996), now in its 9th edition, is a good source of information on pharmacology and, although it may be intimidating due to its size, it is highly readable and extremely informative. Other sources of pharmacologic information are listed in the review by Nies and Spielberg (1996). The text by Vogel, Carter, and Carter (2000) is highly informative and focuses specifically on communication disorders.

Another good source of information is an industry survey, the *Physician's Desk Reference* (PDR). Brand-name manufacturers list various medications. There are no comparative data on product efficacy, safety, or cost. Descriptions of pharmacologic actions of medication are terse and highly technical, and the information is virtually identical to that contained in drug package inserts. The PDR is not intended as a pharmacology text; rather, its primary value lies in its information concerning what indications for use of a drug have been approved by the Food and Drug Administration.

One problem with the PDR is that almost all possible side effects are listed. Thus, when a patient has a particular symptom or sign, and it is important to know whether a prescribed drug is causing it, the PDR often does not provide as much help as one would hope. If the complaint is not listed in the PDR, the likelihood is remote that the symptom or sign is due to the drug. However, if it is listed in the PDR, there is no guarantee that the clinical findings are attributable to the drug. I have found that the PDR often unintentionally frightens patients because of the myriad of side effects it lists. Some patients have been reluctant to take a much needed medication after reading the PDR.

One useful aspect of the PDR is the picture section. The photographs of major drugs help patients to identify the drugs they are taking. It is for this reason that I recommend owning a copy of the PDR.

Another possible source of confusion when interpreting a patient's prescription is the dosage interval. These tend to be reported as abbreviations that may not be obvious. Some abbreviations and their definitions are provided in Table 2.1.

Neurotransmitters

It is the brain that underlies the neuromotor control system of speech, which involves respiratory movements, laryngeal neuromotor dynamics, and articulatory muscles. Medications aimed at treating particular diseases that affect this system affect alleged "chemical inequities." Certain chemicals called neurotransmitters are involved in translation of the neural impulse from the brain to the end organ, whether that end organ be respiratory muscle, laryngeal muscle, articulatory muscle, or other tissue. The complex role of neurotransmitters in the transmission of nerve impulses is elaborated upon in the next sections.

Cholinergic and Adrenergic Nerves. Peripheral nerves consist of motor (*efferent*) nerves that terminate in skeletal muscle (e.g., muscles

Table 2.1
Abbreviations of Terms Associated with Dosages

Abbreviation	Term
ac (a.c.)	Before meals
Ad lib	As needed; as desired
alt. hor.	Every other hour
bid	Two times per day
h.s.	At bedtime
NKA	No known allergies
NPO	Nothing by mouth
pc (p.c.)	After meals
Po, po	By mouth
PRN	As necessary
q.d.	Every day
q. (4) h.	Every 4 hours (number specified)
q.i.d.	Four times per day
q.o.d.	Every other day
t.i.d.	Three times per day

in limbs). Motor fibers interact with muscles through the neuromuscular junction. These motor nerves are under voluntary control.

The nervous system can be divided into voluntary and nonvoluntary components. The nonvoluntary portion includes the autonomic nervous system that, in turn, includes the sympathetic and the parasympathetic nervous system.

The terms *adrenergic* and *cholinergic* reflect the concept that chemicals transmit nerve impulses across the microscopic gap between nerve fibers and the structures they innervate. *Epinephrine* (adrenaline) and a closely related compound called *norepinephrine* (noradrenalin) are important neurotransmitters at peripheral (nonbrain, nonspinal cord) sympathetic, or adrenergic, terminations. *Acetylcholine* is generally associated with parasympathetic, or cholinergic, effects. However, acetylcholine is also an important neurotransmitter at some synapses in both sympathetic and parasympathetic pathways.

Impulses conducted by sympathetic, or adrenergic, nerve fibers usually elicit an active reaction in the effector structure, such as smooth (nonstriated) muscle (e.g., the muscle in the bowel) or glands. This is the reverse of parasympathetic, or cholinergic, fibers, which diminish these activities. Thus, stimulating sympathetic cardiac nerves increases heart rate, whereas stimulation of parasympathetic cardiac nerves decreases heart rate. These effects, however, are not universal: Adrenergic nerves slow gastric and intestinal movement motility, whereas cholinergic nerves accelerate these movements. Likewise, sympathetic nerves cause the bladder wall to relax, whereas the parasympathetic nerves cause bladder contraction.

In Table 2.2 the basic pharmacology of the autonomic nervous system is reviewed.

Activities of the agonists and antagonists are shown in Table 2.2. It should be understood that there is a finely tuned sympathetic and parasympathetic nervous system and that different receptors, end organs, and nerve pathways serve different functions. A drug acting on one set of receptors may have effects on others. The system overall is in a fine balance.

Acetylcholine. Acetylcholine (ACh) is a chemical synthesized by a chemical reaction; that is, it is catalyzed by the enzyme choline acetyltransferase. This process is described by the following reaction:

$$\text{AcetylCoA} + \text{choline} \overset{\text{enzyme}}{\rightleftarrows} \text{ACh} + \text{CoA}$$

As this reaction indicates, ACh is produced by certain chemicals that interact with one another. ACh can also be degraded back into those chemicals. Acetylcholine is found in parts of the autonomic nervous system, the brain (especially the basal ganglia), and the neuromuscular junction (Cooper, Bloom, & Roth, 1996).

The *neuromuscular junction* (motor end plate) is a specialized connection between an axon of a motor neuron and a somatic (striated) muscle fiber. The structure of the neuromuscular junction is such that an action potential (or neural impulse) in the motor axon produces synaptic depolarization of the muscle fiber, thus triggering a muscle action potential and, in turn, making the muscle contract (Hardman & Limbird, 1996).

Table 2.2
Pharmacology of Autonomic Nervous System

	Sympathetic		Parasympathetic
	α-adrenergic Receptors	β-adrenergic Receptors	Muscarinic Cholinergic Receptors
Natural agonists			
Norepinephrine (released by sympathetic nerve endings)	+++	+	—
Epinephrine (released by adrenal medulla)	+	+++	—
Acetylcholine (released by parasympathetic nerve endings)	—	—	+++
Other (artificial) agonists	Methoxamine Phenylephrine	Isoproterenol Methoxyphenamine	Muscarine Pilocarpine Carbachol
Direct effects of agonists on:			
Heart	—	Increased rate and force of contraction	Decreased rate and force of contraction
Blood vessels	Vasoconstriction	Vasodilatation	Vasodilatation
Intestines	Decreased motility	Decreased motility	Increased motility

(continues)

Table 2.2 Continued.

	Sympathetic		Parasympathetic
	α-adrenergic Receptors	β-adrenergic Receptors	Muscarinic Cholinergic Receptors
Antagonists (blocking agents)	Phentolamine Phenoxybenzamine Ergot alkaloids	Propranolol	Atropine Scopolamine
Agents that block enzymatic degradation of transmitter	Monoamine oxidase (MAO) inhibitors Catechol-O-Methyltransferase (COMT) inhibitors		Anticholinesterase

Note. Adapted from *The CIBA Collection of Medical Illustrations: Vol. 1. Nervous System: Part 1. Anatomy and Physiology* (p. 90), by F. H. Netter, 1983, West Caldwell, NJ: CIBA Pharmaceutical. Copyright 1983 by Icon Learning Systems. Adapted with permission.

Reviewing the pharmacology of the neuromuscular junction offers an example of certain basic concepts. The point to observe is not to note every chemical that alters acetylcholine activity. Rather, observe that there is a dynamic process involved in the synthesis, metabolism, release, and reuptake of this neurotransmitter. Different drugs affect this process and, as a result, can alter particular actions of the nervous system. All neurotransmitters—ACh and others—are synthesized and degraded, although each has its own independent chemical processes.

Pharmacological agents can affect transmission at the neuromuscular junction in three major ways. They can (a) alter the amount of ACh that the nerve impulse releases; (b) alter the response of the muscle cell membrane itself to the ACh that has been released; and (c) act upon the enzymes that degrade the ACh after it has been released. Some drugs have only one action, but many have more than one effect.

Five classes of drugs are described in Table 2.3. The choline uptake inhibitors decrease production of ACh in the nerve terminal by blocking the uptake of the choline molecules that are required in its synthesis. This results in decreased ACh synthesis, causing a reduction in the number of ACh molecules reaching the muscle. The net effect is a decrease in the number of muscle fibers activated per nerve impulse, resulting in a lessened strength of muscle contraction.

The ACh release blockers act on the motor nerve terminal by blocking the process through which a nerve impulse liberates ACh into the space between the nerve and muscle. The amount of ACh released may decrease to an amount insufficient to produce an electrical potential in the muscle fibers, thus causing severe weakness.

The ACh antagonists block the electrical depolarizing effect of the acetylcholine on the membrane. Drugs in this class are sometimes referred to as nicotinic antagonists, differentiating them from those blocking the action of ACh at autonomic endings (nicotine mimics the action of acetylcholine at the neuromuscular junction but not at autonomic endings). Many of these antagonists also have a weak depolarizing action on the muscle cells, but their major effect is blocking muscle activation by ACh, thus producing paralysis.

Cholinomimetics mimic the action of ACh, producing a strong, long-lasting muscle cell depolarization, making these cells less sensitive to the ACh subsequently released at the nerve terminal. This process is referred to as desensitization. Accommodation of the muscle cell

Table 2.3
Pharmacology of Neuromuscular Junction

Drug	Effect on Supply of Acetylcholine in Terminal	Effect on Amount of Acetylcholine Released in Terminal by Action Potential	Effect of Amplitude on End Plate Potential	Effect of Muscle Response to Application of Acetylcholine	Direct Effect of Muscle Membrane Resting Potential	Clinical Effect
Choline uptake inhibitors						
Hemicholinium Triethylcholine	Decreased	Decreased (smaller quanta)	Decreased	—	—	Weakness
Acetylcholine release blockers						
Botulinum toxin Low CA^{++} or high Mg^{++}	—	Decreased (fewer quanta)	Decreased			Paralysis (low Ca^{++} concentration may also produce tetany by direct action on nerves)

(continues)

Table 2.3 *Continued.*

Drug	Effect on Supply of Acetylcholine in Terminal	Effect on Amount of Acetylcholine Released in Terminal by Action Potential	Effect of Amplitude on End Plate Potential	Effect of Muscle Response to Application of Acetylcholine	Direct Effect of Muscle Membrane Resting Potential	Clinical Effect
Acetylcholine (nicotinic) antagonists						
D-tubocurarine (curare)	—	—	Decreased	Decreased	Depolarized (in high dosage)	Paralysis
Cholinomimetics						
Nicotine Carbamylcholine Succinylcholine	—	—	Decreased (by desensitization)	Decreased (by desensitization)	Strongly depolarized	Paralysis
Cholinesterase inhibitors						
Physostigmine Neostigmine Edrophonium	—	—			Depolarized slightly in high doses	Muscle power and duration of contraction increased
Organophosphorous compounds (nerve gases)	—		Increased; prolonged	Increased; prolonged	No change	Convulsions

Note. Adapted from *The CIBA Collection of Medical Illustrations: Vol. 1. Nervous System: Part 1. Anatomy and Physiology* (p. 219), by F. H. Netter, 1983, West Caldwell, NJ: CIBA Pharmaceutical. Copyright 1983 by Icon Learning Systems. Adapted with permission.

membrane to the central depolarization eventually blocks muscle action potentials completely, causing paralysis.

Cholinesterase inhibitors decrease the chemical breakdown of ACh, normally achieved by enzymes called *cholinesterases*. ACh released by nerve impulse acts for a longer time on the muscle membrane, producing a larger end plate potential that results in muscle contraction.

Catecholamines. Catecholamines generically refer to a particular type of chemical, one containing a catechol nucleus (a benzine ring with two adjacent hytroxyl substituents) and an amine group. In practice, catecholamines usually imply dihydroxyphenylethylamine (dopamine, DA) and its metabolic products, norepinephrine (NE) and epinephrine (E).

Tyrosine, as are many other (aromatic) amino acids, is actively taken up into the central nervous system and converted to dihydroxyphenylalanine (dopa). This is the most important (rate-limiting) step in this biosynthetic pathway. Dopa is subsequently converted to dopamine (DA), which, in some nerve terminals, is converted to NE.

Dopamine is found in many areas in the brain. The major dopamine pathways are the nigrostriatal, mesolimbic, mesocortical, tuberoinfundibular, and hypothalamic pathways. There is a rich interconnection between cortex, subcortex, and brainstem cells, interacting through dopamine as well as other neurotransmitters. One of the most important pathways of dopamine, apparently involved in Parkinson's disease, is the projection from the substantia nigra, through the nigral striatal pathway, into the caudate and putamen (Cooper et al., 1996).

The *central noradrenergic system* (i.e., the noradrenergic system in the central nervous system, thereby excluding the peripheral nervous system) contains two major clusterings of norepinephrine cell bodies from which axons arise that will innervate targets throughout the entire neuraxis. This is the locus ceruleus, a compact cell group in the bottom part of the pons, and the lateral tegmental noradrenergic neurons, a more loosely scattered group of cells lying outside of the locus ceruleus (Cooper et al., 1996).

The central dopamine-containing systems are more complex in their organization than are the noradrenergic systems. There are many more dopamine cells. The number of dopamine cells in the midbrain alone has been estimated to be between 15,000 and 20,000 on each side, whereas the number of noradrenergic neurons in the entire brainstem is thought to be about 5,000 on each side. There are also several major dopamine-containing cells as well as specialized dopamine neurons that make extremely localized connections within the retina and olfactory bulb. Dopamine, too, has multiple connections throughout the neuraxis (Cooper et al., 1996).

Until recently, dopamine receptors were classified into D-1 and D-2 subtypes. The former displayed "positive linkage" to adenylate cyclase and the latter did not (Stoof & Kebabian, 1981). Adenylate cyclase is an enzyme very important in the metabolic production of cyclic AMP, which, in turn, is most important for the generation of energy in many chemical processes. Further studies have led to the characterization of at least five dopamine receptor subtypes (D-1, D-2, D-3, D-4, D-5) (Purves et al., 1997). Dopamine and dopamine agonists show different selectivity for these subtypes of receptors. At the present time, it is not known whether receptor selectivity of dopamine agonists is maintained *in vivo*, or whether the functional effects (as far as motor activities are concerned) relate to the recently described dopamine receptors. Currently, it is not feasible to use the current classification of dopamine receptors in terms of motor activity in the treatment of Parkinson's disease.

Serotonin. Since the mid-19th century, scientists have been aware that a substance found in the serum of patients can cause powerful contraction of smooth muscle organs. This substance, *serotonin* (5-hydroxytryptamine, 5-HT), has a basic chemical structure underlying it known as an indole. The indole nature of serotonin bears much resemblance to the psychedelic drug LSD, as well as to many other agents that alter mentation. Many of the serotonin pathways originate in the brainstem, primarily in midline nuclei. They go to the cortex and subcortical tissue and have other brainstem connections as well. Serotonin is important in behavior as well as in other brain functions.

In summary, the brain is a conundrum of different pathways and so-called centers, with many of these pathways and centers having particular activities but none acting alone without influence from other centers and other pathways. Together, they enable the brain to program movement as well as other functions. As already noted, medications that allegedly affect one area of the brain sometimes (intentionally or unintentionally) affect other areas. Often times, there are various "side effects" that result from particular pharmacologic properties.

Blocking norepinephrine uptake at nerve endings can produce tremors, tachycardia (abnormally fast heartbeat), and erectile and ejaculatory dysfunction. Blocking serotonin uptake at nerve endings can produce various gastrointestinal disturbances, increase or decrease anxiety (dependent on dose), sexual dysfunction, and an alteration of motor tone (extrapyramidal side effects) (Purves et al., 1997).

A blockade of dopamine uptake at nerve endings can cause psychomotor activation and anti-parkinsonian effects and can aggravate psychosis. Blocking histamine H_1 receptors can cause sedation and drowsiness, weight gain, and hypotension. Blocking muscuranic receptors can produce blurred vision, dry mouth, constipation, increased heart rate, memory dysfunction, and urinary retention (Purves et al. 1997,). Blocking K_1-adrenergic receptors can cause dizziness, low blood pressure, and reflex-induced heart rate. Blocking dopamine (D_2 receptors) can produce various types of movement disorders, sexual dysfunction, and changes in hormones (Purves et al., 1997). For the reader who is interested in pursuing pharmacology further, or who requires more information about major and minor pathways, excellent sources are Cooper et al. (1996), and Vogel et al. (2000).

Disorders of Movement

Extrapyramidal diseases are a group of motor disorders associated with disease in the basal ganglia. From a clinical standpoint, these diseases consist of one or more of the following signs: (a) abnormal involuntary movements, (b) altered skeletal muscle tone, (c) a decrease or increase in movement, and (d) alteration of automatic associated movements.

The involuntary movements seen in extrapyramidal diseases are without purpose. They can be patterned or nonpatterned, predictable or unpredictable, and repetitive or nonrepetitive. The most frequently encountered clinical entities are Parkinson's disease, chorea, dystonia, athetosis, and hemiballismus. Although there are terms that designate these various clinical entities, a thorough understanding of the etiology of these disorders does not exist. Any one of these disorders may result from a wide variety of different types of central nervous system pathologies.

Anatomy of the Extrapyramidal Motor System

The *extrapyramidal system* usually refers to gray matter structures lying deep within the cerebral hemispheres, although other areas may also be involved. Its function is predominantly motor in nature. The extrapyramidal structures are very richly interconnected and include the basal ganglia. The *basal ganglia* consist of the caudate nucleus, putamen, globus pallidus, and several brainstem structures, including the subthalamic nucleus, the substantia nigra, and portions of the reticular formation. The caudate and putamen together are referred to as the *corpus striatum*, or *neostriatum*. The putamen and globus pallidus together are known as the *lenticular* (lens-like) *nucleus* (Chesselet & Delfs, 1996).

Extrapyramidal disorders are characterized either by too much (*hyperkinetic*) or too little (*hypokinetic*) movement.

Hyperkinesia

Hyperkinesias include tremor, tics, chorea, ballismus, dystonia, and athetosis.

Tremor. Tremor is the nonpurposeful, rhythmic, patterned, to-and-fro oscillation produced by contractions of antagonistic and agonistic muscles. There are many types of regular tremors: physiologic, metabolic (enhanced physiologic), tremor at rest, benign essential tremor, intention (cerebellar) tremor, and rubral tremor (Lang, 1996; Riley & Lang, 1996).

Tremor may be classified further as to whether it occurs at rest (*resting tremor*), during sustained posture of an extremity (*postural tremor*), or during intentional acts (*action* or *intention tremor*). The "pill rolling" tremor of Parkinson's disease is the prototype of resting tremor, usually decreasing substantially with voluntary activity of the affected limb. Essential, intention, and rubral tremors are exacerbated by and occur only during movement.

Physiologic tremor is fast (8–12 cycles per second compared to Parkinson's tremor, which is 3–7 cycles per second) and has a low amplitude. It is usually observed in circumstances of fatigue, fear, or emotional stress. Physiologic tremor is often prominent in the extremities, is induced by sustained posture, is a natural phenomenon, and has little pathologic significance.

Hyperthyroidism, emotional stress, and certain medications—steroids and beta-adrenergic agonist medications—can increase the amplitude of physiologic tremor. Hyperthyroidism can cause a fine, rapid tremor (10–20 cycles per second), especially in the hands. This tremor often is confused with the physiologic tremor.

A slower and coarser tremor is observed in patients with a metabolic disturbance such as electrolyte imbalance; withdrawal from alcohol; withdrawal from various drugs; or liver, kidney, or lung disease. Intention tremor, present upon intentional activity, is often seen in cerebellar disease. It is especially prominent when many joints are involved in movements, such as pointing a fully extended arm to an object. Patients with extrapyramidal diseases often have tremor at rest, but the tremor may also have an intentional component. Intentional tremor may be hereditary and familial.

Rubral tremor is a rotatory tremor of the upper portions of the extremities due to a disturbed outflow of impulses from the cerebellum. This tremor usually involves the superior cerebellar peduncle, known as the brachium conjunctivum, usually in an area of the midbrain near the red nucleus.

Tics. Tics are rapid, stereotyped, repetitive, involuntary movements resembling fragments of normal motor acts. As opposed to chorea, tics seldom interfere with ongoing movement and can be suppressed by the patient for variable periods of time. There is an expanding classification of tic disorders, incorporating chronic multiple motor tics, chronic simple tics, transient tics of childhood, and various other disturbances as well. This is well reviewed by Riley and Lang (1996).

Chorea. Chorea (Greek for "dance") varies greatly, depending upon the severity, the site, and the distribution of the underlying brain disturbance. Variability is the cardinal rule; a particular movement is rarely repeated. Choreic movement may be generally distributed all over the body or may be confined to a restricted part of the body. Usually, however, chorea is observed in the face or in outstretched hands. The movements last from approximately 1/10 to 1 second. Those movements involving larger joints appear to be more rapid than those in the fingers and toes. Although dependent upon the severity, voluntary action is often compromised because of the incoordination of the afflicted muscles. When requested to protrude the tongue, the patient with chorea may properly carry out all anticipatory movements but may be very slow in thrusting the tongue forward and may have difficulty maintaining protrusion. Rapid successive movements and intentional acts are impaired (Lang, 1996; Riley & Lang, 1996).

Ballismus. The term *ballismus* comes from the Greek word meaning "jumping about" and refers to violent flinging, flailing, or flipping limb movements. Hemiballismus refers to ballismus in one half of the body. Usually ballismus resembles chorea and is sometimes classified as an extremely violent chorea (Lang, 1996; Riley & Lang, 1996).

Dystonia. Dystonic movements are characterized by slow, long, sustained, powerful, nonpatterned, contorting movements of the axial (trunk, neck) and appendicular (hand, foot) muscles as well as slow, sustained contractions in the platysma (superficial neck muscles), shoulder, and pectoral (chest) muscles. The muscles of the neck, trunk, and upper portions of the extremities are involved most commonly. Involvement may be generalized (dystonia musculorum deformans) or confined to a restricted region such as the neck, face, or tongue (Lang, 1996; Riley & Lang, 1996).

Athetosis. Athetotic movements appear phenomenologically as a mixture of chorea and dystonia. In fact, some authorities deny the existence of athetosis as a separate entity.

Athetotic movements are irregular, nonpatterned, and slow. They are frequently described as writhing, cramp-like, and spasmodic, and they often consist of single movements lacking prompt initiation, smooth continuity of excursion, and smooth termination. Athetotic movements occur when antagonistic muscles contract simultaneously; the resultant movement is caused by differences in the power of the various opposing muscles (McDowell & Cedarbaum, 1988).

Hypokinesia

Akinesia refers to the absence of, and *hypokinesia* (*bradykinesia*) refers to a decrease in, the initiation, implementation, and ease of execution of automatic and volitional movement. When muscle is at rest, it has a particular tone that represents activity provided by the brain, the spinal cord, and the nerves. Too little tone usually means damage to the neurons or the nerves that are supplying the muscle. Two types of increased muscle tone encountered clinically are rigidity and spasticity. *Rigidity* involves simultaneous agonist and antagonist muscle activity; *spasticity* involves only one. If an extremity is rigid, passive movement encounters resistance in flexion as well as in extension. In contrast, resistance to passive movement in a spastic extremity is encountered only in the direction opposite the pull of the muscles with the increased tone. Spastic resistance is not uniform throughout the range of motion; there is increasing opposition up to a point, at which time the resistance suddenly gives, resulting in what is referred to as the "clasped-knife" phenomenon (Chesselet & Delfs, 1996; Lang, 1996; McDowell & Cedarbaum, 1988; Riley & Lang, 1996).

Rigidity of the upper extremity usually involves flexers and extensors (i.e., the pro-gravity and the antigravity muscles), whereas spasticity usually involves only the leg extensors and arm flexers. Increased stretch reflexes (*hyperreflexia*) accompany spasticity but are not observed with rigidity. Basal ganglia diseases and extrapyramidal disorders frequently cause rigidity. In most patients, hypokinesia (or bradykinesia) is a result of rigidity, although sometimes spasticity plays a role (Chesselet & Delfs, 1996; Lang, 1996; McDowell & Cedarbaum, 1988; Riley & Lang, 1996).

Bradykinesia can impair voluntary activity, causing the patient to initiate movements slowly. The patient may freeze upon initiating voluntary acts. This becomes especially evident during walking. Despite good strength, normal fist closure lacks the synergic dorsiflexion of the hand and impairs overall function. In writing, the patient begins well but makes the letters increasingly smaller and often freezes and stops. There is usually limitation of quick successive movements such as rapid skilled finger and foot movements (Lang, 1996; McDowell & Cedarbaum, 1988; Riley & Lang, 1996).

Hyperkinetic Movement Disorders

Dystonia. Dystonia can occur by itself or in association with other complex involuntary movements. It can be classified according to whether an etiology for the disorder is known, as well as according to hereditary pattern, age of onset, and region of the body afflicted. Usually, in the primary dystonias, no underlying pathology or radiologic changes are found. In secondary or symptomatic dystonias, there is a variety of central nervous system disorders. These disorders include trauma (perinatal brain injury, head trauma), focal intracranial pathology (stroke, tumor, or arteriovenous malformation), infection, and metabolic disturbance (Wilson's disease, Hallervorden-Spatz syndrome, hexosaminidase deficiency, lipidoses, gangliosidoses). Other causes of secondary dystonia include toxins such as manganese and various medications (Calne & Lang, 1988; Fahn, 1984, 1988; Fahn, Marsden, & Calne, 1988; Lang, 1996; Marsden, 1988; McDowell & Cedarbaum, 1988; Riley & Lang, 1996).

Focal dystonias appear to represent only a fragment of the dystonic process. They usually begin during adulthood. The most common forms of focal dystonias include torticollis (wry neck), writer's cramp, typist's cramp, musician's cramp, and Meige's syndrome. Meige's syndrome refers to oromandibular dystonias with blepharospasm (involuntary eye closure). This disorder may begin with blepharospasm or spasms and contractions of the muscles of the mouth, jaw, pharynx, and tongue (oromandibular dystonia). This syndrome usually begins between the fourth and the eighth decade, most often in the sixth decade of life. Symptoms are often triggered by bright light, stress, or attempts to read. Some patients wear dark glasses to reduce photic stimulation. As the disorder progresses, eye closure becomes more prolonged and many patients become functionally blind. Spasmodic dysphonia or grunting noises can appear often in this syndrome (Fahn, 1984; Lang, 1996; McDowell & Cedarbaum, 1988; Riley & Lang, 1996).

A combination of dopaminergic and cholinergic overactivity in the basal ganglia are instrumental in causing dystonia. Their therapy, frequently employing dopamine receptor antagonists and anticholinergic drugs, has recently included various newer medications as well, including that of chemodenervation with botulinum toxin (Jankovic & Hallett, 1994).

Multiple therapies for treating dystonia, ranging from pharmacotherapeutic agents to various medications, are reviewed in Table 2.4.

Chorea. Table 2.5 provides the classifications of chorea. *Degenerative (Huntington's) chorea* is inherited as an autosomal dominant disease with complete penetrance. This means there is a 50% chance that each offspring of a person with Huntington's will inherit the disease.

Table 2.4
Pharmacological Therapy for Dystonia

Generic Name	Trade Name	Daily Dosage (mg)	Mechanism of Action
Trihexyphenidyl	Artane	6–40	Anticholinergic
Benztropine	Cogentin	4–15	Anticholinergic
Clonazepam	Klonopin	1–12	Serotonergic; relaxant
Lorazepam	Ativan	1–16	Relaxant
Baclofen	Lioresal	40–120	Antispastic; GABA agonist; substance P antagonist
Primidone	Mysoline	50–800	Antiepileptic; antitremor
Valproate	Depakote	500–1500	Antiepileptic; GABA-T inhibitor
Carbamazepine	Tegretol	1600–1600	Antiepileptic
Levodopa/Carbidopa	Sinemet (CR)	75/300–200/2000	Dopamine precursor
Bromocriptine	Parlodel	10–60 1–10	Dopamine agonist Dopamine agonist
Pergolide	Permax	0.5–5	Dopamine agonist
Pimozide	Orap	2–10	Dopamine blocker
Lithium	Lithobid	600–1800	Antidopaminergic
Tetrabenazine	Nitoman	50–300	Monoamine depleter and blocker
Botulinum Toxin	BOTOX	5–400	Blocks ACh release at neuro-muscular junction units

Note. Adapted from *Advances in Diagnosis, Therapy, and Pathogenesis*, by J. Jankovic, 1996, paper presented at Current Neurology Conference, Baylor College of Medicine, Houston. Adapted with permission.

Huntington's disease has different clinical characteristics and different ages of onset, depending upon the sex of the transmitting parent. Brains of patients who have died from Huntington's disease reveal a significant change in the levels of some neurotransmitters. The most striking change is the reduction in the level of gamma-aminobutyric acid and its synthesizing enzyme, glutamic acid decarboxylase (Cooper et al., 1996; McDowell & Cedarbaum, 1988).

The clinical onset of degenerative chorea is insidious. Some patients complain of abnormal movements whereas others complain of

Table 2.5
Classification of Chorea

Developmental and aging choreas
    Physiological chorea of infancy
    Cerebral palsy
    Buccal-oral-lingual dyskinesia and edentulous orodyskinesia
    Senile chorea (probably several causes)

Hereditary choreas
    Huntington's disease
    Benign hereditary chorea
    Neuroacanthocytosis
    Other CNS degenerations: olivopontocerebellar atrophy, Machado-Joseph's disease, ataxia telangiectasia, tuberous sclerosis, Hallervorden-Spatz's disease, familial calcification of basal ganglia, others
    Neurometabolic disorders: Wilson's disease, Lesch-Nyhan's syndrome, lysosomal storage disorders, amino acid disorders, Leigh's disease, porphyria

Drug induced: neuroleptics (tardive dyskinesia), antiparkinsonian drugs, amphetamines, tricyclics, oral contraceptives

Toxins: alcohol intoxication and withdrawal, anoxia, carbon monoxide, manganese, mercury, thallium, toluene

Metabolic
    Hyperthyroidism
    Hypoparathyroidism
    Pregnancy (chorea gravidarum)
    Hyper- and hyponatremia, hypomagnesemia, hypocalcemia
    Hypo- and hyperglycemia (the latter may cause hemichorea, hemiballism)
    Acquired hepatocerebral degeneration
    Nutritional: beriberi, pellagra, vitamin B12 deficiency in infants

Infectious
    Sydenham's chorea
    Encephalitis lethargica
    Other infectious and postinfectious encephalitides, including Creutzfeldt-Jakob disease

(continues)

Table 2.5 *Continued.*

Immunological
   Systemic lupus erythematosus
   Henoch-Schönlein purpura
Vascular (often hemichorea)
   Infarction
   Hemorrhage
   Arteriovenous malformation
   Polycythemia rubra vera
Tumors
Trauma

Note. Adapted from "Movement Disorder Symptomatology," by A. E. Lang. In *Neurology and Clinical Practice*, edited by W. G. Bradley, R. B. Daroff, G. M. Finichel, and C. D. Marsden, 1996, New York: Butterworth-Heinemann. Copyright 1996 by Butterworth-Heinemann. Adapted with permission.

emotional disturbances. Still others complain of intellectual compromise. Often, there is a combination of these manifestations. There may be a history of an insidious onset of restlessness, progressive clumsiness, and general diminution of motor proficiency. The patient or the patient's family may notice involuntary facial grimaces, twitching of the fingers, or movements of the arms. Dysarthria can be an early symptom. Speech may become severely impaired by the choreoathetotic movements of the tongue, lips, larynx, palate, pharynx, diaphragm, and chest. Facial expression may be contorted, and there may be continuous sucking, grimacing, and lip-smacking movements. Examination reveals abnormal choreic movements that may often be demonstrated by asking the patient to hold hands or feet outstretched.

There is no specific treatment for Huntington's disease. Choreic movements can be reduced with reserpine, haloperidol, or tetrabenazine. Reserpine also has a calming effect on the aggressive behavior of some Huntington's patients, but it usually has less effect than haloperidol. Haloperidol in doses of 1 mg to 10 mg per day lessens the choreic movements. The dosage is gradually increased from a minimal amount (1 mg per day) until symptoms are relieved. Tetrabenazine is still an experimental drug in the United States; most physicians do not have access to it. Sometimes baclofen is used because of its GABA-like action in inhibiting glutamate. Any of these medications may reduce chorea-induced dysarthria, but their effect is often minimal (McDowell & Cedarbaum, 1988).

Drug-induced Chorea. Limb chorea—in combination with athetoid movements of the head, face, mouth, and neck—may be the result of long-term administration of phenothiazines, butyrophenones, and other medications. Choreiform movements are most likely to occur with the use of phenothiazines, such as prochlorperazine, perphenazine, fluphenazine, and triflupromazine. Phenothiazine-induced choreiform movements are most common in young people receiving high doses of these drugs for acute schizophrenia and in elderly females. In 25% of the patients who have developed choreiform movements while taking phenothiazines, these movements have become permanent and may be labeled tardive dyskinesia (Jankovic & Hallett, 1994; McDowell & Cedarbaum, 1988).

Choreiform movements have been noted in many patients with Parkinson's disease who have been treated with levodopa. The occurrence of these movements is dose-related. The dose at which the movements appear varies widely, but it tends to be low in patients with a longer duration of disease. In most instances reported, these movements have stopped with lower doses or upon discontinuation of the medication (Jankovic & Hallett, 1994; McDowell & Cedarbaum, 1988).

Tic Disorders. As already noted, tics are repetitive, stereotyped, involuntary motor acts that resemble normal patterns of muscle movement. They usually do not interfere with voluntary skilled motor performance. They are often volitionally suppressible for long periods of time. They should not be confused with the lightning-like jerks of a single muscle or group of muscles occurring as myoclonus, or with the distal twitch-like movement of chorea (Jankovic & Hallett, 1994; McDowell & Cedarbaum, 1988).

The most notorious of all tic disorders is *Gilles de la Tourette syndrome*. This is a chronic but fluctuating disorder that begins early in life. Onset in adult life is rare. The major symptoms of this disorder are multiple motor and vocal tics. Tourette's syndrome begins between ages 2 and 15 years, the median age of onset being 7 years. Ninety-three percent of the patients are symptomatic by age 11. This syndrome is often misdiagnosed, a median 10-year interval being present between onset of symptoms and establishment of diagnosis. Unlike acute simple tics of childhood, there is a male-to-female ratio of 3:1. In 37% of the patients, tics begin in the head and face. In 8%, the disorder begins with vocal tics. Seventy-five percent of the patients have vocal tics characterized by grunting or barking noises; 62% by squeaks or shrieks; 59% by sniffing or snorting; and 22% by repetitive dysfluencies. *Coprolalia*, or involuntary swearing, occurs in 60% of the patients. In addition to simple tics, 73% of the patients have complicated movements, consisting of touching, hitting, jumping, skipping, squatting, or echopraxia (McDowell & Cedarbaum, 1988).

The tics in Tourette's syndrome, as in other movement disorders, decrease during distraction, disappear during sleep, and increase with tension or anxiety. Unlike other involuntary movements, patients can voluntarily suppress their tics for variable periods of time (Butler, 1984).

It is often difficult to evaluate the effectiveness of a drug in treating tics. This is due to the fluctuating nature of the manifestations of a tic. Dopamine antagonists are often successful therapeutic agents. The original response to haloperidol (dopamine receptor antagonist) helped define the syndrome as a neurological disorder. However, dopamine antagonists are associated with a number of complications, and many physicians attempt to use medications less toxic (Riley & Lang, 1996).

A major problem in treating Tourette's syndrome is sedation and impairment of learning performance. Clonidine is helpful in treating tics and behavioral problems, although this is not being confirmed by all investigators. Clonazepam is a weak but rather benign anti-tic drug that can provide enough additional control for those patients who are less seriously affected. Of the postsynaptic dopamine receptor blockers, pimozide and fluphenazine often produce less sedation than haloperidol and are very effective. Presynaptic dopamine antagonists, such as tetrabenazine, are without as much risk for tardive dyskinesia, but they may not be as effective as the dopamine-receptor blockers (Riley & Lang, 1996). Before beginning pharmacologic treatment, physicians should decide whether treatment is truly necessary. As in treating most movement disturbances, the drug treatment of tics should be determined by the degree of disability and distress experienced by the patient (Riley & Lang, 1996).

Tremor. Essential tremor is characterized by involuntary rhythmic movements of the head, face, jaw, tongue, arms, hands, and, rarely, the legs. It can also involve laryngeal muscles. It can begin at any time but usually begins in adulthood, commonly around the age of 50. It is a gradually progressive disorder, but remissions for long periods of time have been reported. Many patients note that alcohol reduces their tremor (Lang, 1996; McDowell & Cedarbaum, 1988; Riley & Lang, 1996; Rosenfield, 1988c). See Table 2.6 for some of the commonly used beta-blockers in treating essential tremor. Lipid solubility, mentioned in Table 2.6, refers to the solubility of drugs upon entering the brain (the brain is part lipid).

Propranolol—administered as 10 mg three to four times a day, increasing up to 320 mg per day in divided doses—is usually effective in decreasing tremor. The dose should be increased from a small starting dose until tremor or adverse effects, such as bradycardia (slowed heart rate, less than 60 beats per minute), hypotension, dizziness, or fatigue supervene. Propranolol should not be given to patients with known congestive heart failure, bronchospasm, or diabetes. Sometimes propranolol causes sedation, depression, and delirium, so that patients may prefer not to use it. Other effective medications include primidone (Mysoline), beginning at 50 mg three times per day and then gradually increasing the dose until the tremor is reduced or disappears (Koller, 1984; McDowell & Cedarbaum, 1988; Riley & Lang, 1996).

Table 2.6
Beta-Blockers for Treating Essential Tremor

Generic Name	Trade Name	Maintenance Dose	Lipid Solubility	Efficacy
Propranolol	Inderal	80–240 bid	+++	+++
Metoprolol	Lopress	100–200 bid	++	++
Timolol	Blocadren	10–20 bid	++	+
Nadolol	Corgard	80–240 qd	0	++
Atenolol	Tenormin	50–100 qd	0	+
Pindolol	Visken	10–30 bid	++	0

Note. Adapted from *Advances in Diagnosis, Therapy, and Pathogenesis*, by J. Jankovic, 1996, paper presented at Current Neurology Conference, Baylor College of Medicine, Houston. Adapted with permission.

Hyperkinetic Drug-induced Movement Disorders. Many pharmacologic agents can produce extrapyramidal symptoms resembling naturally occurring movement disorders. These symptoms may result from the effects of blocking some of the brain's dopamine receptors, but this has not been proven. Drug-induced hyperkinetic syndromes (tardive dyskinesias), as well as hypokinetic syndromes, have been described.

The most common drug-induced movement disorder is parkinsonism, which will be more fully discussed in the next section. Paradoxically, drugs that cause parkinsonism, a hypokinetic movement disorder, can also cause hyperkinetic disorders. Drug-induced hyperkinesias can present as dystonia or chorea. Treatment is difficult and, unfortunately, often unsuccessful.

Acute dystonic reactions may occur within minutes after patients receive a dopamine-blocking agent. Many of the antipsychotic drugs have dopamine-blocking capabilities. Movements may consist of forced upward ocular deviation or other orofacial dystonias. Anticholinergic therapy or antihistamines may be effective.

Tardive dyskinesia is an increasing problem. These involuntary movements consist of orobuccolingual masticatory movements, with tongue thrusting, grimacing, chewing, and blepharospasm the most common. These oral movements may be associated with choreiform movements of the hands and feet, as well as dystonic postures or laryngeal-pharyngeal dystonic spasms. Tardive dyskinesia occurs in 25% of patients treated with neuroleptic medications. The disorder usually begins several weeks to months after treatment with the offending medication. Fifty percent of the patients are asymptomatic within 6 months after discontinuing the offending drug. The incidence of remission decreases with increasing patient age. Whether the combination of anticholinergic and neuroleptic medications increases the predisposition toward development of tardive dyskinesia has been questioned. It is postulated that tardive dyskinesia results from supersensitivity of postsynaptic dopamine receptors in the striatum or from overactivity of presynaptic dopamine neurons induced by a dopamine-receptor antagonist (Goetz & Klawans, 1984; McDowell & Cedarbaum, 1988; Riley & Lang, 1996).

It is not known why this condition persists after medication has been discontinued. All known dopamine-receptor blocking agents, including antiemitics, prochlorperazine, and metoclopromide, can cause tardive dyskinesia. Many drugs not known to affect dopamine transmission or dopaminergic receptors can produce choreiform dyskinesias, which usually remit after the medication is stopped. These agents include phenytoin (Dilantin), carbamazepine (Tegretol), and, rarely, anticholinergic medications (Goetz & Klawans, 1984; McDowell & Cedarbaum, 1988; Riley & Lang, 1996).

The initial treatment for tardive dyskinesia is to reduce or to eliminate the offending agent. Often this is not possible because of the severity of the underlying psychiatric condition. When dyskinetic symptoms persist or when continuing the offending medication is necessary, treatment of the movement disorder is usually very difficult. Increasing the dose of the neuroleptic drug often masks the symptoms, but this usually exacerbates the underlying pathologic factor. Treatment with presynaptic dopamine-depleting agents (e.g., reserpine) is beneficial in approximately 65% of the patients. Depression is sometimes a side effect. Baclofen and amantadine have been employed also (Goetz & Klawans, 1984; McDowell & Cedarbaum, 1988).

Hypokinetic Movement Disorders

Parkinson's Disease. Parkinson's disease—sometimes known as parkinsonism or Parkinson's syndrome—consists of tremor, rigidity, postural changes, and a decrease in spontaneous movement. This syndrome can be associated with several pathologic processes that can damage the extrapyramidal system (see Table 2.7).

Parkinson's disease usually develops insidiously and progresses slowly. Usually patients cannot tell exactly when the symptoms began. Bradykinesia and rigidity may not occur in the limbs and trunk only, but can appear in speech also. Patients complain that their voices lack volume and force and that they "run out of steam" when they talk for long periods. Some speak in whispers. Articulation may be impaired. Speech is often monotonous with rapid staccato quality. It is as though patients' speech, handwriting, and other motor activities are affected by the same phenomenon that causes the freezing of their gait.

Frequently, early symptoms of Parkinson's disease are unilateral tremor and alteration in facial expression. In early Parkinson's disease, patients may have only a mild unilateral tremor that decreases with activity and decreased arm swing on the same side as the tremor. The tongue may not be weak, but it may have a rapid tremor.

Table 2.7
Classification of Parkinsonism

Primary	Secondary	Pseudoparkinsonism
Idiopathic	Metabolic	"Arteriosclerotic"
Parkinsonism plus	Wilson's disease	"Normal-pressure" hydrocephalus
Olivopontocerebellar degeneration	Chronic nonwilsonian hepatocerebral degeneration	Mass lesions (tumor, subdural hematoma)
Shy-Drager syndrome	Hallervoorden-Spatz syndrome	Tremor syndromes
Striatonigral degeneration	Infectious	
Guamanian parkinsonism-ALS-dementia complex	Acute, postencephalitic	
Azorian motor system degeneration	Toxic	
Progressive supranuclear palsy	Irreversible	
	Carbon monoxide	
	Carbon disulfide	
	Manganese	
	Meperidine analogs (MPTP)	
	Reversible	
	Reserpine	
	Phenothiazine	
	Butyrophenone	
	Neuroleptics	
	Antiemetics	
	Metoclopramide	
	Alpha-methyldopa	

Note. Adapted from "The Extrapyramidal System and Disorders of Movement," by F. H. McDowell and J. M. Cedarbaum, 1988, in *Clinical Neurology*, Vol. 3, rev. ed., p. 18, edited by R. J. Joynt, Philadelphia: Lippincott. Copyright 1988 by Lippincott. Adapted with permission.

Treatment: Anticholinergics. The earliest effective treatment for parkinsonism was a tincture of belladonna, discovered by Charcot. Belladonna and its derivatives have anticholinergic activity. A variety of related anticholinergic compounds since have been synthesized and employed in treating parkinsonism. The exact mechanism of action in these compounds in relieving the symptoms of parkinsonism is not known. Researchers question whether dopamine inhibits and acetylcholine excites the individual cells in the neostriatum (McDowell & Cedarbaum, 1988).

Diminished dopamine activity in Parkinson's disease renders the excitatory effects of acetylcholine more prominent. Before levodopa, anticholinergic agents were often employed alone for therapy in Parkinson's disease. These agents are still useful in some patients, especially when tremor occurs.

Anticholinergic agents rarely produce more than 20% improvement. Despite continued use of these drugs, the symptoms and signs of parkinsonism progress. Sudden discontinuation of them can cause a marked increase in symptoms. The side effects of anticholinergic agents include dry mouth, aggravation of glaucoma, blurred vision, constipation, urinary retention, and psychiatric side effects (delirium, impaired memory, disorientation, anxiety, agitation, and hallucinations).

The most commonly used anticholinergic medications are trihexyphenidyl hydrochloride (Artane), benztropine mesylate (Cogentin), and ethopropazine (Parsidol). The usual starting doses are as indicated in Table 2.8, but patients can have a wide variation of response. Dosages, initially small, are increased until improvement occurs or until side effects prevent further increase (see Table 2.8).

Certain antihistamines, such as diphenhydramine (Benadryl), have anticholinergic side effects and are sometimes helpful if patients cannot tolerate more potent anticholinergics. Antihistamines may cause sedation.

Anticholinergic drugs may help patients who are taking levodopa. Some patients deteriorate markedly if anticholinergics are withdrawn suddenly. Thus, if discontinued, the dose should be reduced gradually.

Treatment: Levodopa and Decarboxylase Inhibitors. Following the discovery of striatal dopamine depletion in patients with parkinsonism, many investigators began treating patients with dihydroxyphenylalanine (dopa) in an effort to replace brain dopamine. Dihydroxyphenylalanine was used instead of dopamine because dopamine does not

Table 2.8
Drugs Used in Treating Parkinson's Disease

Generic Name	Trade Name	Daily Dose (mg)	Mechanism of Action
Deprenyl (Selegiline)	Eldepryl	10	MAO-B inhibitor
Trihexyphenidyl	Artane	4–8	Anticholinergic
Benztropine	Cogentin	0.5–8	Anticholinergic
Amantadine	Symmetrel	100–300	Release of DA, anticholinergic
Levodopa	Larodopa	3,000–8,000	DA precursor
Carbidopa/Levodopa	Sinemet Atamet	30/300– 20/2,000	DOPA decarboxylase inhibitor/ DA precursor
Carbidopa/	Sinemet CR	25/200–	DOPA decarboxylase inhibitor/ DA precursor
Levodopa CR	Permax	250/2,000	DA agonist

cross the blood–brain barrier. Only a particular form of dopa, the levorotatory isomer (L-dopa on levodopa) is effective.

L-dopa greatly decreases hypokinesia and bradykinesia. Postural instability may resist improvement. Some patients become more alert and mental functioning improves after beginning levodopa.

Levodopa treatment is initiated with a small dose that is gradually increased until maximum benefit is achieved or until intolerable side effects occur. These side effects include dyskinesias, loss of efficacy, fluctuations in response, confusion, hallucinations, and drop in blood pressure upon standing (orthostatic hypotension).

Eighty percent of the patients develop dyskinesia at some time during levodopa treatment. These abnormal movements are dose-related side effects and can be relieved by decreasing the dose, but the movements may reappear. Often some dyskinetic movement has to be accepted by the patient as the price of levodopa's therapeutic effect.

Reduced blood pressure (orthostatic hypotension) can occur in 25% of the patients early in the course of treatment with levodopa alone. It is rarely symptomatic and usually disappears as treatment continues. Palpitations and cardiac arrhythmias occur in approximately 10% of the patients.

Abnormal behavior appears in approximately one fifth of the patients early in treatment. This is more common in older patients, those with severe Parkinson's disease, and those with dementia. The most prominent of these abnormalities is delirium with episodes of confusion, agitation, disorientation, and visual hallucination. The episodes are often related to excessive intake of the antiparkinsonian medication, as well as other prescribed drugs such as sedatives, antidepressants, anticholinergic agents, and tranquilizers. Delirium can be precipitated by infection, fever, dehydration, electrolyte imbalance, and frequently by exposing the patient to a new or strange environment. Episodes of delirium seldom occur in nondemented patients. Visual hallucinations are common in patients receiving levodopa but are not threatening to the patient. These mental abnormalities are usually reversed by lowering the dose of levodopa or by eliminating concomitant medications, especially anticholinergics and sedatives (McDowell & Cedarbaum, 1988; Riley & Lang, 1996).

If a patient with Parkinson's disease develops impaired mental status, it is important to determine whether this is due to medication side effects. All medications used to treat Parkinson's disease can compromise cognition, but the ones most likely to do this are the anticholinergic agents. These medications should be decreased or discontinued in patients with altered mental status, and patients should be observed for difficulty in their thinking (McDowell & Cedarbaum, 1988; Riley & Lang, 1996).

Hallucinations are a common problem for patients who have dementia. Dopa, dopamine agonists, and anticholinergic medications can all cause hallucinations, and each should be reduced systematically to determine which contributes to the symptom. Some patients continue to hallucinate while off the medication. Families usually prefer an immobile clearheaded member to one who is mobile but grossly confused.

Loss of intellectual function increases with time and is not recovered until levodopa is discontinued. Effective daily doses of levodopa average 4 g per day, but some patients require as much as 16 g. Currently, levodopa is rarely used alone for treatment of Parkinson's disease, except in the case of an unusual patient who develops an allegic reaction to carbidopa-levodopa tablets or who suffers severe dyskinesia or orthostatic hypotension when using the drugs in combination.

Inhibiting the extracerebral metabolism of levodopa to dopamine is important in the treatment of Parkinson's disease. Drugs accomplish this by inhibiting dopa-decarboxylase, the enzyme that metabolizes levodopa into dopamine. These drugs do not pass the blood–brain barrier. The net effect is a larger amount of unmetabolized levodopa available for transport into the brain, where conversion to dopamine occurs. Thus the total dose of dopa required is lowered and peripheral side effects, due to increased dopamine outside the brain, are markedly reduced. Some adverse effects of levodopa (dyskinesia, agitated confusion, hallucinations) may be more prevalent and more serious when decarboxylase inhibitors are used, because these side effects are directly related to the amount of dopa entering the brain. The dopa-decarboxylase inhibitor used in the United States is alpha-methyldopa hydrazine (carbidopa).

Carbidopa combined in a tablet with levodopa (Sinemet) is marketed in three strengths: 10/100 mg, 25/100 mg, and 25/250 mg. Initial dosage is usually one half to one 25/100 tablet taken three times per day. The dose is slowly increased until maximum benefit is obtained, which usually requires a minimum total dose of 75 mg to 100 mg of carbidopa and 750 mg to 1,000 mg of levodopa.

Patients initially placed on levodopa and then switched to decarboxylase inhibitors with dopa often feel better and have improved appetites. Changing from regular dopa to combinations of levodopa with decarboxylase inhibitors is accomplished by reducing the overall levodopa dose by 75% and by giving the remaining amount in divided doses with carbidopa (McDowell & Cedarbaum, 1988; Riley & Lang, 1996).

The side effects of decarboxylase inhibitors with levodopa are identical to those of levodopa alone. No specific ill effects have been attributed solely to these or decarboxylase inhibitors.

Improvement using dopa alone usually begins to appear at a dosage of 1.5 gm to 2.5 gm per day, or with 100 mg to 400 mg of levodopa with the decarboxylase inhibitor. Improvement is manifested first as a subjective increase in liveliness or ease of movement. Maximal improvement may not occur until the patient has taken a steady dose of levodopa or the levodopa-decarboxylase inhibitor for several weeks.

With few exceptions, levodopa and levodopa with decarboxylase inhibitors can be taken concomitantly with drugs used to treat other illnesses. The combination of levodopa with monoamine oxidase inhibitors (used in treating depression) can cause hypertension. Phenothiazines and reserpine tend to counteract the effects of levodopa. Pyridoxine, found in most vitamin preparations, can interfere with the action of levodopa, but large supplements have to be ingested to produce this action. Vitamin preparations containing large amounts of pyridoxine should be avoided. Because decarboxylase inhibitors act by blocking the binding of pyridoxal phosphate (related to pyridoxine) to decarboxylase enzymes, patients taking the combination need not avoid pyridoxine.

The pharmacokinetics of levodopa are complex and may be altered by its chronic use. There are on-off signs as well as wearing-off signs. Some patients have sudden fluctuations between mobility and immobility; this is known as the *on-off phenomenon*. Patients who have marked fluctuations, or even mild fluctuations, should report this to their physicians. Levodopa is most effective in the first 2 to 5 years of treatment. Later, as the disease progresses, the benefits provided lessen. This is known as the *wearing-off effect*.

Treatment: Amantadine. Amantadine (Symmetrel) is an antiviral agent that also helps relieve symptoms of parkinsonism. The mechanism of action is unknown, but it appears to act by releasing dopamine from striatal neurons. Most of the drug is not metabolized; 90% of it passes from the body into the urine. Thus, the drug should be used cautiously in patients with kidney disease. Amantadine is recommended for patients with mild Parkinson's disease who have not received levodopa.

A dose of 100 mg taken two to three times daily produces rapid benefit, usually within a day, but efficacy diminishes in some patients after several weeks. Amantadine is effective in approximately 60% of the patients and partially relieves rigidity, akinesia, and, to a lesser extent, tremor. Side effects, which are seldom troublesome, include nervousness, insomnia, confusion, hallucinations, dry mouth, nausea, ankle edema, and skin lesions.

Some patients may not respond to amantadine, but the drug should be taken for 10–14 days before assuming that it is ineffective. Amantadine and anticholinergics, when used at the same time, can adversely affect mental function (McDowell & Cedarbaum, 1988; Riley & Lang, 1996).

Treatment: Bromocriptine. Bromocriptine (Parlodel) mimics the action of dopamine. It can relieve akinesia, rigidity, and tremor in many patients with Parkinson's disease. It has less antiparkinsonism effect than levodopa used alone, but may cause less abnormal involuntary movement. It also has a longer duration of action. Nausea and orthostatic hypotension may occur early in treatment, but this is usually avoided by increasing the dosage slowly.

Major disadvantages of bromocriptine, especially in high doses (more than 30 mg a day), are mental disturbance, nightmares, agitation, hallucinations, and paranoid delusions. The latter are more common in older patients. Angina pectoris (chest pain due to lack of appropriate blood supply to the heart), sexual impotence, swelling and redness of the lower extremities, and arterial spasm in the hands and feet causing pain and weakness are rare but have been reported.

The best results of bromocriptine occur early in the treatment, when the drug is used with Sinemet. Low doses of bromocriptine (less than 30 mg a day) combined with Sinemet can ameliorate the wearing-off and on-off effects that sometimes result from prolonged use of levodopa. When bromocriptine is given concurrently, levodopa can be given in lower doses (less than 1,000 mg per day), thus causing fewer dyskinesias and dystonias. However, the toxicity of levodopa and bromocriptine may be additive. This is especially true of their adverse mental effects.

Treatment: Selegiline/Deprenyl (Eldepryl). This treatment is thought to possibly delay disability in the need for levodopa therapy. It is fairly well tolerated at the usual dosage of 5 mg after breakfast and 5 mg after lunch. It occasionally causes nausea, insomnia, and hallucinations. When combined with levodopa, it can enhance the development of levodopa-related dyskinesias. What is known about deprenyl is that it inhibits MAO-B. It is not known whether deprenyl retards the progression of neuronal degeneration as a protective effect or whether the slower rate of disability that ensues following its usage can be explained by this symptomatic effect (Jankovic, 1994).

Adjunctive Drugs in Parkinson's Disease. Depression often accompanies Parkinson's disease. Tricyclic antidepressants such as trazodone (Desyrel) or fluoxetine (Prozac) may be useful. Monoamine oxidase inhibitors used for depression can cause marked swings in blood pressure in patients taking levodopa. Propranolol (Inderal) and other similar medications (known as beta-adrenergic blockers) are useful for decreasing action tremor that may accompany the resting tremor of Parkinson's disease. The use of pallidotomy to treat Parkinson's disease is an effective therapy and has received popular attention (Dogali et al., 1995).

Parkinsonism-plus Syndromes. Parkinsonian symptoms are sometimes the presenting features of parkinsonism-plus syndromes. These neurologic conditions are distinguished clinically from idiopathic Parkinson's disease by the presence of associated signs and symptoms that occur together in various combinations. These signs and symptoms include impaired eye movements; spinocerebellar, corticospinal, and autonomic nervous system dysfunction; motor neuronal degeneration; peripheral neuropathy; and dementia.

The most common of these syndromes is progressive supranuclear palsy (PSP), also known as Steele-Richardson-Olszewski syndrome. Usually the patient's first complaint is difficulty with posture. Gait is slow. There may be axial rigidity and extension of head and neck. Disturbed eye motility usually is present; loss of downward gaze is common, followed by loss of upward gaze. Levodopa may be effective for some patients. Occasionally bromocriptine is helpful (McDowell & Cedarbaum, 1988; Riley & Lang, 1996).

The family of multiple systems degeneration constitutes another group of parkinsonism-plus syndromes. Multiple systems degenerations have three major subgroups: (a) those with predominant cerebellar features (olivopontocerebel lar degeneration); (b) those with predominant autonomic features (Shy-Drager's syndrome), such as orthostatic hypotension without associated rise in pulse; and (c) those in which drug-resistant parkinsonism is the major clinical finding.

Corticobasal degeneration overpresents with an asymmetric motor syndrome of apraxia, dystonia, action myoclonus, and what is known as the "alien hand sign." There is often corticosensory loss. Dementia frequently develops and speech apraxia, as well as oral apraxia associated with dysfluency, occur. Therapy is extremely difficult (Schneider, Watts, Gearing, Brewer, & Mirra, 1997).

Other Parkinsonian Syndromes. The symptoms and signs of postencephalitic parkinsonism are similar to the idiopathic form, but the former usually have more autonomic dysfunction and may have more seborrhea (oily skin), sialorrhea (salivation), and hyperhidrosis (increased perspiration). Blepharospasm (frequent and tight closing of the eyelids) may be prominent.

Many pharmacological agents can cause movement disorders. The disorders appear to result from the actions these drugs have on dopamine receptors, but this is not certain. Hyperkinetic, as well as hypokinetic, syndromes can occur.

The most common drug-induced movement disorder is *parkinsonism*. Parkinsonism can be produced by drugs that deplete the brain of dopamine, interfere with its synthesis and release, block dopamine receptors, or destroy dopaminergic neurons. Reserpine and tetrabenazine deplete the brain of biogenic amines including dopamine. Phenothiazine (e.g., Thorazine), thiothixene (e.g., Navane), and butyrophenone (e.g., Haldol) neuroleptics owe their therapeutic efficacy to the blocking of dopamine receptors. Further, antiemetic (antinausea) preparations such as pro-chlorperazine (Compazine) and metoclopramide (Reglan) may cause parkinsonism.

The clinical syndrome of drug-induced parkinsonism is similar to that of the idiopathic form of the disease, but postural reflexes are less likely to be disturbed in drug-induced parkinsonism and tremor is often prominent. This syndrome is usually reversible upon withdrawal of the offending medication.

The "treatment" for drug-induced parkinsonism is prevention. Rest, using as small a dose as possible of the potentially offending medication, and avoiding use of the stronger parkinsonism-producing agents—especially in the elderly who may have limited dopaminergic reserve—is best. If drug-induced parkinsonism cannot be avoided, small doses of anticholinergic medication such as trihexyphenidyl (2 mg to 6 mg per day) or benztropine (0.5 mg to 2 mg per day) or amantadine (100 mg to 200 mg per day) are useful (Goetz & Klawans, 1984; McDowell & Cedarbaum, 1988; Riley & Lang, 1996).

Any disturbance that causes an increased movement of respiratory muscles, laryngeal muscles, or supralaryngeal articulators can interfere with speech (Darley, Aronson, & Brown, 1975; Hartman & Abbs, 1988). Likewise, any medication that decreases the movement of these muscles can compromise speech. Any of the movement disorders can cause speech compromise. The data pertaining to this realm are continually increasing, as an increasing number of physicians and speech–language pathologists investigate speech motor disturbances.

When a patient presents with speech symptoms or other disturbances, medications are directed at treating the underlying disease state. Thus, a patient who has a known, diagnosed essential tremor, for example, might be prescribed a beta-blocker, whereas a patient with Parkinson's disease might be prescribed a parkinsonian medication. The drug therapy will address the underlying disease state and hopefully will decrease or eliminate the symptoms. Problems arise when there are a presenting speech symptom and associated nonspeech signs, and the symptoms are not recognized. In my experience, this frequently is the case of patients with spasmodic dysphonia. Many of these patients have focal dystonia or essential tremor (Rosenfield, 1988b).

An example of speech problems without nonspeech signs or symptoms is dysfunction of the neuromuscular junction, known as *myasthenia gravis*. Patients with myasthenia gravis have weak muscles because an appropriate amount of acetylcholine does not reach the muscle receptors at the neuromuscular junction. There are different classifications of myasthenia gravis. Some individuals have only double vision or droopy eyelids, whereas others are so weak that they cannot breathe. Often myasthenic patients—whatever their symptoms—improve with a period of rest, which may be as short as 2 to 3 minutes (Rosenfield & Barroso, 1996). The characteristics of speech disturbance due to myasthenia gravis may be poor volume, slurred speech, and hypernasality. As patients continue to talk, they may become short of breath and increasingly hypernasal.

The diagnosis of myasthenia gravis is not always simple—it involves multiple medical and electrical tests. When myasthenia gravis is suspected, the physician should be consulted as soon as possible, especially if the patient complains of shortness of breath. Anticholinesterase medication, such as pyridostigmine bromide (Mestinon), provides an increased amount of acetylicholine at the neuromuscular junction. Therapies may include thymectomy, steroids, and plasmapheresis. Worsening of speech can result if the patient is either on too little or too much medication. Patients with myasthenia gravis should be followed carefully and should be treated by a physician who has experience with this disease. Frequently, there are multiple side effects with the therapies used. This holds especially true for steroids, which have multiple short-term as well as long-term side effects, including weight gain, edema, ulcers, osteoporosis, as well as multiple other problems. Side effects from steroids are pronounced when patients have been on medication over several months but are usually well tolerated in the short term. Any side effects should be reported to the physician.

Speech Motor Control

Normal Speech Motor Output

As previously stated, when a patient takes a drug, the drug does not go only to one particular spot in the brain. Rather, the drug can affect various cerebral sites as well as areas outside the brain, causing behaviors that may or may not be anticipated. Many of these cerebral sites can be involved in production of speech. In order to discuss the realm of speech motor dysfunction further, however, one needs to understand how it is that speech is produced. Our understanding is far from complete. The ensuing discussion pertains only to speech motor output, not aphasia (an acquired disturbance of language).

Mammalian vocalization involves appropriate coordination between respiration, laryngeal activity, and articulatory movements. The lower motor neurons that control the respiratory movements reside in the anterior portion of the cervical, thoracic, and upper lumbar spinal cord. Motor neurons controlling laryngeal closure reside in the nucleus ambiguous, located in the lower part of the brainstem. Neurons directly responsible for articulatory control are the trigeminal motor nucleus, facial nucleus, rostral portion of the nucleus ambiguous, hypoglossal nucleus, and the anterior horn cells of the rostral portion of the cervical spinal cord. This wide array of neural tissue extends from the pons to the lower part of the spinal cord (Jurgens & Ploog, 1981).

Considerable evidence supports the thesis that there is bilateral cortical bulbar input to the periaqueductal gray, an area located in the middle part of the midbrain (the midbrain is the upper part of the brainstem, located above the pons, which, in turn, is above the medulla). There is also major input from the limbic system, a part of the brain that has a strong role in emotions. It is important to note that there are multiple inputs to the lower motor neurons involved with speech motor output. Thus, compromising cortex, subcortex, basal ganglia, thalamus, and multiple areas of the brainstem can independently alter speech. The above-noted compromise can result from lesions (e.g., tumor, stroke, or infection), but it can also result from medications affecting these areas (Jurgens & Ploog, 1981; Rosenfield & Barroso, 1996).

Stuttering

There are very cogent arguments that stutterers have a neurophysiologic predisposition toward stuttering, resulting in speech motor dynamic disturbance. No singular psychiatric theory can explain the fact that (a) the prevalence of stuttering has not decreased (Bloodstein, 1995; Porfert & Rosenfield, 1978), (b) stuttered dysfluencies are not random, (c) there are genetically determined patterns of inheritance for stuttering, and (d) particular fluency-evoking maneuvers (e.g., singing, speaking with loud broad-band noise, speaking during inhalation) eliminate stuttering behaviors. Further, there is no evidence that stuttering has ever been cured by psychiatric intervention (Bloodstein, 1995; Rosenfield, 1984; Rosenfield & Boller, 1985; Rosenfield & Nudelman, 1987).

Stutterers do talk. Stutterers have some fluent output, just as fluent speakers have some dysfluent output. Stress alters the degree and frequency of dysfluent output, as it alters the motor output of all individuals with underlying motor control disturbances. This affect-sensitivity reminds us that speech output is a highly delicate motor coordinative task. Just as emotional stress can exacerbate a parkinsonian tremor or an underlying dystonic disturbance, so can it alter stuttered dysfluencies.

It is in this context that the pharmacotherapy of stuttering is discussed. The degree of emotional stress sometimes can be curtailed through psychotherapy, biofeedback, or pharmacotherapy. Pharmacotherapies that might be effective in treating stuttering are alprazolam (Xanax) and other tranquilizers. Alprazolam might be most effective for reducing speech anxiety in that it can decrease some of the autonomic nervous system responses, such as increased heart rate. For example, if a student who stutters has to give a book report in class and has a rapid heartbeat, that heartbeat itself might cause the student to be more dysfluent. Alprazolam might lessen some of the student's anxiety. It should be stated, however, that no control studies have been conducted with results that support this thesis. There could be a strong placebo effect.

The usual dosage of alprazolam is 0.25 mg to 1.5 mg daily, taken orally. The drug is one of the benzodiazepine derivatives. Other benzodiazepines include chlordiazepoxide (Librium), oxazepam (Serax), diazepam (Valium), clorazepate (Tranxene), and clonazepam (Klonopin). In general, the clinical toxicity of these drugs is low, although they can cause drowsiness and unsteadiness, and there can be physical dependence and withdrawal symptoms.

There have been several investigations pertaining to pharmacotherapies for stuttering. Brady (1991) and Bloodstein (1995) review many of these, but none of the drugs studied has proved unequivocally effective. Several years ago, some schizophrenics who stuttered were treated with the antidopamine medication haloperidol. While taking this medication, they stuttered less. This observation led to multiple studies in which stutterers were given dopamine-blocking agents, such as haloperidol, to determine whether dysfluencies decreased. The results were inconclusive. It may be that the patients on haloperidol who had fewer dysfluencies following medication were somewhat somnolent or slightly fatigued while on the medication, in effect causing them to speak more slowly. Slowed speech is a well-known therapy technique that decreases dysfluencies independently of pharmacologic agents (Bloodstein, 1995; Rosenberger, 1980; Rosenberger, Wheelden, & Kalotkin, 1976).

Haloperidol is primarily a dopaminergic (D-2) antagonist. As noted, its efficacy in treating stuttering has long been queried. It is also effective in reducing vocal and motor tics in patients with Tourette's syndrome. Clomipramine, a tricyclic antidepressant effective in treating obsessive–compulsive disorders, has been successful in reducing repetitive motor behaviors and motor stereotypes. The primary action of clomipramine is that of serotonin reuptake inhibitor. Desipramine is also an antidepressant with effects similar to that of clomipramine but has adrenergic reuptake blockade potency and has only a weak seratonergic effect. These two drugs were studied by Stager, Ludlow, Gordon, Cotelingam, and Rappoport (1995) in treating stuttering. These studies were extremely difficult, but it appears as though there was evidence of improvement when patients took clomipramine when compared to desipramine, thus raising the question whether fluency improvement can relate to serotonergic reuptake inhibition.

To explore further the possible relationship of haloperidol and stuttering, Rosenfield, Freeman, and Jankovic (1983) reasoned that if haloperidol truly reduces stuttering, the effect presumably results from the blocking by haloperidol of CNS dopamine receptors. They questioned whether stutterers who had lost dopamine might actually become more fluent. That is, they reasoned that if stutterers developed Parkinson's disease—which is associated with dopamine depletion in parts of the brain—perhaps their speech would improve.

Rosenfield and colleagues reviewed a large series of stutterers who subsequent to stuttering developed Parkinson's disease. They could not ascertain whether or not their speech improved. In some instances, when speech did improve, it may have been because slowing of speech resulted from the Parkinson's disease itself. It is well known that many patients with Parkinson's disease develop dysfluencies as a result of the disease and that these dysfluencies are different from those caused by developmental stuttering (Cannito, Deal, & DiLollo, this volume; Canter, 1971). Regardless, they were not able to document any improvement in stuttering behavior during the course of treatment for Parkinson's disease.

Personally, I have prescribed different pharmacologic agents for stuttering, thinking that these drugs might be effective in controlling stuttering. These were not prescribed as part of double-blind controlled studies. The stutterers could have had a marked placebo overlay, and all patients were told that there was no guarantee that the medication would control their stuttering, although a pharmacologic rationale for administering the drug did exist. In this context, each of the following drugs was prescribed for multiple stuttering patients: carbamazepine (Tegretol), diphenylhydantoin (Dilantin), clonidine (Catapres), propranolol (Inderal), alprazolam (Xanax), and clonazepam (Klonopin). In a noncontrolled environment, with an admittedly high placebo predisposition, some of these patients reported improvement in answering the telephone, addressing large audiences, introducing themselves, or doing anything else of speech-related importance. Alprazolam and clonazepam were most effective. Finally, to this author's knowledge, there have been no substantiated reports of

Dilantin curing stuttering. There have been some reports of improved speech output under Dilantin, but these have never been substantiated (Bloodstein, 1995).

Hays (1987) wrote a letter stating that bethanechol may help stuttering. Another letter (Goldstein, 1987) contended that carbamazepine helps. A subsequent letter by Rosenfield (1988a) also discussed the efficacy of carbamazepine for stuttering.

Stuttering is so variable that it is difficult to be certain whether a stutterer is better one day or the next, one week or the next, and so on. In this setting, double-blind studies with qualified professionals evaluating the speech output become imperative.

At the present time, there is no definitive indication for pharmacologic therapy in stuttering. In all likelihood, no singular curative drug will be found, because many individuals stutter for different reasons and possibly each one stutters for different reasons at different times. However, there may be a subclass of stutterers who benefit from appropriate medications, especially those that decrease the autonomic responses (such as increased heart rate and hyperventilation) due to anxiety (e.g., alprazolam, clonazepam).

Spasmodic Dysphonia

Spasmodic dysphonia (SD) is a chronic phonatory disorder of unknown etiology that usually appears in adulthood. The speech of SD patients is characterized by choppy breaks in phonation, staccato-like catches, a strained-strangled voice quality, and monopitch. Phonation in SD patients is often accompanied by effortful, jerky, strained sounds that are frequently associated with pain in the laryngeal area.

Interruptions of phonatory airflow in SD presumably result from the intermittent hyperadduction of the vocal folds. Endoscopy usually fails to reveal evidence of nerve or muscle disease. No singular cause of SD has been identified, and there is great argument regarding the possibility of psychogenic disturbance in these individuals.

The nature of the referral base determines the type of SD patients that an individual clinician may see. Neurologists typically see those SD patients who have been seen by multiple speech–language pathologists and several ear, nose, and throat physicians. The majority of patients in our clinic have been seen by several professionals over a long period of time. Neurologic disturbance is evident in two thirds of these patients. Of those patients who have neurologic disturbance, the majority have evidence of dystonia elsewhere (usually face, eyes, head, or neck) or tremor elsewhere (seen in finger-to-nose testing or head movements at rest). Usually these individuals' voices improve with pharmacotherapy, though the symptoms persist. The symptoms that are most distressing are tightness in the larynx and neck and the presence of glottal stops (Rosenfield, 1988b, 1988c, 1994).

Patients with spasmodic dysphonia as a result of underlying phonatory tremor often report that their speech improves when they drink alcohol. This is because alcohol affects the tremor, not because it makes the patient more relaxed. Individuals who have phonatory tremor, and especially those who improve with alcohol, can be treated with a beta-blocker such as propranolol (Inderal). If this fails, sometimes a low-dose regimen of Mysoline or Tegretol is efficacious. In my experience, I have found that the majority of patients respond to propranolol. The symptom that improves the most is glottal stopping. The patients also frequently report a diminished sensation of straining and pain (Rosenfield, 1988b, 1988c, 1994).

Patients with evidence of dystonia—frequently associated with Meige syndrome (oromandibular dystonia associated with blepharospasm)—often respond to a regimen of baclofen (Lioresal). If they fail to respond to this, a combination of trihexyphenidyl (Artane) and lithium may be effective. Frequently, alprazolam (Xanax) or clonazepam (Klonopin) is effective.

Individuals who have no evidence of disease elsewhere may nevertheless be initiated on a regimen of Lioresal, which may reduce the feeling of tightness in their vocal folds. If this fails to help, a regimen of alprazolam (Xanax) or clonazepam (Klonopin) may decrease muscle tension as well as tranquilize the patient.

I believe that all SD patients should be seen by a speech–language pathologist. Sometimes, but not often, patients respond better to speech therapy when they are on medication. If patients do respond to the above medications, they do so in the first 1 or 2 weeks. When patients fail to respond to a medical regimen, one should consider intralaryngeal muscle botulinum toxin injection. Botulinum toxin, as already noted, blocks the release of acetylcholine, a most important neurotransmitter at the neuromuscular junction. Blocking the release of acetylcholine causes the muscle to be weak and thus decreases laryngeal muscle activity (DeBito, Malmgren, & Gacek, 1985; Jankovic, 1988;

Jankovic & Hallett, 1994; Rosenfield, 1988b, 1988c, 1994). For a case study of a spasmodic dysphonic patient treated using combined pharmacotherapy and speech therapy, the reader is referred to Chapter 9.

Summary

The fact that a speech deficit such as stuttering or spasmodic dysphonia worsens under emotional stress does not prove that the disturbance is purely psychogenic (Rosenfield, 1982). Although it is tempting to look to neuropharmacology for a potential mode of treatment, there are many speech motor disturbances that have no real definitive cures. Few clinicians cure stuttering (in adults), spasmodic dysphonia, or speech tremor. However, many excellent therapists can make people considerably better. What is important is to be certain that underlying disease processes have been ruled out and that any medications that might be effective have been tried.

I have discussed some major disease processes as well as basic pharmacology and medication. If a patient has a neurologic disease that is causing speech symptoms, and if the symptoms that are not related to speech respond to medication, then often the speech symptoms will also respond. However, there is sometimes a trade-off in that patients have worsening speech while improving otherwise. Individuals on anticholinergic medication may have improvement in their Parkinson's disease but also have a dry mouth. A simple, effective truism is that any drug can do just about anything to anyone. If a patient is on a medication and after a few weeks develops a speech symptom, question whether that drug has caused the symptom. If a speech–language pathologist who is seeing a patient has questions about a prescribed medication, the pathologist should insist that the patient speak to the referring physician.

Speech–language pathologists, physicians, and other health care personnel have one primary goal: that the patient do well. A working knowledge of pharmacology and its basic mechanisms can help speech clinicians move toward that goal. Taking care of sick patients is not easy, and the more input physicians have from health care personnel who interact with the patients, the more effective medical care they can provide. It is hoped that the information presented in this chapter will contribute to that end.

Acknowledgments

This work was supported by the M. R. Bauer Foundation and the Lowin Medical Research Foundation.

References

Bloodstein, O. (1995). *The handbook of stuttering*. San Diego: Singular.

Brady, J. P. (1991). The pharmacology of stuttering: A critical review. *American Journal of Pyschiatry, 148,* 1309–1316.

Butler, I. J. (1984). Tourette's syndrome: Some new concepts. In J. Jankovic (Ed.), *Neurologic clinics—movement disorders*. Philadelphia: Saunders.

Calne, D. B., & Lang, A. E. (1988). Secondary dystonia. In S. Fahn, C. D. Marsden, & D. B. Calne (Eds.), *Advances in neurology: Vol. 50. Dystonia 2* (pp. 9–33). New York: Raven Press.

Canter, G. J. (1971). Observations on neurogenic stuttering: A contribution to differential diagnosis. *British Journal of Disorders of Communication, 6,* 139–143.

Chesselet, M. F., & Delfs, J. M. (1996). Basal ganglia and movement disorders: An update. *Trends in Neurosciences, 19,* 417–421.

Cooper, J. R., Bloom, F. E., & Roth, R. H. (1996). *The biochemical basis of neuropharmacology*. New York: Oxford University Press.

Darley, F. L., Aronson, A. E., & Brown, J. R. (1975). *Motor speech disorders*. Philadelphia: Saunders.

DeBito, M. A., Malmgren, L. T., & Gacek, P. R. (1985). Three-dimensional distribution of neuromuscular junction in human cricothyroid. *Archives of Otolaryngology, 111,* 110–113.

Dogali, M., Fazzini, E., Kolodny, E., Eidelberg, D., Sterio, D., Devinsky, O., & Beric, A. (1995). Stereotactic ventral pallidotomy for Parkinson's disease. *Neurology, 45,* 753–761.

Fahn, S. (1984). The varied clinical expressions of dystonia. In J. Jankovic (Ed.), *Neurologic clinics—movement disorders* (pp. 541–555). Philadelphia: Saunders.

Fahn, S. (1988). Concept and classification of dystonia. In S. Fahn, C. D. Marsden, & D. B. Calne (Eds.), *Advances in neurology: Vol. 50. Dystonia 2* (pp. 1–8). New York: Raven Press.

Fahn, S., Marsden, C. D., & Calne, D. B. (Eds.). (1988). *Advances in neurology: Vol. 50. Dystonia 2*. New York: Raven Press.

Goetz, C. J., & Klawans, H. L. (1984). Tardive dyskinesia. In J. Jankovic (Ed.), *Neurologic clinics—movement disorders* (pp. 605–614). Philadelphia: Saunders.

Goldstein, J. A. (1987). Carbamazepine treatment for stuttering. *Journal of Clinical Psychology, 48,* 39.

Hardman, J. G., & Limbird, L. E. (1996). *Goodman and Gillman's "The pharmacological basis of therapeutics."* New York: Macmillan.

Hartman, D. E., & Abbs, J. H. (1988). Dysarthrias of movement disorders. In J. Jankovic & E. Tolosa (Eds.), *Advances in neurology: Vol. 49. Facial dyskinesias* (pp. 289–306). New York: Raven Press.

Hays, P. (1987). Bethanecol chloride in the treatment of stuttering. *Lancet, 1,* 271.

Hill, A. B. (1960). *Controlled clinical trials: Conference of Council for International Organization of Medical Sciences.* Oxford, UK: Blackwell Scientific Publications.

Hill, A. B. (1962). *Statistical methods in clinical and preventative medicine.* New York: Oxford University Press.

Ingelfinger, J. A., Mosteller, F., Thibodeau, I. A., & Ware, J. H. (1983). *Biostatistics in clinical medicine.* New York: Macmillan.

Jankovic, J. (1988). Blepharospasm and oromandibular-laryngeal-cervical dystonia: A controlled trial of botulinum A toxin therapy. In S. Fahn, C. D. Marsden, & D. B. Calne (Eds.), *Advances in neurology: Vol. 50. Dystonia 2* (pp. 583–591). New York: Raven Press.

Jankovic, J. (1994). Neuroprotection: A reachable therapeutic goal? In M. B. Stern (Ed.), *Beyond the decade of the brain* (pp. 109–130). Kent, UK: Wells Medical Limited.

Jankovic, J. (1996, November). *Advances in diagnosis, therapy, and pathogensis.* Paper presented at Current Neurology Conference, Baylor College of Medicine, Houston.

Jankovic, J., & Hallett, M. (1994). *Therapy with botulinum toxin.* New York: Marcel Dekker.

Jurgens, U., & Ploog, D. (1981). On the neural control of mammalian vocalization. *Trends in Neuroscience, 4,* 135–137.

Koch-Weser, J. (1972). Serum drug concentrations as therapeutic guides. *New England Journal of Medicine, 287,* 227–231.

Koller, W. C. (1984). Diagnosis and treatment of tremors. In J. Jankovic (Ed.), *Neurologic clinics—movement disorders* (pp. 499–514). Philadelphia: Saunders.

Lang, A. E. (1996). Movement disorder symptomatology. In W. G. Bradley, R. B. Daroff, G. M. Finichel, & C. D. Marsden (Eds.), *Neurology and clinical practice: The neurological disorders.* New York: Butterworth-Heinemann.

Marsden, C. D. (1988). The investigation of dystonia. In S. Fahn, C. D. Marsden, & D. B. Calne (Eds.), *Advances in neurology: Vol. 50. Dystonia 2* (pp. 35–44). New York: Raven Press.

McDowell, F. H., & Cedarbaum, J. M. (1988). The extrapyramidal system and disorders of movement. In R. J. Joynt (Ed.), *Clinical neurology* (Vol. 3, rev. ed., p. 18). Philadelphia: Lippincott.

Netter, F. H. (1983). *The CIBA collection of medical illustrations: Vol. 1. Nervous system: Part 1. Anatomy and physiology.* West Caldwell, NJ: CIBA Pharmaceutical.

Nies, A. S., & Spielberg, S. T. (1996). Principles of therapeutics. In J. G. Hardman & L. E. Limbird (Eds.), *Goodman and Gillman's "The pharmacological basis of therapeutics."* New York: Macmillan.

Porfert, A. R., & Rosenfield, D. B. (1978). Prevalence of stuttering. *Journal of Neurology, Neurosurgery and Psychiatry, 41,* 954–956.

Purves, D., Augustine, G. J., Fitzpatrick, D., Katz, L. C., La Mantia, A. S., & McNamara, J. O. (1997). (Eds.). *Neuroscience.* Sunderland, MA: Sinauer Associates.

Riley, D. E., & Lang, A. E. (1996). Movement disorders. In W. G. Bradley, R. B. Daroff, G. M. Fenichel, & C. D. Marsden (Eds.), *Neurology and clinical practice: The neurological disorders.* New York: Butterworth-Heinemann.

Rosenberger, P. B. (1980). Dopaminergic systems and speech fluency. *Journal of Fluency Disorders, 5,* 255–267.

Rosenberger, P. B., Wheelden, L. A., & Kalotkin, M. (1976). The effect of haloperidol on stuttering. *American Journal of Psychiatry, 133,* 331–333.

Rosenfield, D. B. (1982). A comment on stuttering. *Journal of Fluency Disorders, 7,* 79–80.

Rosenfield, D. B. (1984). Scientific approaches to stuttering. *Critical Reviews in Clinical Neurobiology, 1,* 117–139.

Rosenfield, D. B. (1988a). Carbamazepine treatment for stuttering. *Journal of Clinical Psychology, 49,* 38.

Rosenfield, D. B. (1988b). Spasmodic dysphonia. In J. Jankovic & E. Tolosa (Eds.), *Advances in neurology: Vol. 49. Facial dyskinesias.* New York: Raven Press.

Rosenfield, D. B. (1988c). Spasmodic dysphonia. In S. Fahn, C. D. Marsden, & D. B. Calne (Eds.), *Advances in neurology: Vol. 50. Dystonia 2* (pp. 537–545). New York: Raven Press.

Rosenfield, D. B. (1994). Clinical aspects of speech motor compromise. In J. Jankovic & H. Hallett (Eds.), *Therapeutic botulinum toxin.* New York: Marcel Dekker.

Rosenfield, D. B., & Barroso, A. B. (1996). Difficulties with speech and swallowing. In W. G. Bradley, R. B. Daroff, G. M. Fenichel, & C. D. Marsden (Eds.), *Neurology in clinical practice: Vol. 1. Principles of diagnosis and management* (pp. 129–141). Stoneham, MA: Butterworth-Heinemann.

Rosenfield, D. B., & Boller, F. (1985). Stuttering. In P. J. Binken, G. W. Bruyn, & H. L. Klawans (Eds.), *Handbook of clinical neurology* (pp. 169–173, Vol. 2, No. 46). Amsterdam: Elsevier Science.

Rosenfield, D. B., Freeman, F., & Jankovic, J. (1983, April). *Stuttering and the dopamine system.* Paper presented at the 35th annual meeting of the American Academy of Neurology, San Diego, CA.

Rosenfield, D. B., & Nudelman, H. B. (1987). Neuropsychological models of dysfluency. In L. Rustin, H. Purser, & D. Rowley (Eds.),

Progress in the treatment of fluency disorders. London: Taylor and Francis.

Schneider, J. A., Watts, R. L., Gearing, M., Brewer, R. P., & Mirra, S. S. (1997). Corticobasal degeneration: Neuropathologic and clinical heterogeneity. *Neurology, 48,* 959–969.

Stager, S. V., Ludlow, C. L., Gordon, C. D., Cotelingam, M., & Rappoport, J. L. (1995). Fluency changes in persons who stutter following a double-blind trial of clomipramine and desipramine. *Journal of Speech and Hearing Research, 38,* 516–525.

Stoof, J. C., & Kebabian, J. W. (1981). Imposing roles for D-1 and D-2 dopamine receptors in efflux of cyclic AMP from rat neostriatum. *Nature, 294,* 366–368.

Vogel, D., Carter, J. E., & Carter, P. B. (2000). *The effects of drugs on communication disorders* (2nd ed.). San Diego: Singular.

Chapter 3

Dysarthria Evaluation and Treatment: The Basics

Vicki L. Hammen

Hammen discusses various basic approaches to evaluation and treatment of dysarthria. She outlines perceptual, physiologic, and acoustic aspects of evaluation and treatment.

1. List some general evaluation tools used by dysarthria clinicians.

2. How can being aware of speech production subsystems influence evaluation and treatment of dysarthric patients?

3. What is the relationship between rate control and speech intelligibility?

※　　※　　※

A number of approaches to the evaluation and treatment of dysarthria have been suggested by clinicians and researchers in the field. From the auditory-perceptual methods first described in detail by Darley, Aronson, and Brown (1969a, 1969b, 1975), to the physiologic approach advocated by Netsell (1986), to the acoustic approaches demonstrated by Weismer (1984), there appear to be many ways of looking at the person presenting with dysarthria. How should the clinician decide which one to use? Gerratt, Till, Rosenbek, Wertz, and Boysen (1991) surveyed clinicians in Veteran's Administration medical facilities about their actual and perceived use of perceptual and instrumental measures. They found that clinicians tended to use approaches with which they were comfortable, which was most often auditory-perceptual measures. Does that mean that other methods are not useful? An excellent answer to this question was provided by Rosenbek (1984):

> Perceptual, physiological, and acoustic methods of analyzing dysarthric speech complement one another. Good clinical research programs combine findings from all three. To use only one (most often the perceptual in contemporary clinical practice) is not malpractice. To use more than one is merely enriched practice. (p. 361)

The purpose of this chapter is to provide the reader with information concerning all three aspects—perceptual, physiologic, and acoustic—and to demonstrate their usefulness through selected case studies. It should be noted at the outset that the evaluation and treatment of dysarthria have been covered in greater detail in Yorkston, Beukleman, and Bell (1988); Yorkston, Beukleman, Strand, and Bell (1999); and Duffy (1995). Much of what is included in this chapter is drawn from these excellent resources.

In addition to the issues presented above, another factor in deciding on the specific approach used in evaluation is the goal of the process. For example, if a patient is referred with an unknown neurologic diagnosis, the goal will be to contribute to the differential diagnosis of the patient's disease process. However, if the referral is based on the need for improved intelligibility in an individual 6 months post traumatic brain injury, the goal will more likely be to determine candidacy for intervention and to set appropriate treatment goals. Finally, as professionals are called to be more accountable for their intervention, evaluation can be used to assess outcome. That is, the question that must be answered is, Have the intervention strategies been effective in producing a change in speech performance?

Approaches to the Evaluation of Dysarthria

Perceptual

The perceptual approach to the evaluation of dysarthria was pioneered by Darley et al. (1969a, 1969b, 1975). It is based on the assumption that different types of dysarthria have distinct perceptual characteristics that can be judged via a number of dimensions. The general auditory-perceptual categories for these dimensions include pitch characteristics, loudness, voice quality, respiration, prosody, and articulation. Judges rate speakers with dysarthria using a 7-point, equal-appearing interval scale; 1 is normal and 7 represents very severe deviation from normal. Different types of dysarthria are represented by clusters of deviations in these dimensions. In their original work, Darley and colleagues identified six different types of dysarthria: flaccid, ataxic, spastic, hypokinetic, hyperkinetic, and mixed. Duffy (1995) added two more categories—unilateral upper motor neuron and undetermined. Based on the neurological diagnoses of the patients selected for perceptual judgment, these types of dysarthria are then associated with different lesion sites in the central and peripheral nervous system.

One of the advantages of the perceptual approach is that because dysarthria is by definition a speech disorder, judgments are made on the basis of the speech output of the individual. It can serve as the standard by which intervention is assessed. That is, Has the selected intervention method had an effect on the speech output of the individual? This method requires no more equipment than the clinician's ears. However, the importance of the clinician's skill and experience in judging the speech of a person with dysarthria should not be minimized. Despite its long history of use in the field, relatively little work has been done to establish guidelines for the amount of experience needed to reliably rate dysarthric speech. As reported in their 1975 text, Darley et al. served as the judges for the investigation. Obviously, they were not only highly experienced clinicians, but they also had participated in the development of the dimensions they were rating. Not surprisingly, 80%–95% of the dimensions were within one scale point for both intra- and interjudge reliability measures. Similar results have not been obtained in the two studies that attempted to replicate the findings of Darley et al. (Zeplin & Kent, 1996; Zyski & Weisiger, 1987). Clearly this is an area in need of some solid research efforts. Additionally, the perceptual approach to the evaluation of dysarthria cannot directly test the effects of the neurologic condition on the speech production system.

Physiologic Approach

The perspective taken in the physiologic approach is that the speech production system can be viewed as a series of components that may be impaired as the result of a neurologic condition. This approach has been primarily addressed by Netsell and others (Netsell, 1984, 1986; Netsell, Lotz, & Barlow, 1989). The components within the approach include abdomen–diaphragm, rib cage, larynx, tongue–pharynx, velopharynx, tongue–middle, tongue–anterior, jaw, and lips. Clearly, speech is not the result of only one of these components; rather, it is the interaction of a number of components that produces what is perceived as speech. Netsell and Daniel (1979) addressed the concept of "functional components," which are combinations of the previously listed components that work together to create or valve the speech stream.

One of the advantages of the physiologic approach is that the examiner is seeking evidence of the pathophysiology underlying the dysarthria. The effects of weakness, incoordination, and spasticity on speech production can be assessed directly rather than being inferred. In this way, it represents an approach that is one step closer to the source of the speech disorder. However, it is not without its disadvantages. A number of issues must be considered when employing this approach. First, the direct assessment of the physiologic components underlying speech production requires the use of instrumentation. As with the perceptual method, the validity and reliability of physiologic measures are also dependent on the skill of the clinician to accurately use and interpret the data generated from instrumentation. Secondly, task selection is an important consideration. An ongoing debate concerns the usefulness of nonspeech tasks in the assessment of speech disorders (Luschei, 1991; Weismer & Liss, 1991). Often, nonspeech or non-propositional speech tasks are used as part of a physiologic evaluation. The relationship between performance on such tasks and speech production abilities has not been well established. As discussed by Kent (1994), the distinction between measurement and assessment is a critical one. With the physiologic approach, a number of variables can be *measured*; it is still the responsibility of the clinician to *assess* the impact or importance of that measure with respect to the speech production system of the individual.

Acoustic Approach

The acoustic signal reflects the entire speech production process from sound generation to the modification of the sound through use of the articulators. It, therefore, can serve as a window into the underlying physiology of the system as well as provide confirmation of what our ears are telling us through the auditory-perceptual modality. Temporal and spectral analyses of the speech of persons with dysarthria have been conducted by a number of researchers. Weismer (1984) investigated issues in motor programming of speech by completing a detailed temporal analysis of the speech produced by persons with Parkinson's disease. Kent and colleagues (Kent et al., 1990; Kent et al., 1991; Kent, Weismer, Kent, & Rosenbek, 1989; Weismer, Kent, Hodge, & Martin, 1988; Weismer, Martin, Kent, & Kent, 1992) examined the relationships between the slope of the second formant and speech intelligibility. Acoustic correlates of a subset of the perceptual dimensions used by Darley et al. (1975) were examined by Ludlow and Bassich (1983). In each of these studies, the acoustic signal reflected aspects of the underlying speech impairment associated with the dysarthria type.

Model of Chronic Disorder

In 1980, Wood presented a framework in which the consequences of a disease process are appreciated from three distinct perspectives: impairment, disability, and handicap. Recently, these terms have been modified to impairment, functional limitation, and disability. The definitions of these three aspects of the model are presented in Table 3.1.

From the perspective of dysarthria, *impairment* would be reflected in the neuromuscular disturbances that are the consequence of the neurologic condition. We can observe rigidity and tremor of the oral-facial musculature in persons with Parkinson's disease. Muscle atrophy and weakness are evident in the speech production system following a brainstem stroke. These findings are evidence of an impairment. The physiologic approach outlined above is very useful in evaluating the underlying impairment.

Functional limitation is the impact the impairment has on speech production. In applying this model to dysarthria, the activity under consideration is that of producing speech that is understandable by

Table 3.1
Definitions of the Disease Process Dimensions from the
World Health Organization Framework

Impairment	Any loss or abnormality of psychological, physiological, or anatomical structure or function
Functional Limitation	Any restriction or lack (resulting from an impairment) of ability to perform an activity in the manner, or within the range, considered normal for a human being
Disability	A disadvantage for a given individual, resulting from an impairment or disability (the functional limitation) that prevents the fulfillment of a role that is normal (depending on age, sex, and social and cultural factors) for that individual

listeners. Reduced speech intelligibility, alterations in speaking rate, reduced articulatory adequacy, and abnormal prosody would all reflect a functional limitation.

Lastly, *disability* is the disadvantage the individual experiences as the result of the functional limitation. Wood (1980) described this as an inability to sustain what has been referred to as "survival roles," for example, occupation, social integration, and economic self-sufficiency. As applied to dysarthria, disability may be reflected in the individual's inability to continue in his or her present occupation. For example, a successful businessman with severe dysarthria secondary to amyotrophic lateral sclerosis will likely be prevented from continuing in that role. In this example, disability was reflected in both occupation and economic self-sufficiency. Additional evidence for disability may be the reactions of others to the dysarthria. These reactions may affect the social, vocational, and educational experiences of the person with dysarthria.

The effects of dysarthria can be evaluated across each of the levels of this model. That is, with the appropriate evaluation tools, one can determine the impact of an impairment on disability, or the impact of impairment on functional limitation. The effectiveness of treatment efforts can be assessed in a similar fashion. Can treatment that focuses on the impairment have an effect on the disabling aspects of the dysarthria? To address this issue, appropriate evaluation tools must be selected.

General Evaluation Tools

Despite the approach to motor speech disorders that is adopted, there are a number of tools available to the clinician to evaluate the person with dysarthria. These represent the basic armamentarium of the clinician and include an oral-motor evaluation and speech intelligibility measurement. A summary of the tasks that comprise the general evaluation is presented in Table 3.2.

Oral-Motor Evaluation

Because dysarthria, as defined by Darley et al. (1975), is the result of "disturbances in muscular control of the speech mechanism" (p. 2), assessing the structure and function of the speech production system should be the foundation of evaluation procedures for persons with dysarthria. (Detailed descriptions of such an examination can be

Table 3.2
Summary of General Evaluation Tools

Oral-Motor Examination	• Evaluation of lips, jaw, and tongue
	• Sustained postures
	• Rapid alternating movements
	• Observations of reflexes
	• Perceptual evaluation of speech characteristics
Speech Intelligibility Testing	• *Computerized Assessment of the Intelligibility of Dysarthric Speech* (CAIDS)
	• Phonetic intelligibility test
	• Single words, sentences, connected speech
	• Estimates
Multipurpose Tool: Frenchay Dysarthria Assessment	• Oral-motor evaluation
	• Speech intelligibility estimate

found in Duffy, 1995.) A basic oral-motor evaluation consists of a series of tasks that test the structural and functional integrity of the lips, tongue, jaw, and velopharynx. Observations are made at rest, while holding sustained positions, and during movements. At rest, the symmetry of the structure and the presence of involuntary movements or tremor are noted. During sustained positions—such as tongue protrusion or lip retraction—symmetry, appearance or disappearance of involuntary movements, the resistance of the structure to movement, and the duration the position is held are noted.

When assessing movement capabilities, rapid alternating positions are used, such as lip pucker then retraction or moving the tongue from side to side. One of the standard measurement tasks is to determine diadochokinetic rates, or how many syllable strings can be produced in a specific time interval. Most often the syllables "pa, ta, ka" "pa-ta-ka" are used, but these can be expanded to include blends such as "spra, stra, skra." Additional tasks can evaluate the larynx, for example, having the patient cough, produce an abrupt closure (glottal coup), or sustain phonation. The adequacy of respiratory support can be observed during this portion of the evaluation by noting any shortness of breath, frequent breaths, or stridor.

Finally, the presence of normal and primitive reflexes can be evaluated. These reflexes include gag, cough, jaw jerk, suck, and snout. The absence of normal reflexes and the presence of reflexes that should disappear after infancy can be indicators of the extent and nature of central and/or peripheral nervous system disorders.

Speech Intelligibility Testing

Speech intelligibility can be used as a general severity indicator when evaluating the person with dysarthria. The most often used, published tests of speech intelligibility are the *Assessment of the Intelligibility of Dysarthric Speech* (AIDS) (Yorkston & Beukelman, 1981) and the *Computerized Assessment of the Intelligibility of Dysarthric Speech* (CAIDS; Yorkston, Beukelman, & Traynor, 1984). The only difference between the two versions is that the computerized version can be administered, judged, and scored via a computer. Two subtests, single words and sentences, make up the test. The speaker reads or repeats a series of 50 single words that were generated by selecting one of 12 possible similar words. The single word test can be judged either by open transcription, or by selection of the word from a list of the 12 possibilities. The percentage correct for the 50 words serves as the single word intelligibility score.

The sentence test generates a list of 10 sentences increasing in length from 5 to 15 words for a total of 220 words. The sentences are selected from a pool of 100 sentences for each length. A judge transcribes the sentences, and a percentage of correctly understood words out of the 220 possible is determined. An added feature of the sentence test is the ability to determine reading rate, intelligible words per minute, and a communication efficiency ratio. Each sentence can be timed, and words per minute is calculated to represent reading rate. The number of words understood correctly, divided by the duration of the sample, determines the intelligible words per minute. Finally, the communication efficiency ratio is the intelligible words per minute, divided by 190, which is the reading rate at which nondysarthric speakers were 100% intelligible. These three indices can be useful in tracking the effect of the dysarthria on motor speech performance.

In addition to the published tests of intelligibility, estimates can also be used. In the most general format, a person with dysarthria reads a passage or engages in conversational speech. The clinician then assigns a number to represent the percentage of the passage or conversation that was understandable. Duffy (1995) presented a 10-point rating scale that incorporates dimensions of environment, context, and efficiency into the rating of intelligibility. This type of rating scale provides more information regarding factors that can affect intelligibility than a simple percentage.

Kent et al. (1989) have used their *Phonetic Intelligibility Test* to examine the relationship between perceptual and acoustic evidence of dysarthria. This test consists of 70 words representing 19 different acoustic contrasts that are read or repeated by the speaker. Judges choose a response from a closed set of 4 words that have minimal phonetic contrast. The response of the judge gives an indication of the type of contrast that may be contributing to the intelligibility deficit in a particular person.

Frenchay Dysarthria Assessment

This test combines features of the oral-motor evaluation and intelligibility ratings. Persons with dysarthria perform tasks that address eight different oral-motor features such as lips, tongue, and palate. The person's responses are given a grade on a 5-point scale. Intelligibility is rated from the production of single words, words in a carrier phrase, and conversation. An additional feature of this assessment tool is the inclusion of sections to address sensation and influencing factors such as hearing, sight, mood, and posture. This test has been found to have good inter-judge reliability and validity (Enderby, 1983).

Assessment of Speech Production Subcomponents

The general evaluation tools already discussed can identify the scope and severity of the dysarthria. For example, we may know that the patient being evaluated is 60% intelligible for single words, is 40% intelligible for sentences from the CAIDS, has a slow rate of speech, and has distorted phoneme production during diadochokinetic tasks. However, do we know where to direct our treatment efforts? Should we focus our attention on improving articulatory precision? Is there an aspect of speech production that should be addressed first? The answers to these questions will be found in an evaluation of the individual subsystems underlying speech production. In the following section, methods to specifically evaluate the respiratory, phonatory, velopharyngeal, and articulatory systems will be presented. These methods are applicable for both the physiologic and chronic disease approaches to dysarthria assessment. Table 3.3 contains a summary of the evaluation tools for the speech production subsystems.

Respiratory System

Is there sufficient respiratory function to support speech production? This is the first question that should be asked when evaluating the respiratory system. The clinician should determine whether the person with dysarthria is capable of providing for his or her ventilatory needs or is using a mechanical ventilator. Mechanical ventilation alters the way in which the respiratory system is used during speech production. Hoit, Shea, and Banzett (1994) found shorter speech duration, speaking on inspiratory air, reduced tracheal pressures, and reduced syllables

Table 3.3
A Summary of Evaluation Tasks for Each Speech Subsystem

Respiratory System	• Respiratory support: Presence of tracheotomy? tube? ventilator? Frequency of breathing? laborious?
	• Pulmonary function: Lung volumes and capacities
	• Loudness: Is there sufficient respiratory support for habitual and increased loudness?
	• Respiratory patterning
Laryngeal System	• Vocal quality
	• Vocal intensity: Habitual and variability
	• Fundamental frequency: Habitual and variability
	• Laryngeal airflows and resistance
	• Direct visualization: Videostroboscopy
Velopharyngeal System	• Perceived hypernasality
	• Nasal resonance: Nasometer
	• Nasal air emission: See-Scape
	• Articulatory error patterns, articulation inventories
	• Aerodynamics: Intraoral air pressure, nasal air flow, resistance, orifice size
	• Endoscopy
Articulatory System	• Perceptual ratings, descriptions
	• Articulation inventories
	• Acoustic analysis
	• Movement studies: Strain gauge, X-ray microbeam
	• Force measurement: Iowa Oral Pressure Instrument, FORCE

per breath in their sample of mechanically ventilated individuals. The subjects in their study all had intelligible speech; however, one could predict that a coexisting dysarthria would result in further alterations in the use of the respiratory system.

Persons with dysarthria who are not mechanically ventilated, but who have compromised respiratory support, may show an increased frequency of breaths, laborious breathing, or difficulty sustaining vowel sounds. Hillel, Yorkston, and Miller (1989) found a positive correlation between the duration of sustained vowel production and measured vital capacity in persons with amyotrophic lateral sclerosis.

Pulmonary function testing can be very useful in determining respiratory support for speech through measurement of lung volumes and capacities. Although detailed analyses of pulmonary function require specialized testing equipment and procedures, many speech–language pathologists with access to either a wet or dry spirometer can determine a patient's vital capacity and tidal volumes. Another indirect observation of the adequacy of respiratory support can be through loudness manipulation. That is, is there sufficient respiratory support for habitual and increased loudness levels during conversation? Can the individual increase the volume of air inhaled, and is that done prior to initiating loud voice? Clearly, there are many interactions between the respiratory and other speech production systems. For example, sustained phonation time is dependent not only on respiratory support but also on laryngeal valving.

The evaluation of respiratory patterning can be useful in determining the functional use of respiratory support. Hammen and Yorkston (1994) used the term *respiratory patterning* to reflect a global concept of speech breathing that included breath group length, location, and consistency. They found that speakers with dysarthria had shorter mean breath group lengths, and the distribution of the breath groups was skewed toward very short (two to five words) lengths. Subjects with dysarthria were also much more likely to breathe at an ungrammatical location, such as within a noun or verb phrase. This type of evaluation can be useful in determining underlying factors contributing to reduced intelligibility.

Laryngeal System

The first approach to evaluating the laryngeal system is to identify the perceptual characteristics of the voice. Is the vocal quality breathy, strained, harsh, wet-gurgling? These perceptual observations will lead to hypotheses regarding the patency of the laryngeal valve, which can be tested through a variety of methods. A voice that is predominantly breathy suggests poor vocal fold closure, which allows unmodulated air to flow through the glottis, resulting in a turbulent noise source. This observation can be contrasted with a strained quality, which implies excessive tension in the laryngeal system.

Habitual use of pitch and loudness gives insight into the typical functioning of the laryngeal system. In addition, variation in both frequency and intensity is important for the speaker to be perceived as "natural." Speakers should be evaluated as they read and engage in connected speech tasks. It is especially important to engage in speech tasks that would be likely to elicit variations in frequency and intensity, such as discussion of a favorite hobby or a controversial political topic. In this way, both habitual use and the extent to which the person can vary pitch and intensity when the context requires can be evaluated.

The control of the laryngeal system can be evaluated by asking the person with dysarthria to systematically vary the pitch and the loudness of the voice. Typically this is tested during the production of a sustained vowel sound that is varied either in pitch or loudness. Patients are asked to sing notes up and down the scale until the end points of their range are achieved. It is important to consider such factors as instruction and method of elicitation (step-wise versus glissando) when obtaining phonational range measures as all have been found to affect the range extent (Coulton & Casper, 1996). Loudness is often varied from soft to loud either in a sustained vowel or when producing a single syllable word, such as "Stop!"

Once recordings of the voice are obtained for the tasks outlined above, a number of acoustic examinations of the vocal characteristics are possible. Measurements of fundamental frequency (f_o) and intensity have been part of the acoustic evaluation of dysarthric voices for a number of years (Canter, 1963; Ludlow & Bassich, 1983). In addition to these overall measures, cycle-to-cycle variations in f_o (jitter) and intensity (shimmer) and frequency variations over several seconds (standard deviation of f_o, flutter) have been used to support perceptual judgments of the laryngeal component of the dysarthria (Aronson, Ramig, Winholtz, & Silber, 1992; Ludlow & Bassich, 1983; Ramig, Scherer, Titze, & Ringel, 1988; Strand, Buder, Yorkston, & Ramig, 1994; Zwirner & Barnes, 1992; Zwirner, Murry, & Woodson, 1991).

The patency of the laryngeal valve can be evaluated indirectly through the aerodynamic measurement of laryngeal airflow, intraoral air pressures, and estimated laryngeal resistance. Laryngeal airflow is measured using a pneumotachograph and varies with the degree of vocal fold closure that is achieved during phonation. Intraoral air pressure is sensed with a transducer and tubing that is placed just posterior to the central incisors. Measures of intraoral pressure are used to represent subglottic or tracheal pressures prior to the onset of phonation. The ratio of pressure to airflow constitutes estimated laryngeal resistance (Smitheran & Hixon, 1981). Tasks to elicit these measures are typically sustained vowels or strings of syllables such as, "pae, pa, pi." The advent of microcomputer analysis of physiologic signals has increased the availability of these measures to the practicing clinician. Several instrumentation packages are currently available that provide the user with a number of aerodynamic measures. These include Aerophone (Kay Elemetrics, Inc., 2 Bridgewater Lane, Lincoln Park, NJ 07035-1488), Aerowin (NeuroLogic, Inc., 3105 Creekwood Drive, Lawrence, KS 66049), and other noncommercial systems (Till & Alp, 1991).

Gracco, Gracco, Lofqvist, and Marek (1994) examined the aerodynamic characteristics of the speech of persons with Parkinson's disease. Some of their subjects had lower laryngeal airflow and greater than expected values of laryngeal resistance. The authors suggest that aerodynamic measures may be a useful way to document differing perceptual characteristics in this population. These suggestions were further supported by Theodoros and Murdoch (1996), who found that their measures of laryngeal resistance corresponded well with perceptual judgments of hyperfunction in a group of speakers with a dysarthria secondary to closed head injury. Till and Alp (1991) demonstrated that despite different etiologies, their group of dysarthric subjects all had deviations in managing the laryngeal system as reflected in airflow measures. Finally, Hammen and Yorkston (1994) examined how a group of speakers with dysarthria altered intraoral air pressure when responding to instructions to increase the effort and clarity of speech. They found that the aerodynamic measure of pressure reflected the differences in response style among the subjects in the study. That is, some subjects increased pressure and others did not. The authors suggested that the ability to vary habitual performance may be an important factor in determining candidacy for intervention and that the differences noted in their study could be used to assist in the clinical decision-making process.

Lastly, the laryngeal system can be visualized through the use of endoscopy or videostroboscopy. Recently, videostroboscopy has been used to document the laryngeal abnormalities that frequently occur with Parkinson's disease (Perez, Ramig, Smith, & Dromey, 1996). Additionally, the use of videostroboscopy has been used to investigate the effectiveness of an intensive voice therapy program for persons with Parkinson's disease (Smith, Ramig, Dromey, Perez, & Samandari, 1995).

Velopharyngeal System

As with the laryngeal system, the first approach to evaluating the velopharyngeal system will likely be perceptual. Whether or not a person with dysarthria sounds hypernasal is a fairly basic perceptual distinction. However, the extent to which they are hypernasal is more difficult to determine. A variety of rating scales exists to attempt to objectify the perceptual impression, but these vary in their validity and reliability. Therefore, clinical researchers have sought other means by which to characterize the functioning of the velopharyngeal system.

The most basic of these evaluation systems is to examine patterns of misarticulation. Yorkston, Beukelman, and Honsinger (1989) found that subjects with velopharyngeal inadequacy presented a pattern whereby nasals and glides were perceived more accurately than plosives. Those speakers who had inconsistent or occasional difficulties with velopharyngeal closure did not show a similar pattern. The phonetic intelligibility test (Kent et al., 1989) presented previously in this chapter has a contrast, stop/nasal, which demonstrated much higher error rates as overall intelligibility decreased for a group of speakers with amyotrophic lateral sclerosis.

Although articulation inventories and error patterns can indicate excess nasal resonance, the extent of resonance can be evaluated through the use of the Nasometer (Kay Elemetrics, Inc., 2 Bridgewater Lane, Lincoln Park, NJ 07035-1488). Although documentation of its usefulness in evaluating persons with dysarthria is very limited, this instrument compares levels of oral and nasal resonance for standard paragraphs or conversational speech.

Observations of nasal air emission are possible using a variety of readily available materials. Fogging that occurs on a laryngeal or other small mirror placed under the nostrils can be indicative of excess air flows through the nose during the production of nonnasal sounds.

Some clinics may have a See-Scape available for velopharyngeal assessments. This device consists of a nasal olive and a flowmeter. Escaping air through the nasal cavity causes balls in the flowmeter to rise. Finally, perceptual signs such as nasal snorts can be used in the noninstrumental assessment of velopharyngeal function.

Aerodynamic measures provide another means of evaluating the velopharyngeal system. As described under the laryngeal system section, indirect measures of the patency of velopharyngeal closure can be determined by obtaining airflow and pressure data through the use of special hardware and software. In the case of the velopharyngeal system, it is the nasal airflows and intraoral air pressures that are of interest. The instrumentation setup is similar to that used for laryngeal resistance measures, except that a mask is placed only over the nose. During the production of nonnasal sounds, nasal airflow should be essentially nonexistent. Intraoral air pressures should range from 4 to 10 cm H_2O. As with laryngeal resistance, the ratio of nasal airflow to pressure can indicate the degree of resistance to airflow provided by the velopharyngeal mechanism (Barlow, 1989). These measures are quite sensitive to alterations in velopharyngeal closure and can indicate not only an open versus closed mechanism, but also slow or sluggish movement of the velopharyngeal structures.

In addition to resistance measures, calculation of the extent of velopharyngeal opening can be completed using methods outlined by Warren (Warren, 1979, Warren & DuBois, 1964;). This method uses a similar instrumentation setup but includes a measure of nasal pressure as well. A computer-based hardware and software package is available to facilitate the determination of velopharyngeal opening area, PERCI-SARS from Microtronics Corp. (Warren, Putnam-Rochet, & Hinton, 1997).

Direct observation of the velopharyngeal mechanism is possible through the use of flexible fiberoptic nasoendoscopy. Karnell (1994) is an excellent resource for specific information regarding the skills and techniques necessary for successfully performing and interpreting nasoendoscopy.

Articulatory System

Following diadochokinetics, one of the most common methods of evaluating the integrity of the articulatory system involves the use of perceptual analysis. Descriptive studies of the articulatory characteristics from speakers with dysarthria provide the framework for much of the diagnostic process. However, it is often the case that different types and varying severities of dysarthria can receive the same descriptor; for example, imprecise consonants. As a result of this ambiguity, other approaches to the evaluation of the articulatory system have gained popularity.

Articulation inventories provide a more systematic approach to the perceptual analysis and description of dysarthric speech while still being fairly simple to administer. Logemann, Fisher, Boshes, and Blonsky (1978) completed a detailed analysis of articulation error patterns from persons with Parkinson's disease using the *Fisher-Logemann Test of Articulation Competence* (Fisher & Logemann, 1971) As mentioned earlier, Kent et al. (1989) have developed a phonetic intelligibility test that examines a person's articulatory abilities within the context of specific phonetic contrasts.

Because perceptual analysis is dependent on the acoustic signal created by the speaker, more recently clinicians are using acoustic analysis to assist them in their diagnostic efforts. The advent of affordable microcomputers and more transparent signal analysis software packages allows the use of acoustic analysis in many more clinical settings. Read, Buder, and Kent (1990, 1992) provide an excellent review of some of the commercially available packages.

Weismer and colleagues have studied the impact of dysarthria on a number of acoustic parameters, such as stop closure duration, voice onset time, and trajectories of second formant transitions (Weismer, 1984; Weismer et al., 1988; Weismer et al., 1992). The acoustic signal was sensitive to changes in the ability of the individual to produce clear, intelligible speech.

Examination of the ability of the articulators to move to and from appropriate articulatory targets is the focus of kinematic, or movement, analysis. It is well known that many individuals with dysarthria have difficulties with the speed and range of motion of the articulators. There are two main instrumental approaches to the kinematic analysis of dysarthric speech: strain gauge transduction and X-ray microbeam. The use of a head-mounted, strain gauge system for the examination of articulatory movements has been described by Barlow, Cole, and Abbs (1983). This system involves the attachment of lightweight cantilever beams to the upper lip, lower lip, and jaw. Once attached, strain gauges are capable of tracking both superior-inferior and anterior-posterior movements of the structures of interest. Numerous studies in the literature demonstrate the usefulness of this analysis technique in the differential diagnosis of dysarthria (Abbs, Hunker, & Barlow, 1983; Barlow & Abbs, 1983, 1986; Hunker, Abbs, & Barlow, 1982). Forrest, Weismer, and Turner (1989) used such a system to examine the differences in articulatory function between a group of persons with Parkinson's disease and a group of matched geriatric subjects.

Finally, measures of the force or strength generated by the articulators can give insight into whether the individual with dysarthria can generate sufficient forces to move the articulators to appropriate targets. Although the subjective judgment of the amount of force created by the individual when pressing his or her tongue against a tongue depressor is frequently used by clinicians, new devices are now commercially available that can give objective assessments of the force capabilities of the articulatory system.

The Iowa Oral Performance Instrument (IOPI) uses an air-filled, soft bulb to assess tongue strength and, recently, procedures have been developed to allow assessment of the lips as well. Digital readout of maximum strength is provided, and endurance can be tested through the use of visual feedback provided by a series of lights on the instrument. Solomon, Robin, Lorell, Rodnitzky, and Luschei (1994) found a relationship between measures of tongue strength and speech intelligibility in a group of speakers with Parkinson's disease. This research was expanded by Stierwalt, Robin, Pearl Solomon, Weiss, and Max (1996) to subjects who were dysarthric following traumatic brain injury. In this study, the IOPI was used to assess both strength and fatigue. A significant relationship between intelligibility and the IOPI measures was obtained. Measures of articulatory strength can be useful, objective measures of the integrity of the articulatory system.

A second method of assessing force generation and control in persons with dysarthria has been described by Barlow and Burton (1990). Their paradigm, known as a *ramp-and-hold maneuver*, involves having speakers rapidly generate specific target forces then maintain that level of force for several seconds. Ten repetitions of the maneuver are completed for at least four different target force levels. A software program, FORCE (Neurologic, Inc.), generates the targets for force production and provides data regarding the accuracy and speed to target as well as stability during the hold phase. This information can provide objective assessment of the individual's ability to utilize the force-generating capabilities of the lips, jaw, and tongue. The authors tested the paradigm with a large group of subjects without neurologic impairment and with several individuals who had experienced a traumatic brain injury with resultant dysarthria. Differences between the two sets of subjects were readily apparent. In an extension of that original work, McHenry, Wilson, and Minton (1994) found that similar results could be obtained with fewer tokens, making the procedure more efficient for clinical application.

Treatment of Dysarthria

Yorkston et al. (1988) have stated that the "goal of treatment is to maximize speech intelligibility with minimal decreases in speech naturalness." That is to say, when working with a speaker with dysarthria, the challenge is to devise a treatment plan that will allow the individual to be understood while making every attempt to preserve the prosodic characteristics of speech that contribute to the perception of naturalness.

Another viewpoint on treatment is that the clinician should strive to restore function or to compensate for loss of function within the speech production subsystems. That is, following the evaluation, the speech production subsystems contributing to the dysarthria should be identified and the extent of impairment to the system determined. At that point, decisions can be made regarding the management plan. In some cases, direct improvement of function for one subsystem is necessary before progress can be made in other systems. For example, if it has been determined that an individual has deficits in both the articulatory and velopharyngeal systems, one must determine the impact of one system on the other. When the velopharyngeal system is compromised so that the speaker is severely hypernasal with substantial nasal air emission, it will be difficult, if not impossible, to achieve success within the articulatory system until the velopharyngeal problem is managed. Although the following sections address intervention strategies for each subsystem individually, the interaction between speech production subsystems must always be taken into consideration. A summary of the treatment approaches useful for each subsystem can be found in Table 3.4.

Table 3.4
A Summary of Treatment Approaches Based on Speech Production Subsystems

Respiratory System	• Postural changes
	• Abdominal binders/paddles
	• Eliminating abnormal respiratory patterns
Laryngeal System	• Increased effort/loudness: Lee Silverman Voice Treatment
	• Increased respiratory drive
	• Improved timing of voicing
	• Reduction in hyperfunction
	• Surgical management: Injectibles, thyroplasty
	• Voice amplification
Velopharyngeal System	• Exercise
	• Biofeedback
	• Continuous positive airway pressure (CPAP)
	• Palatal lift
	• Pharyngeal flap surgery
Articulatory System	• Increased strength
	• Contrastive drills
	• Rate control

Respiratory System

Hardy (1983) described the usefulness of postural changes when working with individuals with cerebral palsy. Shifting a speaker from the sitting to supine position places increased gravitational forces on the abdominal region and subsequently the diaphragm. This can result in increased expiratory forces. However, it should be noted that altering the speaker's posture to supine will make inspiration more difficult. Therefore, care must be taken to determine the nature of respiratory system deficits. A person with amyotrophic lateral sclerosis, for example, may have inspiratory muscle weakness that would be exacerbated if the person were placed in a supine position. It is not uncommon to find patients who have dysarthria shifted to one side or forward when attempting to sit in the upright position due to trunk muscle weakness. These positions can limit the range of motion of the respiratory system and, therefore, the extent of expansion when the person inhales for speech purposes. Side supports or other methods of stabilization can be used to assist the speaker in maintaining an upright posture.

Yorkston et al. (1988) report the usefulness of abdominal binders for individuals with expiratory muscle weakness. They state that persons with multiple sclerosis and traumatic brain injury have benefited from the use of a binder. However, the caveat for postural changes also applies to binders; that is, the inspiratory function of the respiratory system is made more difficult. The use of binders, therefore, should be considered only after consultation with the appropriate medical personnel. An alternative to binders is a paddle described by Rosenbek and LaPointe (1985). The paddle can be attached to a wheelchair and can be moved into place as needed to assist in generating expiratory force. The speaker must be able to lean forward to place sufficient pressure on the board and, therefore, the respiratory system. This is often difficult for patients to accomplish. An alternative to the board is the placement of a hand on the abdominal area. Inward pressure during attempts to speak or phonate can assist a person with severe expiratory muscle weakness to experience an increase in respiratory drive.

Another task that can be used to increase respiratory drive is based on the "5 for 5" rule suggested by Netsell and Hixon (1978). That is, persons who are able to generate 5 cm H_2O of intraoral air pressures for 5 seconds will have sufficient respiratory drive to sustain speech. This task is typically accomplished as the patient blows into a straw positioned at the 5 cm level in a water-filled glass, because the desired amount of air pressure would be required to produce an air bubble from a straw at that depth (Hixon, Hawley, & Wilson, 1982). This can be a task that is practiced until the goal of "5 for 5" is met at a predetermined criterion level. A number of modifications to that basic device have been used clinically. For example, relatively transparent sport bottles with screw-on tops and straws are very useful for this task. Centimeter markings can be drawn on the bottle to indicate the target depths.

Once adequate drive from the respiratory system has been established, attention must be placed on eliminating inefficient respiratory patterns. That is, a speaker should initiate speech following a pre-speech breath and should terminate speaking before reaching a very low lung volume level. Breaths should be taken at natural boundaries in speech, rather than within phrases. Length of breath groups (the number of words spoken between breaths) should be adjusted to the capabilities of the person's respiratory system. For many persons with dysarthria, this will mean reducing the number of words per breath group. However, there are those speakers, especially following traumatic brain injury, who will persist in using very short, uniform length breath groups despite adequate respiratory capacities. In both cases, intervention can begin by using reading passages marked to indicate breath groups and progress to more spontaneous speaking tasks. Bellaire, Yorkston, and Beukelman (1986) reported an increase in naturalness for a speaker following intervention focused on breath patterning.

Laryngeal System

Because the respiratory and laryngeal systems are functionally linked, improvements in respiratory drive can have a positive impact on laryngeal function as well. Perhaps the most dramatic behavioral approach for improving laryngeal function has been reported by Ramig and colleagues (Dromey, Ramig, & Johnson, 1995; Ramig, Bonitati, Lemke, & Horii, 1994; Ramig, Countryman, Thompson, & Horii, 1995; Ramig, Pawlas, & Countryman, 1995) through use of the Lee Silverman Voice Therapy program. This program consists of an intensive course of therapy (16 one-hour sessions over 4 consecutive weeks) that focuses on increasing vocal loudness levels, maximum phonation times, phonational range, and vocal steadiness. Subjects who successfully complete the program demonstrate improvements in vocal intensity levels and variation of fundamental frequency (Ramig et al., 1995). Improvements in the aerodynamic characteristics of voice production, such as subglottic air pressure, have also been demonstrated (Ramig & Dromey, 1996).

Another aspect of phonatory function important for speech intelligibility is the timing of voicing. The onset and offset of voicing to produce voiced and voiceless phonemes in continuous speech requires considerable precision. Therefore, teaching the person with dysarthria to clearly distinguish voiced and voiceless phonemes strictly through manipulation of the laryngeal system may be an insurmountable challenge. Other pertinent cues, such as increasing intraoral air pressure and bursts for voiceless plosives, can also be taught in order to improve laryngeal and articulatory timing (Rosenbek & LaPointe, 1985). Yorkston et al. (1988) describe an "intelligibility task" to address phonatory timing problems. In this task, voiced and voiceless cognate words are presented to the speaker while the listener remains "blind" to the target word. Following the speaker's production of the target word, the listener reports what was perceived. A match between the target and the perceived word indicates whether phonatory timing was appropriate for the distinction. If a misperception occurs, the speaker can attempt the production again, modifying it as needed.

When there is a flaccid paralysis of the laryngeal musculature, medical or surgical intervention may need to be considered. There are two primary methods for improving vocal fold closure: the use of injectibles and thyroplasty. *Thyroplasty* is a surgical procedure in which a window is cut into the thyroid cartilage at the level of the paralyzed vocal cord. Typically, a silastic block, or shim, is placed between the thyroid cartilage and the inner perichondrium of the thyroarytenoid muscle, which displaces the muscle medially toward the midline. Injections of collagen, autologous fat, or Teflon into the affected vocal fold will increase its bulk and reposition the impaired fold toward the midline. Ford and Bless (1991) and Coulton and Casper (1996) provide excellent descriptions of these approaches to managing vocal fold paralysis. Improvements in glottal closure following either procedure can result in improved vocal quality and loudness.

Visual feedback of vocal intensity, frequency, and steadiness is available through the use of a variety of commercial products, such as Visi-pitch and Speech Viewer (Kay Elemetrics, Inc.). Feedback and knowledge of results have been shown to improve performance in persons with and without dysarthria (Adams, 1994; Rubrow, 1984).

If, despite all efforts to increase phonatory loudness and quality, the person with dysarthria continues to experience reduced vocal loudness, a prosthetic device should be considered. A number of voice amplifiers are available through local and national electronics stores as well as from specialty catalogs, such as those available for laryngectomy supplies. Some speakers with dysarthria use the device whenever they engage in conversation, whereas others will only need the device when they are in challenging situations, such as speaking to a group or when background noise is present. Matching the needs of the individual with the amplification system is a critical component in selecting the appropriate prosthetic device.

Velopharyngeal System

Impairments to the velopharyngeal system can have both upstream and downstream effects on speech production. That is, phonation times (downstream) can be reduced because of the "leak" existing at the level of the velopharynx. Imprecise articulation (upstream) can be exacerbated by excess nasal resonance caused by ineffective velopharyngeal closure. Therefore, considerable efforts are made to manage this system when it is found to be impaired.

Behaviorally based intervention for velopharyngeal dysfunction has been the subject of disagreement over the years. Methods that have been attempted with essentially disappointing results are blowing, sucking, and digital manipulation. Some suggest that if the neuromotor problem is such that velopharyngeal closure is not possible, behavioral therapy to improve muscle strength is futile (Noll, 1982). Others, such as Dworkin (1991), recommend a series of exercises to be performed over a prescribed period of time, thereby allowing the person with dysarthria to try to improve neuromuscular functioning while also establishing a time frame for reevaluation of the process. These exercises focus on increasing intraoral air pressure in a hierarchy of speaking tasks through the use of biofeedback tools such as See-Scape and audio recordings. Certainly one critical issue in the use of behavioral methods is that many exercises employed in these programs involve the maintenance of a static position for the velopharyngeal system, for example, blowing. Frequently, the problems experienced by the speaker with dysarthria include the inability of the system to make the rapid alterations in velopharyngeal position and closure that is required in connected speech.

However, recent reports by Kuehn and Wachtel (1994) and Liss, Kuehn, and Hinkel (1994) have suggested that use of continuous positive airway pressure (CPAP) can reduce the hypernasality occurring with dysarthria. According to Kuehn and Wachtel (1994), CPAP provides resistance within the nasal airways by delivering air into the nasal passages through an air pressure flow mask. The velopharyngeal musculature must then generate increased forces to overcome the resistance. Issues such as the intensity and frequency of treatment session are being explored (Liss et al., 1994), but CPAP represents an exciting avenue for the behavioral management of the velopharyngeal dysfunction associated with dysarthria.

When behavioral methods do not improve velopharyngeal closure and reduce hypernasality, prosthetic and surgical methods to manage the system provide other alternatives. Yorkston et al. (1988) report that the first use of a prosthesis to improve velopharyngeal closure in a speaker with dysarthria appeared nearly 40 years ago (Gibbons & Bloomer, 1958). The most commonly used device is a palatal lift prosthesis, which is fabricated by a prosthodontist. Resembling the retainers used in orthodontic treatment, a palatal lift includes a posterior extension that provides passive elevation of the soft palate. A number of researchers have examined the usefulness of the palatal lift prosthesis in the management of dysarthria (Aten, McDonald, Simpson, & Gutierrez, 1984; Gonzalez & Aronson, 1970; Hardy, Netsell, Schweiger, & Morris, 1969; Yorkston et al., 1988; Yorkston et al., 1999). There are a number of candidacy requirements that need to be taken into account when a palatal lift is considered for a patient with dysarthria. These include severity, impairment of other speech production systems, patient cooperation, course of the disorder, swallowing function, and presence of dentures. Additional details regarding candidacy can be found in Gonzalez and Aronson (1970), Rosenbek and LaPointe (1985), Yorkston et al. (1988), and Yorkston et al. (1999).

Finally, surgical intervention for velopharyngeal impairments in the form of pharyngeal flaps has been infrequently reported in the literature. Johns (1985) described a single case that demonstrated improved speech intelligibility and reduced hypernasality following a superiorly based pharyngeal flap surgery. Generally, however, the results of such surgeries have been less than optimal.

Articulatory System

The articulatory system represents the converging point for all the speech production subsystems; therefore, intervention should not be focused only on this system without considering the other subsystems. When the clinician is faced with the imprecise articulation that frequently occurs with dysarthria, improved function of the articulators is often the first treatment approach pursued. Most frequently this is addressed through the use of strengthening exercises. Controversy over the need for increasing the strength of the lips, tongue, and jaw for speech purposes exists and has been discussed in detail by Duffy (1995), Rosenbek and LaPointe (1985), Yorkston et al. (1988), and Yorkston et al. (1999). The heart of the controversy lies in reports that speech uses only 10%–30% of the maximum forces that the lips and tongue are capable of generating. Therefore, one can conclude that considerable muscle force must be lost before weakness becomes the critical component in the impaired articulation experienced by persons with dysarthria. However, as mentioned earlier, Stierwalt et al. (1996) presented data that showed a relationship between tongue strength as measured by the IOPI and speech intelligibility. It is likely that this debate will continue for some time. If the clinician believes that weakness is contributing to the patient's dysarthria, exercise programs that have been described in detail by Dworkin (1991) and Linebaugh (1983) may be useful.

Another approach to reducing the impairment within the articulatory system has its roots in traditional articulation therapy. Activities that involve stimulating the correct production through observation and imitation, manual assistance in achieving and maintaining articulatory placements, and exaggeration of articulatory gestures have all been recommended for use in dysarthria treatment (Darley et al., 1975; Netsell & Rosenbek, 1985; Rosenbek & LaPointe, 1985). Duffy (1995), Yorkston et al. (1988), and Yorkston et al. (1999) provide instructions on how to conduct contrastive stress drills in therapy with persons with dysarthria. The procedures are essentially similar to those described as the voicing drill under the laryngeal system. Often, the goal for a speaker during these drills is to develop compensatory approaches to articulation that result in adequate perception of the target phoneme.

Finally, improvement within the articulatory system and, therefore, intelligibility, may be achieved through the reduction of speaking rate. Yorkston et al. (1988) and Yorkston et al. (1999) describe rate control as one of the long-standing approaches to improving intelligibility. Clinicians frequently request that their patients with dysarthria slow down. Several approaches to rate reduction have been reported over the years, ranging from finger tapping and metronomes to computer-based systems. Some of the approaches require external devices to assist people with dysarthria to reduce their speech rate. One of the earliest published accounts of a rate control device was the pacing board

(Helm, 1979). The board provided clearly marked slots that were to be touched as the person spoke a word or syllable. Helm reported successfully using this device with a person with Parkinson's disease and hypokinetic dysarthria. Another frequently used device is an alphabet board (Crow & Enderby, 1989; Yorkston et al., 1988; Yorkston et al., 1999). The person with dysarthria is instructed to point to the first letter of each word. Two benefits are obtained from this strategy. First, the speaker is forced to slow down to accomplish the task, and, secondly, the listener is given the first letter of the target word as a context cue.

Another popular external device that is used to control speaking rate is delayed auditory feedback (DAF). Numerous reports of improved articulation and intelligibility following DAF can be found in the literature (Adams, 1994; Downie, Low, & Lindsay, 1981; Hanson & Metter, 1980, 1983; Yorkston et al., 1988; Yorkston et al., 1999). The speaker wears a microphone that sends the speech signal to the DAF device. The device then adds a delay to the signal that can be controlled by the clinician or speaker. The delayed speech signal is then fed to the speaker through earphones. The effects of DAF on dysarthric speech are usually quite rapid and dramatic. Speakers typically slow the speaking rate down as they attend to the delayed speech signal. Although DAF can be effective for a considerable period of time, some speakers do adapt to DAF and require adjustments in the delays or a shift to another rate control strategy.

Computerized rate control requires the speaker to read text presented on the monitor at a rate governed by the movement of an underlining cursor through the passage (Beukelman, Yorkston, & Tice, 1997). The rate of cursor movement can be set by the clinician, and additional time at syntactic boundaries can be allotted. Improvements in intelligibility following computerized rate control have been reported for persons with ataxic and hypokinetic dysarthria (Hammen, Yorkston, & Minifie, 1994; Yorkston, Hammen, Beukelman, & Traynor, 1990).

Visual feedback can also provide a means to reduce speaking rate. Berry and Goshorn (1983) presented a case in which they used an oscilloscope screen to give feedback regarding rate and loudness to a speaker with ataxic dysarthria. The speaker was instructed to fill up the screen when reading a series of sentences. The time base of the oscilloscope could be altered to reduce the speaker's rate.

Finally, it should be noted that some interventions for other speech subsystems can affect speaking rate and, potentially, articulation. For example, modification of breath patterning can slow speaking rate, and efforts to increase vocal loudness such as LSVT will likely reduce speech rate and increase articulatory drive.

Case Studies

To conclude this chapter and to illustrate the benefits of integrating the various approaches to evaluation and treatment of dysarthria, two case studies will be presented. The examples chosen have been adapted from Hammen (1995). Both patients were dysarthric as the result of a traumatic brain injury.

CASE 1

GW, a 21-year-old female, sustained a traumatic brain injury 21 months prior to the evaluation. Her medical history included a right subdural hematoma and a right frontal lobe and brainstem damage; she had been comatose for 5 months. GW had received both in-patient and out-patient speech–language pathology services at a variety of medical centers. Therapy efforts had focused on the use of a communication board, as it was believed that her sustained phonation was not long enough to support speech as a primary mode of communication. The patient's mother indicated that verbal communication was the avenue of choice and that GW was primarily using speech at home. During the motor speech evaluation, the patient demonstrated the perceptual characteristics of flaccid dysarthria, including a weak, breathy voice and slow articulatory movements. The patient was found to be severely dysarthric, and she frequently failed to complete movements to articulatory contacts. Hypernasality, the typical perceptual characteristic of reduced velopharyngeal competency, was suggested but was not obvious due to the severe breathiness. An analysis of articulatory error patterns showed both vowel and consonant productions to be imprecise. Single word intelligibility was 0% on the *Computerized Assessment of the Intelligibility of Dysarthric Speech* (Yorkston et al., 1984). Perceived accuracy of consonant production was 12% and vowel production was 31% on a phoneme identification task. Her vital capacity was 1.4 liters, which was approximately half of the expected capacity for a person of her age and height. It was hypothesized that the decreased duration of sustained phonation and weak consonant productions were due to velopharyngeal insufficiency.

In order to determine candidacy for the palatal lift, aerodynamic measures of intraoral pressure, nasal airflow, and velopharyngeal resistance were obtained using the Aerowin (Neurologic, Inc.). Intraoral air pressure was found to be on the order of 0.62 cm H_2O (normal range is 4–9 cm H_2O). Nasal airflows averaged 305 cc/sec during the production of nonnasal syllable strings such as "pa-pa-pa." Minimal nasal airflow (i.e., less than 50 cc/sec) should be produced during these speech tasks. When the nostrils were pinched closed, thereby preventing nasal air escape despite velopharyngeal insufficiency, GW was able to generate intraoral air pressures of 4–5 cm H_2O.

The differential diagnosis of GW's dysarthria within the physiologic model suggested reduced respiratory drive; poor laryngeal valving; velopharyngeal insufficiency; and weak, slow oral musculature. Using Wood's (1980) model, GW's neuromotor impairment was reflected in articulatory weakness. This impairment resulted in a functional limitation evidenced by severe unintelligibility and a slow, laborious speaking rate. It was observed that GW rarely initiated social conversation, making this a disabling component.

Because GW had a severely impaired velopharyngeal system, it was not expected that attempts to improve phonatory function (e.g., sustained phonation) or oral articulation (e.g., increasing the precision of articulation) would result in improved performance. In fact, vigorous efforts to improve speech production in this patient appeared to have resulted in fatigue and frustration.

Due to the severity of her velopharyngeal weakness, a palatal lift prosthesis followed by speech therapy was recommended. Speech therapy efforts would focus on increasing vocal loudness and labial closure. The need for modifications to the palatal lift were monitored through the use of aerodynamic measures and perceptual assessments in the form of analysis of articulatory error patterns. Following a year of prosothodontic management and behavioral intervention, GW was able to produce intraoral air pressures of 2.0 cm H_2O with nasal airflows of 67 cc/sec with the palatal lift in place. Sustained phonation increased to 14.72 seconds. The perceived accuracy of consonant production was 27% and vowels were 81% accurate. GW also became more willing to participate in and initiate social conversations.

This first case demonstrates that intervention addressing one aspect of the impairment (velopharyngeal muscle weakness) can affect other speech production systems (respiratory, phonatory, and articulatory). It can also reduce the functional limitation of the dysarthria (by increasing speech intelligibility) and affect the disability (by reducing participation in social conversations). The second case will illustrate how perceptual impressions may mask the actual underlying problems.

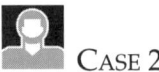 CASE 2

When seen for an evaluation, JP, a 20-year-old male, was approximately 24 months postonset of a traumatic brain injury following a motor vehicle accident. The referral indicated that his current speech–language pathologist was concerned that the perceived hypernasality was preventing JP from making further gains in speech intelligibility, vocal quality, and speech naturalness. Behavioral intervention for the dysarthria had focused on increasing awareness of hypernasality and increasing oral opening to reduce the hypernasality.

The motor speech evaluation indicated a mixed dysarthria, characterized by imprecise consonant and vowel production; inconsistent articulatory breakdowns; a harsh, loud vocal quality; and increased nasal resonance. The physiologic assessment of JP's speech production system included measures of vital capacity, respiratory patterning, velopharyngeal and laryngeal aerodynamics, and tongue force. JP's vital capacity was 3.3 liters, which was considered adequate for his age and height. Sustained phonation was in excess of 20 seconds, also within the normal range. Respiratory patterning analyses indicated that the number of words produced per breath was reduced. Intraoral air pressures averaged 11 cm H_2O during the production of plosives and nasal airflows averaged 58 cc/sec. Velopharyngeal resistance (a ratio of intraoral air pressure and nasal airflow) was within the expected range. Laryngeal resistance, obtained using procedures outlined by Smitheran and Hixon (1981), was 178 ohms, indicating very high resistance. Tongue force was measured with two different systems, the IOPI and FORCE. Results from both systems showed substantially reduced tongue forces, and FORCE indicated substantial difficulty controlling the rate and extent of force generated by the tongue.

Clearly, the results of the physiologic evaluation procedures indicated that the velopharyngeal system was not impaired. However, there was an impression of increased nasal resonance. One explanation was that JP was driving his speech production system harder in response to the substantial weakness in his tongue. Individuals with dysarthria frequently report trying to improve production as a means of compensating for the effects of the dysarthria (Yorkston, Bombardier, & Hammen, 1993). However, for JP, his attempts to improve production resulted in overdriving the respiratory and laryngeal systems. This overdriving resulted in increased laryngeal resistance, exaggerated nasal resonance, and fewer words per breath. The loud voice and harsh vocal quality can be attributed to increased laryngeal resistance. Although JP's speech was intelligible, the consonant imprecision noted during the motor speech evaluation was thought to be the result of respiratory overdriving. Fricatives, affricates, and some stops were produced with so much effort that the following vowel was masked on occasion.

Traditional cues to reduce overdriving had not been effective previously, so a physiologic approach to reducing respiratory and phonatory effort was selected. A paradigm employing biofeedback of intraoral air pressure as a gauge of how hard he was driving the speech production system was used. JP was given a targeted level of intraoral air pressure not to be exceeded during the production of single words containing plosives. No additional cues were given. After several weeks of biofeedback training, he was able to maintain intraoral air pressures in the range of 5–7 cm H_2O during the production of voiceless plosives. Improvements in vocal quality and resonance were achieved with this physiologic approach to intervention, and JP felt he was using less effort to speak.

Although the perceptual approach to evaluation suggested an impairment of the velopharyngeal system for JP, no such impairment was indicated during the physiologic assessment. In addition, this method suggested an approach to intervention that was effective and directed at the source of the perceived speech problems.

Summary

As indicated at the outset of this chapter, the perceptual, physiologic, and acoustic approaches to the evaluation and treatment of dysarthria are complementary. The integration of these approaches in the planning and execution of intervention will maximize the likelihood of improving the functional communication of the person with dysarthria.

References

Abbs, J. H., Hunker, C. H., & Barlow, S. M. (1983). Differential speech motor subsystem impairments with suprabulbar lesions: Neurophysiological framework and supporting data. In W. R. Berry (Ed.), *Clinical dysarthria* (pp. 21–56). San Diego: College-Hill.

Adams, S. G. (1994). Accelerating speech in a case of hypokinetic dysarthria: Descriptions and treatment. In J. A. Till, K. M. Yorkston, & D. R. Beukelman (Eds.), *Motor speech disorders: Advances in assessment and treatment* (pp. 213–228). Baltimore: Brookes.

Aronson, A. E., Ramig, L. O., Winholtz, W. S., & Silber, S. R. (1992). Rapid voice tremor, or "flutter," in amyotrophic lateral sclerosis. *Annals of Otology, Rhinology, and Laryngology, 101,* 511–518.

Aten, J. L., McDonald, A., Simpson M., & Gutierrez R. (1984). Efficacy of modified palatal lifts for improving resonance. In M. McNeil, J. Rosenbeck, & A. Aronson (Eds.), *The dysarthrias* (pp. 231–341). San Diego: College-Hill.

Barlow, S. M. (1989). A high-speed data acquisition system for clinical speech physiology. In K. M. Yorkston & D. R. Beukelman (Eds.), *Recent advances in clinical dyarthria* (pp. 39–52). Boston: College-Hill.

Barlow, S., & Abbs, J. (1983). Force transducers for the evaluation of labial, lingual and mandibular motor impairments. *Journal of Speech and Hearing Research, 26*, 616–621.

Barlow, S. M., & Abbs, J. H. (1986). Fine force and position control of select orofacial structures in the upper motor neuron syndrome. *Experimental Neurology, 94*, 699–713.

Barlow, S. M., & Burton, M. K. (1990). Ramp-and-hold force control in the upper and lower lips: Developing new neuromotor assessment applications in traumatically brain injured adults. *Journal of Speech and Hearing Research, 33*, 660–675.

Barlow, S., Cole, K., & Abbs, J. (1983). A new headmounted lip-jaw movement transduction system for the study of motor speech disorders. *Journal of Speech and Hearing Research, 26*, 283–288.

Bellaire, K., Yorkston, K. M., & Beukelman, D. R. (1986). Modification of breath patterning to increase naturalness of a mildly dysarthric speaker. *Journal of Communication Disorders, 19*, 271–280.

Berry, W. R., & Goshorn, E. L. (1983). Immediate visual feedback in the treatment of ataxic dysarthria: A case study. In W. R. Berry (Ed.), *Clinical dysarthria* (pp. 253–266). Austin, TX: PRO-ED.

Beukelman, D. R., Yorkston, K. M., & Tice, R. L. (1997). *Pacer/tally rate measurement software*. Lincoln, NE: Tice Technology Services.

Canter, G. J. (1963). Speech characteristics of patients with Parkinson's disease: I. Intensity, pitch and duration. *Journal of Speech and Hearing Research, 28*, 221–229.

Coulton, R. H., & Casper, J. K. (1996). *Understanding voice disorders: A physiologic perspective for diagnosis and treatment* (pp. 211–234). Baltimore: Williams & Wilkins.

Crow, E., & Enderby, P. (1989). The effects of an alphabet chart on the speaking rate and intelligibility of speakers with dysarthria. In K. M. Yorkston & D. R. Beukelman (Eds.), *Recent advances in clinical dysarthria* (pp. 99–107). Boston: College-Hill.

Darley, F. L., Aronson, A. E., & Brown, J. R. (1969a). Cluster of deviant speech dimensions in the dysarthrias. *Journal of Speech and Hearing Research, 12*, 462–496.

Darley, F. L., Aronson, A. E., & Brown, J. R. (1969b). Differential diagnostic patterns of dysarthria. *Journal of Speech and Hearing Research, 12*, 246–269.

Darley, F. L., Aronson, A. E., & Brown, J. R. (1975). *Motor speech disorders*. Philadelphia: Saunders.

Downie, A. W., Low, J. M., & Lindsay, D. D. (1981). Speech disorders in parkinsonism: Usefulness of delayed auditory feedback in selected cases. *British Journal of Disorders of Communication, 16*, 135–139.

Dromey, C., Ramig, L. L., & Johnson, A. B. (1995). Phonatory and articulatory changes associated with increased vocal intensity in Parkinson disease: A case study. *Journal of Speech and Hearing Research, 38*, 751–764.

Duffy, J. R. (1995). *Motor speech disorders*. St. Louis: Mosby.

Dworkin, J. P. (1991). *Motor speech disorders: A treatment guide*. St. Louis: Mosby.

Enderby, P. (1983). *Frenchay Dysarthria Assessment*. Austin, TX: PRO-ED.

Fisher, H., & Logemann, J. (1971). *The Fisher–Logemann Test of Articulation Competence*. Austin, TX: PRO-ED.

Ford, C. N., & Bless, D. M. (1991). *Phonosurgery: Assessment and surgical management of voice disorders*. New York: Raven Press.

Forrest, K., Weismer, G., & Turner, G. S. (1989). Kinematic, acoustic, and perceptual analyses of connected speech produced by parkinsonian and normal geriatric adults. *Journal of the Acoustical Society of America, 85*(6), 2608–2622.

Gerratt, B. R., Till, J. A., Rosenbek, J. C., Wertz, R. T., & Boysen, A. E. (1991). Use and perceived value of perceptual and instrumental measures in dysarthria management. In C. A. Moore, K. M. Yorkston, & D. R. Beukelman (Eds.), *Dysarthria and apraxia of speech* (pp. 77–93). Baltimore: Brookes.

Gibbons, P., & Bloomer, H. H. (1958). The palatal lift: A supportive-type prosthetic speech aid. *Journal of Prosthetic Dentistry, 8,* 363–369.

Gonzalez, J., & Aronson, A. (1970). Palatal lift prosthesis for treatment of anatomic and neurologic palatopharyngeal insufficiency. *Cleft Palate Journal, 7,* 91–104.

Gracco, L. C., Gracco, V. L., Lofqvist, A., & Marek, K. P. (1994). Aerodynamic evaluation of parkinsonian dysarthria: Laryngeal and supralaryngeal manifestations. In J. A. Till, K. M. Yorkston, & D. R. Beukelman (Eds.), *Motor speech disorders: Advances in assessment and treatment* (pp. 65–79). Baltimore: Brookes.

Hammen, V. L. (1995). Differential diagnosis of dysarthrias: The physiologic approach. *Special Interest Division: Neurophysiology and Neurogenic Speech and Language Disorders, 5,* 6–9.

Hammen, V. L., & Yorkston, K. M. (1994). Effect of instruction on selected aerodynamic parameters in subjects with dysarthria and control subjects. In J. A. Till, K. M. Yorkston, & D. R. Beukelman (Eds.), *Motor speech disorders: Advances in assessment and treatment* (pp. 161–173). Baltimore: Brookes.

Hammen, V. L., Yorkston, K. M., & Minifie, F. D. (1994). Effects of temporal alterations on speech intelligibility in parkinsonian dysarthria. *Journal of Speech and Hearing Research, 37,* 244–253.

Hanson, W., & Metter, E. J. (1980). DAF as instrumental treatment for dysarthria in progressive supranuclear palsy: A case report. *Journal of Speech and Hearing Disorders, 45,* 268–276.

Hanson, W., & Metter, E. J. (1983). DAF speech rate modification in Parkinson's disease: A report of two cases. In W. Berry (Ed.), *Clinical dysarthria.* Austin, TX: PRO-ED.

Hardy, J. (1983). *Cerebral palsy.* Englewood Cliffs, NJ: Prentice Hall.

Hardy, J., Netsell, R., Schweiger, J., & Morris, H. (1969). Management of velopharyngeal dysfunction in cerebral palsy. *Journal of Speech and Hearing Disorders, 34*, 123–137.

Helm, N. A. (1979). Management of palilalia with a pacing board. *Journal of Speech and Hearing Disorders, 44*, 350–353.

Hillel, A. D., Yorkston, K., & Miller, R. M. (1989). Using phonation time to estimate vital capacity in amyotrophic lateral sclerosis. *Archives of Physical Medicine & Rehabilitation, 70*(8), 618–620.

Hixon, T., Hawley, J., & Wilson, J. (1982). An around-the-house device for the clinical determination of respiratory driving pressure: A note on making simple even simpler. *Journal of Speech and Hearing Disorders, 47*, 413.

Hoit, J. D., Shea, S. A., & Banzett, R. B. (1994). Speech production during mechanical ventilation in tracheostomized individuals. *Journal of Speech and Hearing Research, 37*(1), 53–63.

Hunker, C., Abbs, J., & Barlow, S. (1982). The relationship between Parkinson rigidity and hypokinesia in the orofacial system: A quantitative analysis. *Neurology, 32*, 749–756.

Johns, D. F. (Ed.). (1985). *Clinical management of neurogenic communication disorders*. Boston: Little, Brown.

Karnell, M. P. (1994). *Videoendoscopy: From velopharynx to larynx*. San Diego: Singular.

Kent, R. D. (1994). The clinical science of motor speech disorders: A personal assessment. In J. A. Till, K. M. Yorkston, & D. R. Beukelman (Eds.), *Motor speech disorders: Advances in assessment and treatment* (pp. 3–18). Baltimore: Brookes.

Kent, R. D., Kent, J. F., Weismer, G., Sufit, R. L., Rosenbek, J. C., Martin, R. E., & Brooks, B. R. (1990). Impairment of speech intelligibility in men with amyotrophic lateral sclerosis. *Journal of Speech and Hearing Disorders, 55*, 721–728.

Kent, R. D., Sufit, R. L., Rosenbek, J. C., Kent, J. F., Weismer, G., Martin, R. E., & Brooks, B. R. (1991). Speech deterioration in amyotrophic lateral sclerosis: A case study. *Journal of Speech and Hearing Research, 34*, 1269–1275.

Kent, R. D., Weismer, G., Kent, J. F., & Rosenbek, J. C. (1989). Toward phonetic intelligibility testing in dysarthria. *Journal of Speech and Hearing Disorders, 54*, 482–499.

Kuehn, D. P., & Wachtel, J. M. (1994). CPAP therapy for treating hypernasality following closed head injury. In J. A. Till, K. M. Yorkston, & D. R. Beukelman (Eds.), *Motor speech disorders: Advances in assessment and treatment* (pp. 207–212). Baltimore: Brookes.

Linebaugh, C. (1983). Treatment of flaccid dysarthria. In W. Perkins (Ed.), *Dysarthria and apraxia*. New York: Thieme-Stratton.

Liss, J., Kuehn, D., & Hinkel, K. (1994). Direct training of velopharyngeal musculature. *National Center for Voice and Speech: Status and Progress Report, 6*(5), 43–52.

Logemann, J. A., Fisher, H. B., Boshes, B., & Blonsky, E. R. (1978). Frequency and co-occurrence of vocal tract dysfunctions in the speech of a large sample of Parkinson's patients. *Journal of Speech and Hearing Disorders, 43*, 47–57.

Ludlow, C. L., & Bassich, C. J. (1983). The results of acoustic and perceptual assessment of two types of dysarthria. In W. R. Berry (Ed.), *Clinical dysarthria*. San Diego: College-Hill.

Luschei, E. S. (1991). Development of objective standards of nonspeech oral strength and performance. In C. A. Moore, K. M. Yorkston, & D. R. Beukelman (Eds.), *Dysarthria and apraxia of speech* (pp. 3–13). Baltimore: Brookes.

McHenry, M. A., Wilson, R. L., & Minton, J. J. (1994). Management of multiple physiology system deficits following traumatic brain injury. *Journal of Medical Speech Language Pathology, 2*, 58–74.

Netsell, R. (1984). Physiological studies of dysarthria and their relevance to treatment. In J. C. Rosenbek (Ed.), *Seminars in language* (pp. 279–292). New York: Thieme-Stratton.

Netsell, R. (1986). *A neurobiologic view of speech production and the dysarthrias*. San Diego: College-Hill.

Netsell, R., & Daniel, B. (1979). A physiologic approach to rehabilitation for adults with dysarthria. *Archives of Physical Medicine and Rehabilitation, 60*, 502–508.

Netsell, R., & Hixon, T. J. (1978). A noninvasive method of clinically estimating subglottal air pressure. *Journal of Speech and Hearing Disorders, 43,* 326–330.

Netsell, R., Lotz, W. K., & Barlow, S. M. (1989). A speech physiology examination for individuals with dysarthria. In K. M. Yorkston & D. R. Beukelman (Eds.), *Recent advances in clinical dysarthria* (pp. 3–37). Boston: College-Hill.

Netsell, R., & Rosenbek, J. C. (1985). *Treating the dysarthrias: Speech and language evaluation in neurology: Adult disorders.* New York: Grune & Stratton.

Noll, J. D. (1982). Remediation of impaired resonance among patients with neuropathologies of speech. In N. Lass, L. McReynolds, J. Northern, & D. Yoder (Eds.), *Speech language and hearing: Vol. III: Pathologies of speech and language.* Philadelphia: Saunders.

Perez, K. S., Ramig, L. O., Smith, M. E., & Dromey, C. D. (1996). The Parkinson larynx: Tremor and videostroboscopic findings. *Journal of Voice, 10,* 354–361.

Ramig, L. O., Bonitati, C., Lemke, J. H., & Horii, Y. (1994). Voice therapy for patients with Parkinson's disease: Development of an approach and preliminary efficacy data. *Journal of Medical Speech–Language Pathology, 2,* 191–210.

Ramig, L. O., Countryman, S., Thompson, L. L., & Horii, Y. (1995). A comparison of two forms of intensive speech treatment for Parkinson disease. *Journal of Speech and Hearing Research, 38,* 1232–1251.

Ramig, L. O., & Dromey, C. (1996). Aerodynamic mechanisms underlying treatment related to changes in SPL in patients with Parkinson disease. *Journal of Speech and Hearing Research, 39,* 798–807.

Ramig, L. O., Pawlas, A. A., & Countryman, S. (1995). *The Lee Silverman Voice Treatment (LSVT): A practical guide to treating the voice and speech disorders in Parkinson disease.* Iowa City, IA: National Center for Voice and Speech.

Ramig, L. A., Scherer, R. C., Titze, I. R., & Ringel, S. P. (1988). Acoustic analysis of voice patients with neurological disease: Rationale and preliminary data. *Annals of Otology, Rhiniology, and Laryngology, 97,* 164–171.

Read, C., Buder, E. H., & Kent, R. D. (1990). Speech analysis systems: A survey. *Journal of Speech and Hearing Research, 33*(2), 363–374.

Read, C., Buder, E. H., & Kent, R. D. (1992). Speech analysis systems: An evaluation. *Journal of Speech and Hearing Research, 35*(2), 314–332.

Rosenbek, J. (1984). Treating the dysarthric talker. *Seminars in Speech and Language, 5*, 359–384.

Rosenbek, J. C., & LaPointe, L. L. (1985). The dysarthrias: Description, diagnosis, and treatment. In D. F. Johns (Ed.), *Clinical management of neurogenic communication disorders*. Austin, TX: PRO-ED.

Rubrow, R. (1984). Role of feedback, reinforcement and compliance on training and transfer in biofeedback-based rehabilitation of motor speech disorders. In M. R. McNeil, J. C. Rosenbek, & A. E. Aronson (Eds.), *The dysarthrias: Physiology, acoustics, perception, management* (pp. 207–230). San Diego: College-Hill.

Smith, M. E., Ramig, L. O., Dromey, C. D., Perez, K. E., & Samandari, R. (1995). Intensive voice treatment in Parkinson's disease: Laryngovideostroboscopic findings. *Journal of Voice, 9*, 453–459.

Smitheran, J., & Hixon, T. (1981). A clinical method of estimating laryngeal airway resistance during vowel produciton. *Journal of Speech and Hearing Disorders, 46*, 138–146.

Solomon, N. P., Robin, D. A., Lorell, D. M., Rodnitzky, R. L., Luschei, E. S. (1994). Tongue function testing in Parkinson's disease: Indications of fatigue. In J. Till, K. Yorkston, & D. Beukelman (Eds.), *Motor speech disorders: Advances in assessment and treatment* (pp. 147–160). Baltimore: Brookes.

Stierwalt, J. A. G., Robin, D. A., Pearl Solomon, N., Weiss, A. L., & Max, J. E. (1996). Tongue strength and endurance: Relation to the speaking ability of children and adolescents following traumatic brain injury. In D. A. Robin, K. M. Yorkston, & D. R. Beukelman (Eds.), *Disorders of motor speech: Assessment, treatment, and clinical characterization* (pp. 241–256). Baltimore: Brookes.

Strand, E. A., Buder, E. H., Yorkston, K. M., & Ramig, L. O. (1994). Differential phonatory characteristics of four women with amyotrophic lateral sclerosis. *Journal of Voice, 8*(4), 327–339.

Theodoros, D. G., & Murdoch, B. E. (1996). Differential patterns of hyperfunctional laryngeal impairment in dysarthric speakers following severe closed head injury. In D. A. Robin, K. M. Yorkston, & D. R. Beukelman (Eds.), *Disorders of motor speech: Assessment, treatment, and clinical characterization* (pp. 205–227). Baltimore: Brookes.

Till, J. A., & Alp, L. A. (1991). Aerodynamic and temporal measures of continuous speech in dysarthric speakers. In C. A. Moore, K. M. Yorkston, & D. R. Beukelman (Eds.), *Dysarthria and apraxia of speech* (pp. 185–203). Baltimore: Brookes.

Warren, D. W. (1979). PERCI: A method for rating palatal efficiency. *Cleft Palate Journal, 16,* 279–285.

Warren, D. W., & DuBois, A. B. (1964). A pressure-flow technique for measuring velopharyngeal orifice area during continuous speech. *Cleft Palate Journal, 1,* 52–71.

Warren, D. W., Putnam-Rochet, A., & Hinton, V. A. (1997). Aerodynamics. In M. R. McNeil (Ed.), *Clinical management of sensorimotor speech disorders* (pp. 81–106). New York: Thieme Medical.

Weismer, G. (1984). Acoustic descriptions of dysarthric speech: Perceptual consequences and physiological inferences. *Seminars in Speech and Language, 5,* 293–314.

Weismer, G., Kent, R. D., Hodge, M., & Martin, R. (1988). The acoustic signature for intelligibility test words. *Journal of the Acoustical Society of America, 84*(4), 1281–1291.

Weismer, G., & Liss, J. M. (1991). Age and speech motor control. In D. Ripich (Ed.), *Handbook of aging and communication* (pp. 205–226). Austin, TX: PRO-ED.

Weismer, G., Martin, R., Kent, R. D., & Kent, J. F. (1992). Formant trajectory characteristics of males with amyotrophic lateral sclerosis. *Journal of the Acoustical Society of America, 91,* 1085–1098.

Wood, P. H. N. (1980). Appreciating the consequences of disease: The classification of impairments, disability, and handicaps. *The WHO Chronicle, 43,* 376–380.

Yorkston, K. M., & Beukelman, D. R. (1981). *Assessment of intelligibility of dysarthria speech.* Austin, TX: PRO-ED.

Yorkston, K. M., Beukelman, D., & Bell, K. (1988). *Clinical mangagement of dysarthric speakers*. San Diego: College-Hill.

Yorkston, K. M., Beukelman, D. R., & Honsinger, M. J. (1989). Perceived articulatory adequacy and velopharyngeal function in dysarthric speakers. *Archives of Physical Medicine & Rehabilitation, 70*, 313–331.

Yorkston, K. M., Beukelman, D. R., Strand, E. A., & Bell, K. R. (1999). *Management of motor speech disorders in children and adults* (2nd ed.). Austin, TX: PRO-ED.

Yorkston, K. M., Beukelman, D. R., & Traynor, C. D. (1984). *Computerized assessment of intelligibility of dysarthric speech*. Austin, TX: PRO-ED.

Yorkston, K. M., Bombardier, C., & Hammen, V. L. (1993). Dysarthria from the viewpoint of individuals with dysarthria. In J. A. Till, K. M. Yorkston, & D. R. Beukelman (Eds.), *Motor speech disorders: Advances in assessment and treatment* (pp. 19–35). Baltimore: Brookes.

Yorkston, K., Hammen, V., Beukelman, D., & Traynor, C. (1990). The effect of rate control on the intelligibility and naturalness of dysarthric speech. *Journal of Speech and Hearing Disorders, 55*, 550–560.

Zeplin, J., & Kent, R. D. (1996). Reliability of auditory-perceptual scaling of dysarthria. In D. Robin, K. M. Yorkston, & D. R. Beukelman (Eds.), *Disorders of motor speech: Assessment* (pp. 145–154). Baltimore: Brookes.

Zwirner, P., & Barnes, G. J. (1992). Vocal tract steadiness: A measure of phonatory and upper airway motor control during phonation in dysarthria. *Journal of Speech and Hearing Research, 35*, 761–768.

Zwirner, P., Murry, T., & Woodson, G. E. (1991). Phonatory function of neurologically impaired patients. *Journal of Communication Disorders, 24*(4), 287–300.

Zyski, B. J., & Weisiger, B. E. (1987). Identification of dysarthria types based on perceptual analysis. *Journal of Communication Disorders, 20*, 367–378.

Chapter 4

A Top-Down Approach to Treatment of Dysarthric Speech

Deanie Vogel, Lynda Miller, and Jane Mertz Garcia

Vogel, Miller, and Garcia describe a knowledge-driven approach that provides the cognitive scaffolding for treatment of dysarthric speech. They show how providing insight into the characteristics involved in a top-down approach to treatment for dysarthria may improve speech intelligibility and the patient's overall ability to communicate. In addition, they provide anecdotal information and examples from the literature of how this approach can be effective in the treatment of dysarthria.

1. *List potential benefits of a top-down approach for treatment of dysarthria.*

2. *How can primary-level and secondary-level pragmatics be used in treating the dysarthric patient?*

3. *The authors discuss how discourse analysis can be used to counsel the dysarthric patient. How can awareness of the different types of discourse benefit the patient?*

4. *How have results of recent systematic investigations supported the use of a top-down approach to the treatment of dysarthric speech?*

※ ※ ※

In their landmark papers published in 1969 (a,b), Darley, Aronson, and Brown identified deviant speech dimensions and differential diagnostic patterns of dysarthric speech. These important

119

papers revolutionized the thinking about dysarthria and spawned many new investigations of dysarthria. For an extensive review of this literature, the reader is directed to additional sources such as Darley, Aronson, and Brown (1975) and Duffy (1995).

Since the publication of the papers by Darley and his colleagues, several different approaches to dysarthria management have been postulated. A *symptomotology approach* is one in which a symptom (e.g., inadequate velopharyngeal closure) is treated and the effect on a sign (e.g., hypernasality) is observed. Yorkston and colleagues (Yorkston, Beukelman, & Bell, 1988; Yorkston Beukelman, Strand, & Bell, 1999) described treatment of disordered speech intelligibility, and Rosenbek and LaPointe (1985) wrote of assessment and treatment of impaired respiration, phonation, resonance, articulation, and prosody. Ramig and colleagues (Dromey, Ramig, & Johnson, 1995; Ramig, 1998, 2000; Ramig, Bonitati, Lemke, & Horri, 1994; Ramig, Countryman, O'Brien, Hoehn, & Thompson, 1996) have concentrated on the treatment of the underlying vocal pathology and have focused treatment on an increase of the amplitude of output and the perception of effort. (See Chapter 3 in this book for further discussion.)

Dysarthria clinicians should be aware that a return to normal speech is not a realistic goal for many dysarthric speakers. Thus, compensated intelligibility (Rosenbek & LaPointe, 1985) may be more realistic, especially for dysarthric speakers who are able to use spoken communication but whose speech is not completely intelligible. Some specific techniques used to attempt to achieve compensated intelligibility involve normalizing muscle tone to increase strength and movement precision, management with a palatal lift prosthesis or laryngoplasty, engaging in phonetic and vocal loudness drills, and attempting to control speaking rate.

Historically, dysarthria clinicians have tended to focus on the speaker and the dysarthric speech rather than on the listener and the communication interaction. In this chapter, a knowledge-driven, top-down approach to communication is described, involving the study of the relationships between language and the context in which it is used. The top-down process and its characteristics are defined and contrasted with the signal-oriented, bottom-up approach in which the organization of language is largely ignored. Suggestions for using components of a top-down approach for improving the communication of dysarthric patients are presented.

Top-Down and Bottom-Up Processing

The term *top-down* is generally used to refer to the cognitive process of using available information to construct a gestalt, or whole. In this perspective on cognitive processing, the whole serves as an overall form into which supporting details can be fit. The supporting details are added after the general pattern has been constructed and are used to corroborate the general pattern. As Wallach and Miller (1988) pointed out, "Top-down processing is analogous to deductive thinking. In deductive thinking one formulates a general hypothesis and infers specific outcomes on the basis of the general principle" (p. 20).

Recent conceptualizations of top-down processing have focused on metacommunicative functions (van Kleeck, 1994) that describe communication accompanying language and carrying a significant portion of the communicative message. Metacommunicative functions communicate information about how the speaker's utterances are to be interpreted, how speakers feel about their messages and their listeners, and various speaker intentions (van Kleek, 1994). These metacommunicative functions are communicated most often through nonlinguistic means, such as eye movement, facial expression, body posture and movements, and the suprasegmentals of intonation.

Although children typically learn the various metacommunicative aspects of communication as part of their acquisition of language, it is not unusual for adults to engage in the learning of new cultural variations on metacommunicative functions. Moreover, for adults with dysarthria, focusing on the "meta" aspects of communication may offer a powerful way to regain some facility with conversation and social intercourse.

Metacommunication includes several subcomponents, including metapragmatic and metalinguistic functions. *Metapragmatic functions* refer to the speaker's or listener's awareness of the social rules for the uses of language, whereas *metalinguistic functions* refer to an individual's conscious focus on language and its various forms and functions. These metacommunicative functions will be discussed in more depth later in this chapter.

In contrast to top-down processing, the term *bottom-up* has been used to refer to the cognitive process of using available information to collect a group of details before constructing a general pattern. The details serve as the salient features from which a larger concept is built.

Bottom-up processing is analogous to inductive thinking in that it involves accumulating examples until a general conclusion can be reached (Wallach & Miller, 1988). Traditional dysarthria therapies involve more bottom-up than top-down processing.

In developing knowledge of and facility with language and communication, children typically engage in inductive learning. They hear assorted pieces of language form, various ways of encoding content, and examples of usage, all of which rarely suggest the organizational aspects of the language they are hearing. From these bits and pieces, children gradually construct their own methods of choosing words, forming sentences, translating them into the sound system of their language, and using them in appropriate and relevant ways.

Many language users, as they grow into adults, continue to engage in inductive learning about language and communication and may never use top-down thinking in considering the linguistic and nonlinguistic aspects of communicating. They may use language with facility but have little or no insight into how it works. As bottom-up learners, they are relatively adept at choosing appropriate sound combinations, words, and sentence structures for their messages, but they remain unaware of the patterns underlying these aspects of communicating through language. For many adults, language is something that just happens; talking about it, or reflecting on its myriad parts, is foreign and unfamiliar, and the idea that communication patterns can be analyzed may be surprising to them.

For other language users, deciphering the general patterns and rules of language and communication from their ongoing experiences is a natural process. These language users actively search for the organizational patterns characterizing communication and language. They find the top-down characteristics salient and obvious, and they use them in their own understanding of how to use both linguistic and nonlinguistic means to communicate. For top-down learners, the general patterns stand as organizational themes from which to deduce specific examples to incorporate into their communicating. In adulthood, top-down learners most likely have developed a considerable ability to reflect on communication and how language and its parts function in various communicative contexts. Usually, they can talk about language and its parts and understand the interactions of linguistic and nonlinguistic form, content, and use.

A third type of processing consists of a combination of top-down and bottom-up processing. This is *interactive processing* and is the process language users employ when comprehending language. Interactive language users analyze the peripheral input delivered via the input signal while consulting their central knowledge stores in order to arrive at an interpretation of the signal.

Regardless of whether the clinical intervention is focused on the motor speech mechanism or on the language system of the user, the dysarthria clinician can introduce the bottom-up, top-down, and interactive aspects of communication. It may be beneficial to begin treatment by attempting to discover what the dysarthric patient knows about language and communication in order to determine whether the patient is a top-down, bottom-up, or interactive learner. A conversation about communication can yield a great deal of information that can be used to focus treatment. For the dysarthric patient whose knowledge of communication and language is primarily bottom-up, focusing on the top-down aspects of language and communication may constitute a significant portion of the treatment sessions. For these bottom-up learners, the initial task may focus on helping the patient become aware of general patterns of language and communication that are independent of the speech signal.

A significant corollary of discovering how clients prefer to process communicatively is for clinicians to become aware of which approach they, themselves, prefer. The clinician who would rather use a bottom-up approach may not want to introduce a top-down aspect to intervention. For this reason, Miller (1992a, 1992b) advocates that clinicians analyze their own preferences as well as those of their clients. The patient who regards the goal of dysarthria therapy as improvement in speech, rather than progress in overall communication, needs information about general patterns of communication and language. Top-down characteristics must be described. Meanings of words such as topic must be explained, because the patient who does not understand what a topic is will be less than adept at understanding how to maintain one. Furthermore, these patients with an inductive orientation to language use may not be aware of how to get a turn in a conversation; how, either verbally or nonverbally, to signal turn-taking shifts in a conversation; or how to send a message to their listeners that a humorous remark is on the way.

Dysarthric patients who are not bottom-up learners may benefit from a top-down orientation, as well. These individuals should be made aware of how to use alternative strategies that may not be immediately obvious, even to more top-down-oriented communicators.

The clinician's task is somewhat easier when treating patients who, before becoming dysarthric, developed an understanding of the top-down characteristics of language. These individuals may only need to be reminded of those characteristics and how to manipulate them effectively.

The Top-Down Characteristics of Language

Traditional descriptions of language focus on the patterns associated with semantic, morpho-syntactic, phonological, and pragmatic components. Although it is true that there is a general pattern characteristic of each of these primary linguistic components, it is also true that general patterns of language exist at a secondary level of analysis. This secondary level was distinguished from the primary level by Miller (1988), who termed it the "level of higher-order language," on the basis that this level of awareness develops as a function of the acquisition of the primary-level structures, forms, and uses of language. Higher-order language constitutes what are currently referred to as metapragmatics and metalinguistics.

Dysarthric individuals may find it possible to increase their speech intelligibility and the overall quality of their communication by focusing on the higher-order levels of language. By manipulating some of the top-down aspects of language, many dysarthric individuals can significantly alter the degree to which their messages are interpreted accurately. The top-down characteristics of primary and higher-order levels of language processing are described in the sections that follow.

Top-Down Characteristics of the Primary Level of Language Processing

Typically, the primary level of language processing consists of semantics, syntax and morphology, phonology, and pragmatics. (Note, however, that some portions of the pragmatic component of language will be described as secondary-level aspects.)

Semantics

The most salient, general semantic characteristic is that things-in-the-world are named. Although this may seem obvious, what may not be so obvious is that many things-in-the-world have more than one name. Often, alternate names or synonyms for a particular word comprise phonological sequences that are much easier for a dysarthric patient to produce than the word the patient has intended to say. For example, a dysarthric patient attempting to tell us about his neighbor's spring planting produced several unintelligible attempts at the word *rosebush*. Finally, he substituted the word *roses* for the intended word; this turned out to be easier for him to produce than the word *rosebush*. Moreover, the word *roses* served the same general purpose as the word *rosebush*. The patient's word substitution was understood, the communication was successful, and the conversation could continue.

Another general characteristic of the semantic component of language is that, usually, there is a specific word to refer to each specific thing-in-the-world. Using that specific word rather than a more general referent substantially increases the likelihood that the word will be understood. A corollary of the specific word for a specific referent is that, usually, intelligibility is maximized when speakers use a word according to its denotative or explicit functions, rather than relying on its connotative or associative functions. What this means is that usually literal meanings are easier to understand than figurative meanings, except in certain circumstances where idiomatic or metaphoric expressions are more common. The use of figurative language and its relationship to the treatment of dysarthria will be discussed further in a subsequent section that describes the characteristics of the secondary-level language components.

A third characteristic of the semantic component is that mature language users recall overall sentence meanings more often than they recall particular syntactic forms (Owens, 1988). The implication for the dysarthric individual with compromised ability to produce connected strings of sounds and syllables intelligibly is that for comprehension, syntactic structure may not be as important as semantic meaning. This is of considerable importance for the clinician, especially when treating the severely dysarthric patient who is using a method of communication that is an alternative to speech. Counseling the patient to construct brief messages consisting of only nouns or nouns and verbs rather than using long, complete sentences is a common practice in dysarthria therapy. What may not be so common is the practice of making the patient aware that for effective communication, meaning is more important than syntax.

The semantic content of sentences is an important feature for the dysarthria clinician to consider. Some sentences may convey message content that facilitates comprehension of impaired speech intelligibility. For example, in some cases, single words are more readily identified (understood) when they are produced within a meaningful sentence context than when they are read or spoken in isolation. Dongilli (1994) studied eight flaccid dysarthric speakers whose speech intelligibility ranged from mild to profoundly impaired. He compared the intelligibility of words read in isolation with the intelligibility of the same words embedded within high probability test sentences from the Speech Perception in Noise (SPIN) test (Kalikow, Stevens, & Elliott, 1977). Dongilli found that for all but the speakers who were profoundly impaired, words read in sentences were more intelligible than words read in isolation. This finding appears to support the contention that for all but the speakers who were most severely impaired, sentence content information enhances the understanding of dysarthric speech.

Although sentence context may increase the understanding of specific words spoken by speakers with dysarthria, it is not known just how semantic components contribute to the understanding of the overall message. One hypothesis is that some sentences contain intrinsic message cues that differentially contribute to listener understanding. Berry and Goshorn (1983) demonstrated that predictability of sentence information is such a cue. Their subject was a dysarthric speaker who read high and low predictive sentences from the SPIN test and demonstrated that the high predictive sentences were the more intelligible.

Garcia and Cannito (1996b) also found the level of sentence predictiveness to be an influential factor in the understanding of dysarthric speech. Their patient was a speaker with severe dysarthria who read some sentences containing either high or low predictive message content. The sentences with high predictive message content were found to be 60% intelligible, whereas sentences containing low predictive messages were only 15% intelligible. The discrepancy in the speaker's intelligibility scores appeared to be related to the degree of predictive content in the sentences. Garcia and Cannito concluded that highly predictive sentences encoded spoken messages containing greater semantic cohesion that assisted listeners in understanding unintelligible speech. Consequently, the predictability of sentence content information may be an important factor in comprehension of dysarthric speech. Results of a subsequent study conducted by Garcia and Dagenais (1998) supported this conclusion.

From a treatment standpoint, it is important to realize that the potential benefit of semantic content information within sentence length utterances will be influenced by the severity of the dysarthria. For example, in comparing the importance of word versus sentence length utterances for understanding dysarthric speech, there may be a "point where the signal is so distorted that intelligibility cannot be influenced regardless of efforts to increase listeners' knowledge through increased utterance length" (Dongilli, 1994, p. 184). As a result, speakers with profoundly impaired speech intelligibility may benefit from treatment that de-emphasizes the importance of lengthy sentence responses and emphasizes the semantic aspects of single words.

Morpho-Syntax

The syntactic and morphological aspects of language are closely linked and are often considered to be part of the same grammatical system. The most general characteristic of the grammatical component of language is that there are patterns that underlie sentence structure and word endings. The most basic sentence structures are the following: the simple, active declarative (*John kicked the ball.*), the imperative (*Get the ball out of the flowers!*), the negative (*I don't want any coffee right now.*), and the interrogative (*Is that a black tie?*). Less obvious sentence structures are the nonreversible passive (*The book was picked up by the woman.*), the reversible passive (*The boy was chased by the girl.*), the "wh" question (*Why do you want to go today?*), and the embedded clause (*The man who came by the office yesterday is the guy I was telling you about in the park that day.*). We hypothesize that listeners of dysarthric speech would find sentences using basic structures easier to interpret than sentences consisting of less obvious sentence structures.

Although the effects of different sentence structures on the understanding of dysarthric speech have not been studied extensively, one study (Carter, Yorkston, Strand, & Hammen, 1996) did investigate the influence of syntactic context on understandability of dysarthric speech. Syntactic context was considered to be the part of a sentence that does not add meaning or suggest information about message intent; for example, the number of words or the number of functor words in a sentence. Carter et al. (1996, p. 74) found that sentence intelligibility scores of speakers with severe dysarthria (35%–39% intelligible) improved by approximately 11% when listeners were given cues about the grammatical structure of the sentences. Moreover, the investigators speculated that the predictability of specific grammatical structures, such as stated subject-verb-object sentence forms, also improved sentence intelligibility scores. These findings imply that dysarthric speakers may benefit from clinical instruction that encourages the use of simple, but predictable, sentence types.

Patterns of word endings signal specific meanings, as in the following example: *The cats played in the trees*. Here, the underlined segments indicate a plural, a past tense, and another plural. These particular endings illustrate regular patterns in English and are found in the majority of plural and past tense markers. As a general rule, regular and higher-frequency irregular forms are more likely to be predicted correctly by listeners—that is, communicated more effectively—than lower-frequency irregular markers. Many English words with irregular markers, however, are quite recognizable. The words *ate*, *sang*, *drank*, *hit*, *bought*, *made*, *children*, *mice*, *feet*, and *sheep* are examples. Although, to date, there have been no systematic investigations with dysarthric subjects, we predict that words with regular morphological forms and high-frequency irregular markers are more likely to be understood by listeners of dysarthric speech than are words with exceptions to regular usage.

Phonology

A primary characteristic of the phonological system that is relevant to improving communication for the dysarthric speaker is that sounds and sound combinations that can be seen (e.g., labials and labiodentals) and heard (e.g., vowels and voiced consonants) are more understandable than sounds that are less visible and audible. This is especially true under conditions in which the speech signal is degraded (as it is in dysarthria). Garcia and Cannito (1996a) found that when speech was presented in a video-only viewing format, judges had difficulty interpreting dysarthric speech, but their understanding improved when they were provided with speech-reading cues about phonetic gestures.

When a degraded speech signal is presented to listeners, visual and auditory information presented simultaneously is better understood than information presented through the auditory modality alone (see Binnie, Montgomery, & Jackson, 1974; Erber, 1975; Hubbard & Kushner-Vogel, 1981; Summerfield, 1987). In fact, visual information appears to be increasingly important to speech intelligibility as the clarity of the auditory signal diminishes (Massaro, 1987). A few studies have examined the contribution of visual input to the comprehension of dysarthric speech. Garcia, Dagenais, Terrell, and Mallory (1992) studied listener understanding of words and sentences read by a speaker with moderate dysarthria. These investigators reported that listener understanding was significantly better for both words and sentences in an auditory and visual combined condition than in a condition where the listeners were exposed to the auditory signal alone. Barkmeier (1988) described similar findings for sentence production for a group of dysarthric speakers. Barkmeier also found that the influence of the visual signal decreased as experience in listening to dysarthric speech increased.

The results of these studies have implications for the dysarthria clinician. The clinician can point out the differences between highly visible and audible sounds and sound combinations and those that are less so, in order to illustrate the sounds that may increase speech intelligibility and communicative effectiveness for the dysarthric speaker.

It is important to realize that the phonological system of some dysarthric persons may be so impaired that the potential benefits of semantic or syntactic predictability for comprehension is limited. Consequently, there is a "need for a minimal level of intact phonetic information for the listener to maximize contextual clues" (Sitler, Schiavetti, & Metz, 1983, p. 34). No doubt this is especially true when listening to dysarthric speech without concomitant visual information.

A second general characteristic of the phonological system is that short sound sequences are more understandable than long sound sequences. Perhaps this is true because the shorter sequences place a lighter load on the working memory of the listener. The clinician can demonstrate how to use phonologically short phrases while underscoring the idea that both the phonological and grammatical systems are involved in the selection of the message. Of course, in the case of the dysarthric talker with profoundly impaired speech intelligibility, it is highly likely that the potential benefits of semantic or syntactic cues will be limited. This is especially true when the dysarthric speech is produced without concomitant visual information, for example, as during a telephone speaking situation, or when the dysarthric talker attempts to speak with someone who is in another room (Yorkston, Bombardier, & Hammen, 1994).

Primary-Level Pragmatics

Pragmatics involves the psychosocial uses of language and constitutes one of the most pervasive processes in communication. Pragmatic functions occur at both the primary and secondary levels of language processing. At the primary level, pragmatics involves three functions: joint and mutual attending; initiating, maintaining, and shifting topics; and appropriate turn-taking.

Joint and Mutual Attending. It is imperative that the patient with compromised speech intelligibility use both verbal and nonverbal methods to signal joint and mutual attending. *Joint attending* involves sharing attention with others during conversation. Nonverbal signals for joint attention include appropriate eye gaze (the listener watches the speaker much more frequently and closely than the speaker watches the listener); facial expression; body orientation; head nods; and other body gestures such as hand, arm, head, leg, and foot movements. The clinician can help the dysarthric speaker develop a set of clear nonverbal signals to use to alert the listener that the speaker is engaging in joint attention.

Mutual attending occurs when communication partners are engaged in observing an event, person, object, relationship, or attribute, or in participating in an event or process. Nonverbal means for mutual attending are similar to those required for joint attending, but the actual movements, expressions, orientations, and statements may be somewhat different. For instance, to indicate mutual attending, conversation partners may need to engage in major shifts of body position or other overt behaviors to signal their partner to use eye contact, or to employ specific statements to check understanding or participation.

Initiating, Maintaining, and Shifting Topics. Topic initiation, maintenance, and shifting are crucial to successful communication. To communicate a message effectively, the speaker must know how to engage the listener's attention. Listeners attend best when speakers initiate new topics in interesting and appropriate ways; when they maintain the topic through interesting, relevant, and appropriate comments; and when they shift topics appropriately. Introducing new topics without providing appropriate background, maintaining a topic beyond the listener's interest and attention level, and shifting topics abruptly—all result in a communicative exchange that is in danger of deteriorating, unless the speaker can initiate speedy and appropriate repairs.

Monsen (1983) underscored the importance of providing the listener with information regarding the topic or situation in which the utterance was spoken. For a person with dysarthria, providing the listener with this knowledge when initiating or shifting conversational topics would appear to be imperative for successful communication. Results of several studies have shown that when listeners are provided context cues (e.g., category name, situational setting), subsequent word and sentence understanding improves for some dysarthric speakers (Carter et al., 1996; Dongilli, 1994; Garcia & Cannito, 1996a, 1996b; Hammen, Yorkston, & Dowden, 1991; Yorkston, Dowden, & Beukelman, 1992).

It is important to note that although semantic context cues can improve comprehension of long as well as short utterances, the amount of gain is of a lesser magnitude for long utterances. For dysarthric speakers with more moderate to severe intelligibility impairments, approximately 7%–12% improvement has been reported for sentence understanding by listeners who are provided with prior knowledge of the communicative context (Carter et al., 1996; Dongilli, 1994; Garcia & Cannito, 1996a, 1996b).

Turn-Taking. Crucial to successful communicating is the ability to engage in appropriate turn-taking. Knowing how to get a turn, how to maintain a turn once it is obtained, and how to relinquish the turn appropriately is essential for successful communication in conversation. The ability to signal effectively is absolutely necessary for getting a turn, especially in a large conversational group. The individual who wants a turn must signal this desire effectively to the person who is speaking. The signal may be an eye gaze, a breathing pattern, a facial expression, a body movement, a gesture, or a verbal interjection. To be successful at getting a turn, often, the potential speaker has to interject quickly—and this can be difficult for dysarthric individuals who may have to become proficient at using nonverbal signals to get a turn in a conversation.

Maintaining a turn once it is obtained requires that the speaker produce relevant, interesting, and appropriate comments during the conversation. Also, maintenance must follow a timetable; that is, the speaker must maintain a turn for a certain amount of time, then relinquish the turn. Although there are no explicit guidelines for maintaining a turn in conversation, there seems to be an implicit understanding of the optimum time interval. Dysarthric speakers who are trying to produce more understandable speech by reducing their speaking rate may have to shorten their messages or alert their communication partners that they may need more time to speak than the listener may have anticipated.

Many a dysarthria clinician has advised many a dysarthric talker to slow down by pausing between syllables and words in order to increase the understandability of speech. Following this advice may present a problem for the dysarthric talker who is attempting to maintain a turn in conversation. Conversation partners may interpret the pause as an intention of the dysarthric talker to yield the turn in the conversation, and they may begin to speak while the dysarthric talker is pausing. The clinician can introduce nonverbal signals for the patient to use to communicate an unwillingness to relinquish a turn. Examples of such signals are a hand gesture that provides a signal to stop or an exaggerated averting of eye gaze to indicate that the speaker is not yet ready to relinquish the turn.

Yorkston and colleagues (Yorkston et al., 1988; Yorkston et al., 1999; Yorkston, Strand, & Kennedy, 1996), focusing on both dysarthric speakers and their listeners, offered suggestions for preventing communication breakdown in conversations with dysarthric persons. These authors wrote of the value of encouraging listeners to use gestures immediately to signal that the dysarthric individual's message has not been understood. This gives the dysarthric speaker some time to decide whether to stop and repair the message or to continue with the expectation that added context will improve the communication. Yorkston and colleagues also recommended instructing the patient to either repeat the misunderstood portion of the utterance, perhaps with elaboration, or to spell out the message slowly, letter by letter. Finally, in a most cogent and clinically relevant paper, Yorkston et al. (1996) created a checklist for communication partners of dysarthric speakers containing strategies for dealing with communication breakdown.

Clinicians who are curious about intervention structured around the primary-level pragmatic characteristics may be interested in the pragmatics program developed by Hoskins (1987). Although designed for use with adolescents, this program is easily modifiable for use with adults, as well.

Top-Down Characteristics of the Higher-Order Level of Language Processing

There are three secondary level processes of language: metalinguistic processing, metapragmatics and metacommunication, and discourse knowledge. A discussion of these language processes and their application to dysarthria therapy is provided in the next section.

Metalinguistic Processing

To be metalinguistic is to be able to reflect on language, its parts and their functions and uses. The person with metalinguistic ability is cognizant of the various aspects of language; for example, an unfamiliar word, a humorous-sounding word, an unusual wording in a phrase, or a notable comment. Our description of the primary metalinguistic awareness will be from a top-down perspective, although from a metalinguistic viewpoint, one can consider language from a top-down perspective, a bottom-up perspective, or from a combination of the two.

Arbitrary Relationship Between Words and Referents

With few exceptions, words are arbitrarily related to the referents for which they stand. How things are called is largely a result of which peoples traded with each other as the language was being used or, often, of who conquered whom. Typically, the victor's language became dominant, and words from the dominant language infiltrated the entire populace. As a result of this arbitrary relationship between words and referents, the referents have names that are understood through convention, only.

Some words represent communications that are understood universally. *OK* is an example of universal agreement on a word to signify a certain meaning. Many dysarthria clinicians encourage their patients to communicate the message *OK* with a gesture. For example, the patient can be encouraged to touch the tip of the index finger of one hand to the tip of the thumb on the same hand and point the remaining three fingers upward. Additionally, some clinicians encourage their patients to use a "thumbs up" gesture to communicate that "everything is okay." Understanding that referents and words are separate entities allows the language user to employ synonyms, homonyms, and homophones as well as verbal humor and figurative language forms.

Levels of Meaning in Language. Meaning exists on a variety of levels in language. For example, in every communicative interaction there is an underlying level of intent, and what is spoken may or may not directly signal that intent. In fact, much underlying intent is communicated indirectly. In addition to the underlying level, there is also a *denotative*, or *literal*, *level of meaning* in language, in which words stand for referents in an explicit and specific manner. In contrast to the denotative level, there exists a *connotative level of meaning* through which speakers can use a word to stand for referents in a more associative, or implied, manner. Slang words are typical examples of connotative meanings, such as when the word *bad* is used to mean *good* or *sharp*. Also, there are *figurative meanings* beyond the merely connotative; examples are idioms, similes, and metaphors. To use figurative language effectively, both the speaker and the listener must know the relationship between the words used and the speaker's intended referents.

Verbal humor provides an example of how levels of meaning are used to communicate. For example, in a riddle, the listener is led into a certain set of circumstances in which the punch line is fairly predictable. Then, the listener is confronted with a punch line that capitalizes on multiple meanings at the syntactic, lexical, or phonological level. For instance, in an old riddle the question is, *When is a door not a door?* and the answer is, *When it is ajar*. The humor is based on the punch line, which capitalizes on the fact that, although they sound alike, the phrase *a jar* and the word *ajar* have different meanings. These meanings, of course, depend upon the way in which the listener segments (i.e., identifies and assigns the word boundaries).

Another example of verbal humor is the pun. Once a visiting professor of anatomy from a foreign country asked us to define the word *pun*. Knowing that he had recently visited the famous city in Nevada, we gave the following example:

- ▶ Q. What happens when you damage the 10th cranial nerve? (CN X)
- ▶ A. You get a Lost Vagus.

Our friend recognized the phonological similarities between *lost vagus* and *Las Vegas*, and so he laughed. Put another way, the verbal humor was understood by the listener because he had developed metalinguistic awareness of the various levels of meaning in English. As in the case of figurative language, users of a language do not understand verbal humor unless they have developed this metalinguistic awareness of meanings.

Figurative language may present a greater inferential processing burden for the listener: When it is combined with the degraded speech signal produced by a dysarthric speaker, it well may be incomprehensible. Thus, the dysarthric person may do well to minimize or even avoid figurative language, particularly in conversation with individuals who are not accustomed to hearing dysarthric speech. Dysarthric patients can be counseled that the success or failure of their communication may depend upon whether or not their listeners are familiar with various meanings of words or phrases that the dysarthric speaker may use. This is especially important when the speaker is attempting to communicate with persons from different cultural and/or linguistic backgrounds. Figure 4.1 illustrates the consequences that can occur in this situation.

Dysarthric persons who can predict that their listeners may not be familiar with a particular term can help avoid a communication breakdown by substituting a term that may be more familiar to the listener. We know of a situation where a dysarthric patient, a former bartender, told his clinician that "sparkling water" was one ingredient he included when mixing a particular drink. The clinician misperceived the term *sparkling water* and thought the patient had said *talcum powder*, probably because *sparkling water* was not a term used in the geographical area where the conversation took place. The clinician explained this possible reason for the miscommunication to the surprised patient,

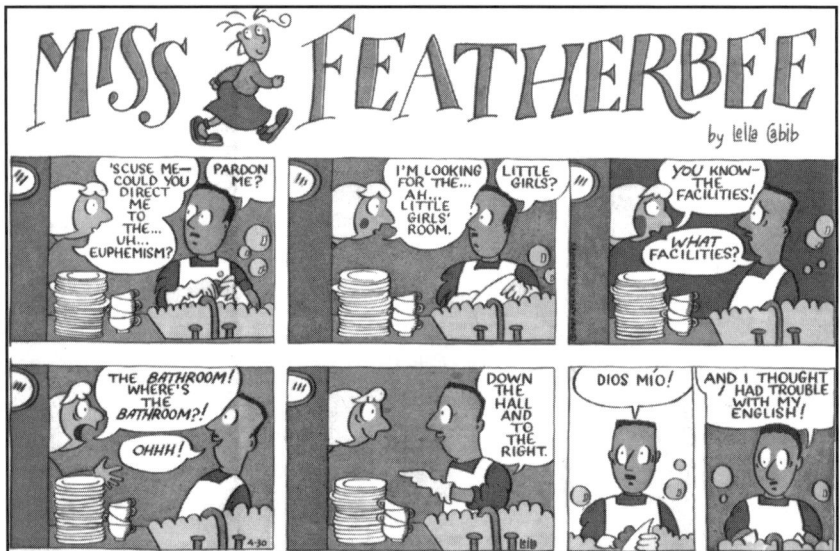

Figure 4.1. Miscommunication that can result from assuming that the listener knows alternate meanings of a term. Copyright 1989 by Asterisk Features. Reprinted with permission.

who agreed that his use of the unfamiliar term and its misinterpretation had the potential to lead to disastrous consequences!

Taking the Listener's Perspective. Although taking the listener's perspective can be considered a pragmatic function, once the speaker is conscious of the process, it becomes a metalinguistic awareness. Being aware of the listener's perspective allows the speaker to manipulate language, form, content, and function to accommodate the different needs of various listeners. Taking the listener's perspective also enables the speaker to make good guesses about the use of which language structures, contents, and functions will result in successful communication with a particular listener. The listener's perspective will be discussed further in the section on secondary-level pragmatics.

Metalinguistic awareness can increase communication effectiveness. The dysarthric speaker who understands that words and referents are arbitrarily related may be better able to choose words that the listener will understand. Furthermore, dysarthric speakers can be counseled that if they do not know the education level or socioeconomic status of their communication partners, using common semantic and syntactic forms as well as common phonological structures will allow them to communicate with the highest possible degree of speech intelligibility. By taking the listener's perspective, the dysarthric speaker can alert the listener to the speech deficit and can ask for an agreement to violate underlying communication rules, such as by extending speaking time in conversation. Finally, dysarthric speakers can provide cues about their communicative content; for example, they can alert their listener when a humorous comment is forthcoming, thus providing the listener with an extra cue about the communicative intent.

Dysarthria clinicians who would like additional information about intervention programs designed to develop metalinguistic knowledge are referred to the work of Wallach and Miller (1988) and van Kleeck (1984a, 1984b, 1994) who devote considerable space to discussing the development of metalinguistic knowledge. Much of the information in these publications is adaptable for use with adult dysarthric individuals.

Metapragmatics

Most language users readily develop the primary-level pragmatic functions naturally. For most children, these functions are acquired by 6 years of age. A secondary layer of pragmatic functions emerges, as well. This secondary level develops throughout childhood and adolescence and is highly influenced by the social and cultural conventions of the linguistic community. As in metalinguistic awareness, there are some general characteristics of metapragmatics; these are described in the following sections.

Use of Verbal and Nonverbal Means to Communicate Intention. Part of being a successful communication partner stems from the ability to use various verbal and nonverbal means to communicate underlying intentions. For instance, to be clear and explicit, a speaker will use semantic, syntactic, and phonological structures that state the intended message directly. The verbal message, "Please close the window; I'm cold" may be made clearer if it is accompanied by the gestures associated with shivering (e.g., rubbing the arms). Additionally, an intention to tease can be communicated both verbally and nonverbally. For example, the speaker could announce:

> "I'm going to tease you now. What do you mean, you can't go to the store in shorts! It's 100° in the shade, and you can't go out wearing shorts because someone might see your legs."

These statements, when accompanied by exaggerated hand and body movements and an emphasis on appropriate syllables and words, signify further that the speaker's intention is to tease.

Nonverbal communication "accounts for between 65 and 93% of the communication we have with one another in face to face interactions" (Hickson & Stacks, 1993, p. 14). Nonverbal factors can be maximized to enhance the communicative effectiveness of dysarthric speakers. For example, pointing to the first letter on an alphabet board for each spoken word (i.e., the alphabet board supplementation procedure; Beukelman & Yorkston, 1977) provides communication partners with additional content information that helps them understand dysarthric speech. This can result in improved speech production for the dysarthric speaker by slowing down the rate of speech (Crow & Enderby, 1989; Beukelman & Yorkston, 1977; Yorkston et al., 1999).

Hand gestures occur naturally while speaking and serve to augment speech (Ekman & Friesen, 1969, 1972; McNeill, 1985, 1992). Results of recent investigations have indicated that message comprehension improves when gestures accompany dysarthric speech (Garcia & Cannito 1996a, 1996b; Garcia, Cannito, & Dagenais, 2000; Garcia & Dagenais, 1998). For example, in a study of the effects of gestures on understanding the communication of a dysarthric speaker, Garcia and Cannito (1996b) asked a severely flaccid dysarthric speaker to produce sentences with and without scripted gesticulations. Garcia and Cannito found that intelligibility improved by nearly 25% when gestures accompanied speech. In a subsequent analysis, Garcia and Cannito (1996a) compared the communicative value of gestured information across audio + video, audio-only, and video-only presentation conditions. Results revealed that subjects correctly understood approximately 26% of the sentence information presented without the auditory signal. The investigators concluded that the speaker had conveyed semantic information nonverbally as well as verbally and that listeners use visual information for message comprehension.

In another study, Garcia and Cannito (1994) investigated the influence of hand gestures on listeners' perceptions of dysarthric speakers. Listeners were asked to complete the Questionnaire for Attractiveness (Barkmeier, Jordan, Robin, & Schum, 1991) after they observed a video of a dysarthric patient. Garcia and Cannito found that hand gestures did not adversely affect how the listeners perceived the dysarthric individual; in fact, the presence of the gestures resulted in positive perceptions. For example, the dysarthric patient was perceived as a healthier and more assertive communicator when gestures accompanied his speech than when he spoke without accompanying gestures.

Degree of Directness in Communicating Intention. Every linguistic community has developed methods for communicating underlying intention in indirect ways. An example is the politely indirect way of making an imperative statement. For example, the polite request, "Would you mind closing the window?" stands for the imperative, "Close the window"; the polite statement, "I don't mind if I do have another piece of cake" can actually stand for, "I want more cake." Idiomatic expressions provide another way of indirectly communicating intention. Again the speaker must be certain that the listener is familiar with the idiom. For example the idiom, "You're pulling my leg" to indicate that someone is teasing communicates the intended message only if the listener knows the intended meaning of the idiom.

Effective communication demands that speakers and listeners agree on the underlying meaning of the indirect communication. If the speaker uses an idiomatic expression that is unfamiliar to the listener, the message will not be communicated effectively unless the underlying intention is explained by the speaker. Indirect communication of intention is, by definition, more susceptible to communication breakdown than is direct communication for the simple reason that it is not direct. Cultural conventions demand indirect communication of intention. Thus, speakers who do not indirectly communicate underlying intention are noticed precisely because they are not adhering to a cultural convention. There seems to be a trade-off between cultural acceptance and the probability that the communication will be effective.

Making Assumptions About Listeners. Speakers must make assumptions about what their listeners know in order to use the appropriate language form and content and, therefore, to communicate successfully. In order to maximize the probability of a message being understood and interpreted accurately, speakers must make decisions about which words, sentence constructions, phonological sequences, and prosodic features to use; how much information to include; and how much background to provide. These decisions are based on the speaker's assumptions about such listener conditions and attributes as the following:

1. Listener's age, gender, and appearance (including hair color, clothing, and skin color)

2. Listener's speech and what it implies (e.g., level of education and ethnicity or nationality, and whether these are similar or different from those of the speaker)

3. Geographic location of the conversation

4. Speaker's perception of who functions as the authority in each communicative interaction

Adherence to and Violation of Community Conventions for Cooperating in Communicating. In each linguistic community, speakers adhere to common conventions in order to communicate effectively. At the same time, speakers consistently violate the conventions in commonly agreed upon ways. Such violations carry as much communicative information as adherence. In fact, within each linguistic community, there are institutionalized violations of the communicative conventions. Some understood rules for communicating cooperatively are (a) tell the truth, (b) be brief, (c) be relevant, (d) be unambiguous, (e) ask only for information that you want, and (f) give only information you believe is wanted.

Many indirect means of communicating intentions violate communicative conventions. For instance, the intention underlying the question, "How are you?" spoken to a colleague at work on a Monday morning usually is to extend a simple greeting and not to obtain a comprehensive account of the state of the colleague's health and well-being. The question itself, then, violates the rule to ask only for information you want.

One of the maxims associated with cooperating in communicating is to be informative. One way to express that information is new or important is through prosody. For example, we use prosody to mark sarcasm. When we say, "You really look terrific" but we mean, "You really look terrible," we are using prosody to mark and communicate meaning. Dysarthric persons who are also dysprosodic lose this ability.

Another aspect of prosody for expressing salient or new information is the use of intonation. Again, dysprosody can impede this function. If a listener does not know what part of a word to focus on, a message will be more difficult to interpret than it would be if the listener were aware of this important information. For a more complete discussion of how prosody can be used in the treatment of motor-speech disorders, see the discussion by Seddoh and Robin in Chapter 8 of this volume.

Focusing on the secondary level of pragmatic functions may constitute a crucial part of the dysarthric patient's treatment sessions. The clinician can instruct the patient in how to discriminate between direct statements of intent and indirect means of communicating by presenting examples of each. Rather than making assumptions about what listeners know, dysarthric speakers can focus on asking for explicit information. With this information in hand, they can then tailor their own remarks to be direct and explicit. The clinician can advise the patient to limit or eliminate low-frequency idiomatic expressions and metaphoric forms, concentrating instead on the direct, literal terms or frequently used idioms and metaphors that will be understood by most potential communication partners.

For a discussion of intervention for higher-level pragmatics with school age children, see Wallach and Miller (1988). Hoskins (1987) outlined a general program that includes both primary- and secondary-level pragmatics, which may be of interest to clinicians treating dysarthric patients. In addition, Scott (1994) and Westby (1994) have described metapragmatic functions across cultural groups.

Discourse Knowledge

Communication takes place in a variety of situations and contexts. Speakers and listeners converse with varying levels of familiarity, about topics ranging from the everyday to the esoteric. The study of discourse processes and knowledge focuses on how speakers and listeners organize their communication in various types of conversations. These conversations differ with the context in which they take place. The type of discourse used in a coffee shop between good friends is different from that used between teacher and students, and both are different from the type used in a corporate office between a middle-level manager and an upper-level executive. Not only do each of these conversations employ different types of discourse, but each type carries with it a separate set of rules and conventions for participating.

Everyday Discourse. Everyday discourse is the most frequent and familiar type of conversational form. Most people engage in everyday conversations without thinking about the rules and conventions underlying their utterances or those of their conversation partners. Even though it is the most familiar conversational form, everyday discourse is characterized by a variety of features that, if omitted or altered, significantly influence the understandability of a conversation. The primary characteristics of everyday conversations are the following:

1. Informal language and conversational style are familiar to participants (e.g., "Hey, how's it going?" "What's up?" or "Wow, it was an awesome experience, you know?").

2. Participants share assumptions about experiences and knowledge upon which language content and context are based; therefore, there is no need to use language to provide background.

3. Meaning is available in the immediate, nonverbal context; therefore, there is no need for participants to explain terms or to use descriptors extensively to convey meaning.

4. Frequently, language use is specific to the immediate context. For example, "Hand it to me" or "Bring it here" is understood easily because the desired object can be seen by both the listener and the speaker.

5. Turn-taking is relatively equal among participants according to cultural conventions.

6. There are frequent, ongoing checks for at-the-moment understanding; that is, participants frequently ask for confirmation that their messages were understood. Often the speaker accomplishes this by asking the listener questions such as, "Do you understand?" or "Am I being clear?"
7. Topics of conversation are familiar to participants. There is no need for extensive use of language to convey meaning.
8. Typically, language structures are short and concise (e.g., "I want one" or "Is it there?").

Job-Related Discourse. Conversing in a job setting may be a relatively formal and unfamiliar process for a new employee who must learn the vocabulary, topics, and context that form the bases for conversation in the work setting. Usually, after becoming familiar with both the co-workers and the context within which conversations will occur, new employees can begin to engage in everyday conversations at work. And of course, there can be situations in a job setting in which information must be conveyed in a more formal style. The job itself may require the employee to use everyday discourse in combination with job-related discourse.

Everyday conversation may be the easiest type of discourse for the dysarthric talker because of the familiarity, informality, and characteristically short structures of everyday discourse. The clinician can make the patient aware that it is easier to converse with persons who share experiences and knowledge than with people who do not share the same background. It is well known that communication is more effective when the dysarthric speaker's message can be anticipated by the listener, regardless of how the message is produced. The clinician can inform the patient that successful communication is largely dependent upon how well the listener anticipates the message, which, in turn, depends upon how much the listener knows about the dysarthric individual. The patient should be made aware that making the message redundant or providing background information can also improve communication.

Dysarthric speakers who are planning to return to their previous work will likely have already made the transition into everyday discourse in their job settings. For these speakers, job-related discourse will probably be as familiar as everyday discourse. The dysarthric patient who must enter a new job situation, however, will be confronted with a new set of conversational requirements. Prior to starting the new job, the clinician can help the patient to learn and practice the job-related discourse in order to prepare for communicating in the new setting.

Determining Familiarity. The dysarthria clinician can assist the patient in assessing familiarity with partners, topics, and contexts. Being able to determine familiarity will aid the dysarthric speaker in predicting correctly whether or not participation in a conversation will be successful. Dysarthric patients who have learned to judge familiarity can then concentrate on tailoring the length and complexity of the linguistic structures to the listener. In situations in which it appears that speech will not be adequate for effective communication, patients can inform their conversation partners that they will be gesturing, writing, typing, drawing, using an augmentative communication device, or communicating in whatever ways are most effective. Attending to the top-down characteristics of the discourse type in progress may enable the patients to avoid the frustration that can accompany unsuccessful communication attempts. Dysarthric patients who are able to prevent frustration or failure while engaging in conversation have a level of control over the communicative interchange that they would not have if they were unaware of how discourse functions. This is especially important because patients who are able to exert some control in their communicative interactions can reduce much of the anxiety and stress that occurs when dysarthria interferes with the ability to produce understandable speech.

From the listener's standpoint, increased familiarity with a dysarthric speaker and his or her speech may enhance understanding of less intelligible speech. In fact, Tjaden and Liss (1995a, 1995b) found that listeners understood more of a dysarthric speaker's sentence information when they were provided with a specific familiarization procedure before hearing the dysarthric speech. On the other hand, Yorkston and Beukelman (1983) and Garcia and Cannito (1996a) reported no appreciable benefit of listener familiarization. However, in these studies, the listeners were young adults; many were college students who did not know the speaker and were unfamiliar with dysarthric speech, in general. Possibly, the results of the studies would have been different if the communication partners were familiar with the speaker and the dysarthric speech, or if the listeners shared background knowledge with the dysarthric speaker.

Case Study

The following case study illustrates how a top-down approach to dysarthria therapy was used.

 TOP-DOWN APPROACH TO DYSARTHRIA

D.M., a 40-year-old bilingual Spanish–English-speaking male, was admitted to a rehabilitation hospital. Eleven years prior to his admission, he had sustained a gunshot wound to the right temporal-parietal lobe and subsequently had undergone a complicated course that included hematoma evacuation, tracheostomy placement, and multiple episodes of seizures.

D.M. was unemployed. For approximately 10 of his posttrauma years, he had lived in a long-term care facility. Cranial nerve deficits included a mild central VIIth. His gait was ataxic, and he had a left hemiparesis. Oral mechanism exam revealed facial flaccidity, absent gag reflex, severe lip weakness with reduced range and mobility, reduced speed and mobility of the tongue, and chronic tongue deviation to the right with the tongue tip lodged in the right cheek. He did not move his tongue on command.

The patient's speech was severely dysarthric. Disturbances in speech alternate motion rate (production and timing of the syllables /pa/, /ta/, and /ka/) were observed. Speech intelligibility in sentences was measured with the *Assessment of the Intelligibility of Dysarthric Speech* (Yorkston, Beukelman, & Traynor, 1984) and was judged to be an average of 0.9% (2 out of 220 words transcribed correctly by two judges). A disturbance in rhythm and stress was noted; often he produced two words as if they were one. For example, when repeating the sentence, "Tie my shoe," he said, "Tiemy shoe." When instructed to count to five, he said, "Onetwo, threefour, five."

D.M. was pleasant and cooperative. His comprehension of verbal instructions was good. Reading comprehension of single words was within normal limits; however, his writing was not intelligible enough for consistent, clear communication.

To improve D.M.'s overall communication, we introduced the alphabet board supplementation technique (Beukelman & Yorkston 1977), pacing with a metronome (Dworkin, Abkarian, & Johns, 1988), and a pacing board (Helm, 1979). None of these were effective. Nor was instructing him to mark on a page, one stroke per spoken syllable, or to swing his arm from side to side while producing a syllable or a word with each arm swing. We tried many techniques to improve his speech intelligibility, but the techniques we tried did not work. D.M.'s speech remained too unintelligible for effective communication.

D.M. could type using one finger of his right hand. He typed two-word sentences legibly enough to communicate a message effectively. He answered questions by indicating *yes* or *no* with appropriate head gestures, and often his verbalizations of "yeah" or "no" were interpretable. Occasionally, when asked a question and given a choice of two words, he produced a response that was understood.

With D.M's participation, we constructed a communication board consisting of printed words and symbols for communicating in everyday conversation. Among these words were "excuse me," "thank you," "nurse," "doctor," "more," "less," "A.M.," and "P.M." In order to expand his communication capabilities, we introduced drawing for communication (Lyon, 1995; Lyon & Helm-Estabrooks, 1987). Figure 4.2 is an example of how, by drawing, he communicated about his favorite spectator sport.

We asked D.M. what he knew about communication, and he typed, "Many ways." It was then that we decided to introduce components of a top-down approach.

We made suggestions about how D.M. could alert his listeners before beginning a conversation. D.M. was bilingual and communicated frequently in both English and Spanish. We suggested that D.M. inform his listeners about which language he would be using and that he could do this either by typing "English" or "Spanish," or by pointing to the appropriate word on his

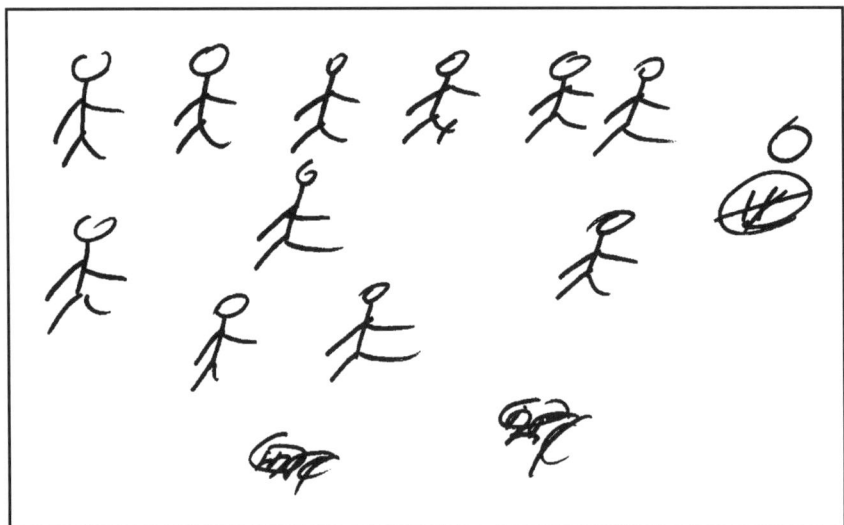

Figure 4.2. D.M.'s drawing to communicate his favorite spectator sport.

communication board. Also, we suggested that before beginning communication, he inform his communication partners whether he would be speaking, drawing, writing, using his communication board, or using a combination of methods. The words *drawing, speaking, writing, board,* and *all* were written on a card, and he practiced pointing to the appropriate words before beginning a conversation.

D.M. demonstrated how he could use gestures for alerting his conversation partners that he wanted a turn in the conversation. For example, he raised his left hand to indicate "stop" and, later, he snapped his fingers to get attention.

We suggested that he shorten his written messages, writing the name of an object or action rather than attempting sentences longer than two words. He found that with shorter messages, he was able to communicate more efficiently and effectively.

After 11 years of relative inactivity, D.M. was ready to return to work. Prior to his accident, he had worked in a tax preparation office, and he was interested in returning to similar work. After being introduced to the concept of job-related discourse, he spent some time reviewing the terminology he had used in his previous work setting and thinking about how he would communicate those terms most effectively if he worked in a tax office again.

Eventually, D.M. began to use an electronic pocket computer on which he typed short messages. During our first meeting after receiving the computer, he pointed to the display on which he typed, "I talk again." D.M. was motivated to communicate as effectively as possible, and he demonstrated that he could access a knowledge-driven, top-down approach to improve his communication. Although he remained severely dysarthric, and his speech may never be fully intelligible, his ability to communicate improved significantly as a result of his becoming aware of the characteristics of a top-down approach to treatment of his dysarthric speech.

Summary

In this chapter we have taken the position that for optimum communicative effectiveness, it is essential to make the dysarthric patient aware of how language is communicated. That is not to say that we are discounting the importance of a bottom-up approach to dysarthria therapy (i.e., instrumental procedures, palatal lift fitting, and additional behavioral therapies). Certainly we recognize that many techniques are basic to treating the dysarthric patient. However, we have observed that a top-down approach to treatment of dysarthric speech has therapeutic value and that it can provide the cognitive scaffolding for an effective communication experience for the dysarthric patient.

Furthermore, we believe that a combination of bottom-up and top-down processing is analogous to normal interactive processing in which top-down and bottom-up information sources interact in ongoing communication. Therefore, the combination of the top-down and bottom-up approaches should be used to improve communication for the dysarthric patient.

We recognize now, as we did previously (Vogel & Miller, 1991), that the success of the dysarthric patient's ability to use top-down information may be compromised as a result of aging, dementia, and left hemisphere (aphasia) or right hemisphere impairment. To the extent that dysarthria is complicated by these co-occurring deficits, top-down approaches may be contraindicated or may require specific types of modification for certain patients. Although research in this area is evolving, and results appear to be promising, at this time we can offer no absolutes for every dysarthric patient based on the results of systematic investigations. Nevertheless, we urge the dysarthria clinician to consider the top-down approach with patients who demonstrate that they understand the characteristics and can use the approach effectively.

Epilogue: A Preliminary Model of Interactive Processing

Garcia and Vogel have developed a preliminary Model of Interactive Processing (see Figure 4.3) illustrating the multiple factors that interact and contribute to communication as the sender (dysarthric speaker) relays a message to the receiver (listener). An explanation of this model follows.

The Model of Interactive Processing recognizes the distinctiveness of each speaker. Communication characteristics are unique to each person and can be shaped by numerous factors, such as multilingual and cultural influences. Additional influencing factors include the neurologic disease or condition underlying the speech impairment; age of the speaker; impairment in general motor control; and the co-occurrence of other communicative disorders such as aphasia, right hemisphere communication impairment, or dementia. The interaction of these factors contributes to an overall perception of severity that is

A Top-Down Approach 149

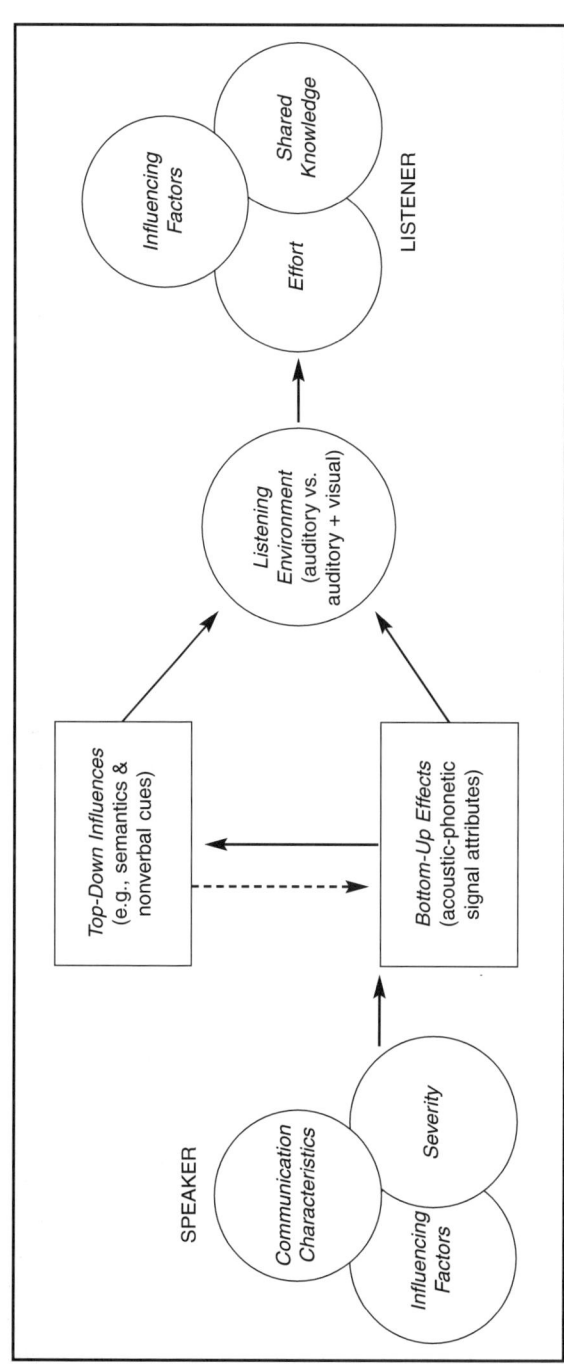

Figure 4.3. Model of Interactive Processing.

typically characterized in terms of the degree of intelligibility impairment and/or changes in the naturalness of speech. In typical interactions speakers communicate messages composed of both bottom-up effects and top-down influences. The bottom-up effects are the specific acoustic-phonetic attributes of the spoken signal. Top-down influences are multifaceted and include, for example, predictive semantic and syntactic content or nonverbal factors (e.g., facial affect; hand gestures). The model also recognizes that top-down influences and bottom-up effects often interact. In other words, top-down influences may indirectly cause speakers to modify their speech in a positive or negative manner. Signals are then communicated through different types of listening environments, which provide receivers with auditory or auditory plus visual information.

The Model of Interactive Processing also recognizes the importance of the listener. The two-way arrows indicate the active role of listeners in applying bottom-up and top-down processing strategies in different listening environments. In addition, the heterogeneity of listeners must be considered. Influencing factors might include variables such as the listener's age and preexisting communication concerns (e.g., hearing loss).

Finally, the model recognizes that shared knowledge and familiarity with the dysarthric speaker are important variables that contribute to communication proficiency. When speech is difficult to understand, listeners may be more prone to "give up" and quit listening, or to terminate the communication interaction as quickly as possible. As a consequence, each interaction depends on some degree of listening effort, especially for messages that are difficult to understand.

References

Barkmeier, J. (1988). *Intelligibility of dysarthric speakers: Audio-only and audio-visual presentations.* Unpublished thesis, University of Iowa, Iowa City.

Barkmeier, J., Jordan, L. S., Robin, D. A., & Schum, R. L. (1991). Inexperienced listener ratings of dysarthric speaker intelligibility and physical appearance. In C. Moore, K. M. Yorkston, & D. R. Beukelman (Eds.), *Dysarthria and apraxia of speech: Perspectives on management* (pp. 65–75). Baltimore: Brookes.

Berry, W. R., & Goshorn, E. L. (1983). Immediate and visual feedback in the treatment of dysarthria: A case study. In W. R. Berry (Ed.), *Clinical dysarthria* (pp. 253–266). Boston: College-Hill.

Beukelman, D. R., & Yorkston, K. M. (1977). A communication system for the severely dysarthric speaker with an intact language system. *Journal of Speech and Hearing Disorders, 42,* 265–270.

Binnie, C. A., Montgomery, A. A., & Jackson, P. L. (1974). Auditory and visual contributions to the perception of consonants. *Journal of Speech and Hearing Research, 17,* 619–630.

Carter, C. R., Yorkston, K. M., Strand, E. A., & Hammen, V. (1996). The effects of semantic and syntactic content on the actual and estimated sentence intelligibility of dysarthric speakers. In D. Robin, K. M. Yorkston, & D. R. Beukelman (Eds.), *Disorders of motor speech: Assessment, treatment and clinical characterization* (pp. 67–87). Baltimore: Brookes.

Crow, E., & Enderby, P. (1989). The effects of an alphabet chart on the speaking rate and intelligibility of speakers with dysarthria. In K. M. Yorkston & D. R. Beukelman (Eds.), *Recent advances in clinical dysarthria* (pp. 99–108). Boston: College-Hill.

Darley, F. L., Aronson, A. E., & Brown, J. R. (1969a). Clusters of deviant speech dimensions in the dysarthrias. *Journal of Speech and Hearing Research, 52,* 462–469.

Darley, F. L., Aronson, A. E., & Brown, J. R. (1969b). Differential diagnostic patterns of dysarthria. *Journal of Speech and Hearing Research, 52,* 346–369.

Darley, F. L., Aronson, A. E., & Brown, J. R. (1975). *Motor speech disorders.* Philadelphia: Saunders.

Dongilli, P., Jr. (1994). Semantic context and speech intelligibility. In J. Till, K. M. Yorkston, & D. R. Beukelman (Eds.), *Motor speech disorders: Advances in assessment and treatment* (pp. 175–191). Baltimore: Brookes.

Dromey, C., Ramig, L. O., & Johnson, A. B. (1995). Phonatory and articulatory changes associated with increased vocal intensity in Parkinson's disease: A case study. *Journal of Speech and Hearing Research, 38,* 751–764.

Duffy, J. R. (1995). *Motor speech disorders: Substrates, differential diagnosis, and management*. St. Louis: Mosby.

Dworkin, J. P., Abkarian, G. G., & Johns, D. F. (1988). Apraxia of speech: The effectiveness of a treatment regimen. *Journal of Speech and Hearing Disorders, 53*, 280–294.

Ekman, P., & Friesen, W. V. (1969). The repertoire of nonverbal behavior: Categories, origins, usage and coding. *Semiotica, 1*, 49–98.

Ekman, P., & Friesen, W. V. (1972). Hand movements. *Journal of Communication, 22*, 353–374.

Erber, N. P. (1975). Auditory-visual perception of speech. *Journal of Speech and Hearing Disorders, 40*, 481–492.

Garcia, J. M., & Cannito, M. P. (1994, November). *Attractiveness ratings of a dysarthric speaker: Influence of illustrative gestures*. Paper presented at the annual convention of the American Speech–Lanaguage Association, New Orleans.

Garcia, J. M., & Cannito, M. P. (1996a). Influence of verbal and nonverbal context on the sentence intelligibility of a dysarthric speaker. *Journal of Speech and Hearing Research, 39*, 750–760.

Garcia, J. M., & Cannito, M. P. (1996b). Top-down influences on the intelligibility of a dysarthric speaker: Addition of natural gestures and situational context. In D. Robin, K. Yorkston, & D. Beukelman (Eds.), *Disorders of motor speech: Assessment, treatment and clinical characterization* (pp. 89–103). Baltimore: Brookes.

Garcia, J. M., Cannito, M. P., & Dagenais, P. A. (2000). Hand gestures: Perspectives and preliminary implications for adults with acquired dysarthria. *American Journal of Speech–Language Pathology, 9*(2), 107–115.

Garcia, J. M., & Dagenais, P. A. (1998). Dysarthric sentence intelligibility: Contribution of iconic gestures and message predictiveness. *Journal of Speech–Language Hearing Research, 41*, 1282–1293.

Garcia, J. M., Dagenais, P., Terrell, P., & Mallory, A. (1992, November). *Normal and dysarthria speech intelligibility using audio versus videotaped presentation*. Poster session presented at the annual convention of the American Speech-Language-Hearing Association, San Antonio.

Hammen, V. L., Yorkston, K. M., & Dowden, P. (1991). Index of contextual intelligibility: Impact on semantic context in dysarthria. In C. Moore, K. Yorkston, & D. Beukelman (Eds.), *Dysarthria and apraxia of speech: Perspectives on management* (pp. 43–53). Baltimore: Brookes.

Helm, N. A. (1979). Management of palilalia with a pacing board. *Journal of Speech and Hearing Disorders, 44,* 350–353.

Hickson, M. L., & Stacks, D. W. (1993). *Nonverbal communication: Studies and applications* (3rd ed.). Dubuque, IA: William C. Brown.

Hoskins, B. (1987). *Conversations.* Allen, TX: Developmental Learning Materials.

Hubbard, D. J., & Kushner-Vogel, D. (1981). A comparison of speech intelligibility between esophageal and normal speakers via three modes of presentation. *Journal of Speech and Hearing Research, 23*(4), 909–916.

Kalikow, D. N., Stevens, K. N., & Elliott, L. L. (1977). Development of a test of speech intelligibility in noise using sentence materials with controlled word predictability. *Journal of the Acoustical Society of America, 61,* 1339–1351.

Lyon, J. G. (1995). Communicative drawing: An augmentative mode of interaction. *Aphasiology, 9,* 84–94.

Lyon, J. G., & Helm-Estabrooks, N. A. (1987). Drawing: Its communicative significance for expressively restricted aphasic adults. *Topics in Language Disorders, 8*(1), 61–71.

Massaro, D. W. (1987). *Speech perception by ear and eye: A paradigm for psychological inquiry.* Hillsdale, NJ: Erlbaum.

McNeill, D. (1985). So you think gestures are nonverbal? *Psychological Review, 92,* 350–371.

McNeill, D. (1992). *Hand and mind: What gestures reveal about thought.* Chicago: University of Chicago Press.

Miller, L. (1988, November). *Components of language processing: An intervention model for academic success.* Paper presented at the annual meeting of the American Speech-Language-Hearing Association, Boston.

Miller, L. (1992a). *What we call smart*. San Diego: Singular.

Miller, L. (1992b). *Your personal smart profile: A qualitative approach for describing yourself in your everyday life*. Austin, TX: Smart Alternatives.

Monsen, R. (1983). The oral speech intelligibility of hearing impaired talkers. *Journal of Speech and Hearing Disorders, 48*, 286–296.

Owens, R. E., Jr. (1988). *Language development: An introduction* (2nd ed.). Columbus, OH: Merrill.

Ramig, L. O. (1998). Speech and voice disorders in Parkinson disease and their treatment. In L. Cherney (Ed.), *Topics in geriatric rehabilitation*. Gaithersberg, MD: Aspen.

Ramig, L. (2000). Voice Treatment for Parkinson's disease. In J. Stemple (Ed.), *Voice therapy* (pp. 76–84). San Diego: Singular.

Ramig, L. O., Bonitati, C. M., Lemke, J. H., & Horii, Y. (1994). Voice treatment for patients with Parkinson disease: Development of an approach and preliminary efficacy data. *Journal of Medical Speech–Language Pathology, 2*(3), 191–210.

Ramig, L. O., Countryman, S., O'Brien, C., Hoehn, M., & Thompson, L. (1996). Intensive speech treatment for patients with Parkinson's disease: Short and long-term comparison of two techniques. *Neurology, 47*, 1496–1504.

Rosenbek, J., & LaPointe, L. L. (1985). The dysarthrias: Description, diagnosis and treatment. In D. F. Johns (Ed.), *Clinical management of neurogenic communicative Disorders* (pp. 97–152). Austin, TX: PRO-ED.

Scott, C. M. (1994). A discourse continuum for school-age students. In G. P. Wallach & K. G. Butler (Eds.), *Language learning disabilities in school-age children and adolescents*. New York: Merrill.

Sitler, R. W., Schiavetti, N., & Metz, D. E. (1983). Contextual effects in the measurement of hearing-impared speakers' intelligibility. *Journal of Speech and Hearing Research, 26*, 30–35.

Summerfield, Q. (1987). Some preliminaries to a comprehensive account of audio-visual speech perception. In B. Dodd & R. Campbell (Eds.), *Hearing by eye: The psychology of lip-reading* (pp. 3–51). Hillsdale, NJ: Erlbaum.

Tjaden, K., & Liss, J. M. (1995a). The influence of familiarity of judgments of treated speech. *American Journal of Speech–Language Pathology, 4,* 39–48.

Tjaden, K. K., & Liss, J. M. (1995b). The role of listener familiarity in the perception of dysarthric speech. *Clinical Linguistics and Phonetics, 9,* 139–154.

van Kleeck, A. (1984a). Assessment and intervention: Does "meta" matter? In G. P. Wallach & K. G. Butler (Eds.), *Language learning disabilities in school-age children* (pp. 179–199). Baltimore: Williams & Wilkins.

van Kleeck, A. (1984b). Metalinguistic skills: Cutting across spoken and written language and problem-solving abilities. In G. P. Wallach & K. G. Butler (Eds.), *Language learning disabilities in school-age children.* Baltimore: Williams & Wilkins.

van Kleeck, A. (1994). Metalinguistic development. In G. P. Wallach & K. G. Butler (Eds.), *Language learning disabilities in school-age children and adolescents.* New York: Merrill.

Vogel, D., & Miller, L. (1991). A top-down approach to treatment of dysarthria. In D. Vogel & M. P. Cannito (Eds.), *Treating disordered speech motor control: For clinicians by clinicians.* Austin, TX: PRO-ED.

Wallach, G. P., & Miller, L. (1988). *Language intervention and academic success.* Austin, TX: PRO-ED.

Westby, C. E. (1994). The effects of culture on genre, structure and style of oral and written texts. In G. P. Wallach & K. G. Butler (Eds.), *Language learning disabiities in school-age children and adolescents.* New York: Merrill.

Yorkston, K. M., & Beukelman, D. R. (1983). The influence of judge familiarization with the speaker on dysarthric speech intelligibility. In W. R. Berry (Ed.), *Clinical dysarthria* (pp. 155–163). San Diego: College-Hill.

Yorkston, K. M., Beukelman, D. R., & Bell, K. R. (1988). *Clinical management of dysarthric speakers.* Austin, TX: PRO-ED.

Yorkston, K. M., Beukelman, D. R., Strand, E. A., & Bell, K. R. (1999). *Management of motor speech disorders in children and adults* (2nd ed.). Austin, TX: PRO-ED.

Yorkston, K. M., Beukelman, D. R., & Traynor, C. D. (1984). *Assessment of intelligibility of dysarthric speech*. Austin, TX: PRO-ED.

Yorkston, K. M., Bombardier, C., & Hammen, V. L. (1994). Dysarthria from the viewpoint of individuals with dysarthria. In J. Till, K. M. Yorkston, & D. R. Beukelman (Eds.), *Motor speech disorders: Advances in assessment and treatment* (pp. 19–35). Baltimore: Brookes.

Yorkston, K. M., Dowden, P. A., & Beukelman, D. R. (1992). Intelligibility measurement as a tool in the clinical management of dysarthric speakers. In R. Kent (Ed.), *Intelligibility in speech disorders: Theory, measurement and management* (pp. 265–285). Philadelphia: John Benjamins.

Yorkston, K. M., Strand, E. A., & Kennedy, M. R. T. (1996). Comprehensibility of dysarthric speech: Implications for assessment and treatment planning. *American Journal of Speech–Language Pathology, 5*, 55–66.

Chapter 5

Dysarthria: A Breakdown in Interpersonal Communication

Rosemary Lubinski

Lubinski writes of dysarthria as a breakdown in the patient's social system focusing on the effect of the speech disorder on the patient, the family, and the clinician.

1. What are typical ways that dysarthric individuals react to and cope with their communication disorder?

2. How is the family of a dysarthric individual affected by the patient's communication disorder?

3. What is the role of the speech–language pathologist in meeting the psychosocial needs of individuals with dysarthria and the patients' family members?

4. What are reasons that a speech clinician may experience burnout when working with dysarthric patients?

5. What are some ways to enhance the physical and social environments of dysarthric patients that will have an impact on the patients' opportunities to communicate?

❋ ❋ ❋

Although the multifaceted nature of dysarthria has become better understood in recent years, more attention continues to be directed toward investigating respiratory, laryngeal, and supralaryngeal structures and functions than to the psychosocial impact of reduced intelligibility on dysarthric individuals, their families, and other caregivers. The speech rehabilitation literature generally espouses the philosophy that if only the individual could speak more clearly or communicate ideas with an assistive device, the individual's psychosocial needs would be automatically relieved. Approaches include some combination of managing the underlying pathology, symptom modification, or supplementation or substitution of an alternative/assistive communication system. This philosophy has innate appeal, but it neglects to understand the unique nature of each individual who has dysarthria and the complex physical and psychosocial environment that influences the thinking, feelings, and motivation of the individual. Furthermore, today's health care financing climate values explicit, operationally defined therapy outcomes and rapid intervention. There is little time to understand who the clients are and the scope of characteristics that they bring to the therapy endeavor.

This chapter focuses on dysarthria acquired in adulthood, which is usually associated with progressive neurological disease, trauma, or stroke. Specifically, the chapter explores dysarthria as a breakdown in the individual's social system and communication opportunities. It is divided into four main sections, all of which stress diagnostic and therapeutic implications for the speech–language pathologist providing service to dysarthric individuals and their significant others. The first two sections of the chapter focus on understanding the impact of dysarthria on the individual and the family. The third section describes the impact of institutionalization on the dysarthric person. The final section discusses the stress that the speech–language pathologist may incur when working with dysarthric individuals, particularly those with progressive, degenerative disorders.

Several themes are evident throughout the chapter. The first is that dysarthria should be considered from a broad psychosocial perspective if quality speech–language pathology services are to be meaningful to the individuals served. A second theme is that treatment effectiveness should be measured from at least two perspectives: the traditional assessment of intelligibility *and* improved quality of life for the individual and caregivers. A third theme is that more research is needed regarding the psychosocial impact of dysarthria. There is little research specific to this aspect of dysarthria management. Finally, an underlying theme throughout the chapter is that speech–language pathologists have an important role in identifying the psychosocial needs of their clients and providing appropriate intervention or referral. Keeping in mind the scope of practice and skills of the speech–language pathologists, these issues must not be ignored if quality communication service is to be provided.

Impact of Dysarthria on the Individual

The ability to communicate effectively is a skill that many adults take for granted. Although we, as adults, may desire a richer vocabulary or more sophisticated social communication skills, we assume that we will be able to produce the sounds of our language clearly and effortlessly. The mastery of our phonological system is a developmental skill accomplished early and relatively easily in our lives with little conscious attention to individual sounds or how these sounds are produced physiologically. It is not until an adult encounters a chronic illness, trauma, or stroke that affects the motor-speech system that he or she realizes how complex the mechanism is that produces sounds and how devastating the psychosocial effects of the impairment can be.

Phonology and Social Development

Although unintelligible speech may be tolerated in young children, mastery over the sound system is encouraged and, eventually, expected. The reciprocal nature of conversation is difficult until the young child's sound system at least minimally matches that of the linguistic environment. Before the match occurs, parents and other adults anticipate what the child may be trying to say; they guess, look for cues in the environment, say something encouraging, and, sometimes, give up trying to converse with the child. As the child's sound system matures and matches with the linguistic environment, more opportunities for social interaction and social role development arise, more stimulation is given, vocabulary and syntax develop, and the child gains communicative competence. Communicative opportunities and communicative competence become enmeshed. Although the cognitive and sensory abilities of the child are contributors to this competence, mastery over the sound system to an acceptable level is crucial for others to perceive the child as a viable communication partner.

The sound system becomes the building block for further communication skill learning and refinement throughout childhood and, indeed, throughout the life span. Adults are evaluated in work and social contexts on their ability to articulate sounds clearly. Fortunately, it is unusual for adults to experience difficulty with their phonological system; that is, failure in their ability to produce intelligible speech. Thus, when the phonological system becomes impaired, individuals may experience not only communicative distress, but also some degree of breakdown in their emotional well-being and social system. For adults, unintelligible speech may alter vocational opportunities and satisfaction, independence and decision making, socialization with family and friends, and the pursuit of interests. When such goals are thwarted, natural consequences include frustration, anger, and withdrawal.

Psychosocial Impact of Dysarthria

The literature reveals little research specific to the psychological, social, and emotional consequences of dysarthria. Thus, we must extrapolate such information from research regarding the impact of chronic illness, aphasia, and other long-term disabilities on the psychosocial functioning of adults. Although for these populations there are commonalties, we must appreciate their diversity in etiology and impact. Antonak and Livneh (1995) caution that reaction and adaptation to a disability associated with a chronic illness are likely to be different from reaction and adaptation to a disability with an etiology of sudden onset. They posit that the typical reactions to disability are shock, anxiety, denial, depression, internalized anger, externalized hostility, and acknowledgment. A person's final adjustment to a disability may take different constellations and phases. Thus, although some broad generalizations regarding the psychosocial consequences of dysarthria are possible, diversity and distinctiveness are more likely than homogeneity of symptoms.

The reaction to chronic illnesses by adults has received much research attention, some of it focusing on chronic neurological disorders, sensory disabilities, and disease-related health disabilities. Some studies have documented reactions from point of identification through the progression of the diseases, but a few describe the effects of various types of intervention. Caplan and Schecter (1987) stated that individuals with chronic illnesses may exhibit confusion, emotional numbing, depression, grief, anxiety, paranoia, and denial. Goodstein (1983) added such emotional feelings as fear surrounding loss of control, independence, and affection and fear of recurrence of illness or death itself. In addition, changes in cognitive functioning may impair judgment, critical thinking ability, and appropriate pragmatic skills.

Table 5.1 shows the large repertoire of possible reactions of individuals to sudden onset of communication problems associated with stroke and head trauma. Some of these are primary reactions, such as depression, but others are coping mechanisms in themselves, such as denial. What may be most important about this array is the sheer number

Table 5.1
Common Reactions to Stroke and Head Trauma

Anger

Anxiety

Catastrophic responses

Decreased sexual activity

Denial

Depression

Dysphoria

Emotional lability

Exaggeration

Fears

Frustration

Hopelessness

Hostility

Indifference

Irritability

Lack of initiative

Mania

Overprotectiveness

Paranoid reactions

Projection

Rationalization

Regression

Rejection

Withdrawal

and variety of reactions. Furthermore, what is not seen in such a listing is the timing, intensity, co-occurrence, and impact of the reactions on the individual or caregivers. Dysarthric individuals, as any persons with a disability, may display a wide range of coping styles and mechanisms. Henderson and Bryan (1984) stated that persons with disabilities are "more vulnerable to stress than persons without disabilities . . . and react more intensively" (p. 125). These authors described three major coping or defense mechanisms that are likely to be used by the disabled person: (a) deception, such as repression, projection, and displacement; (b) substitution devices, such as compensation and reaction formation; and (c) avoidance devices, including fantasy and regression. Safilios-Rothchild (1970) provided another source of discussion about the effects of disability by examining the sociology and social psychology of disability at the personality, societal, and cultural levels.

Furthermore, for those persons experiencing progressive disorders, uncertainties about increasing incapacity and fear of reduction in speech intelligibility complicate the emotional turmoil. These factors can contribute to gradual or precipitous withdrawal from social, occupational, leisure, and other activities. The patient may experience a sense of loss over behaviors that were once easily executed and taken for granted and are now irretrievable. Part of the fear may be attributable to the uncertainty of not knowing how and to what degree their communication will deteriorate. Progressive phonological incompetence, combined with other physical or psychological deterioration, can be devastating regardless of the individual's original level of motivation and positive self-esteem. The reader is advised to see Livneh and Antonak (1994) for a critical review of psychosocial reactions to disability in general and Wahrborg (1991) for a detailed description of psychosocial reactions to brain damage and aphasia.

As individuals with dysarthria lose their speech intelligibility, they become increasingly aware that society values communicative competence. Thus, previous social roles become difficult to maintain, and new social roles may be unattainable. The dysarthric person has become part of a minority group of disabled adults and may incur some or all the negative reactions and stereotyping ascribed to the disabled in our society. Sussman (1977) described these individuals with disabilities as "marginal." Certainly those adults who cannot express themselves clearly and easily are marginal members of our society inasmuch as they do not fit our society's definition of effective adult communicators.

When dysarthria occurs in a person age 65 years or older, the individual is placed in double jeopardy. This individual faces the negative attitudes directed toward the aged in addition to those directed toward individuals with disabilities. The older dysarthric person presents unique and, perhaps, even more difficult diagnostic and rehabilitative dilemmas because of this double handicap. The older dysarthric person is likely to have one or more chronic illnesses, is likely to be dependent on others for assistance in activities of daily living, and is likely to face a variety of personal and social changes or losses, including those that occur with retirement, death of a spouse, and relocation. Numerous other factors—such as ethnic background, gender, living environment, financial status, and easy access to desired communication partners—further affect how the older dysarthric individual will cope with changes in health, physical functioning, and communication ability.

Furthermore, communication partners may not know how to interact with a disabled adult, especially one with compromised speech intelligibility. Researchers have documented the negative attitudes toward the disabled stemming from such factors as ignorance of the problem, anxiety, fear of embarrassment, and stereotypes of individuals with disabilities (Dunn, 1987). These attitudes are reflected in the reduction of communication opportunity for the dysarthric individual. Dunn (1987) stated that individuals who are not handicapped do not know the "rules" for interacting with the person with a disability. This fact can be extended to the area of communication with the dysarthric individual who may have sustained both physical and communication disabilities. In fact, the dysarthric person may pose a dual threat for communication partners in that the possible presence of a visible physical disability coupled with the speech disorder may heighten communication anxiety and discourage interaction. Many dysarthric persons are physically disabled from stroke or progressive neurological disease and require assistance with ambulation and activities of daily living. The more visible and debilitating the disability, the less likely that others will want to encourage interaction. Conversation may be limited to obligatory topics and terminated as quickly as possible.

Communication partners may not have a repertoire of strategies to help decode unintelligible messages or to facilitate more intelligible speech. If the dysarthric person fails to speak clearly, the communication partner may feel helpless and may minimize communication contact to prevent further failure and frustration. Some communication partners may be uncomfortable guessing content or demonstrating their own paucity of communication-enhancing strategies. Responses may be limited to stereotypical phrases, such as "uh hum," "well," and "right."

Dysarthria as Stress

Dysarthria is a source of communication stress for the individual and for communication partners. *Stress* is defined as the "physical, mental or emotional reaction resulting from an individual's response to environmental tensions, conflicts and pressures" (Greenberg & Valletutti, 1980). Stress may occur during the actual, or even in the anticipated, interaction with the dysarthric individual. This stress may arise from the frustration created by an unsuccessful attempt at sending or receiving a message. It may stem from the conflict between wanting to express oneself successfully and the fear of failure to do so. Or it may originate from internal and societal expectations that articulatory proficiency equals communicative competence. Dysarthria—particularly severe dysarthria—by its very nature may create chronic stress that will be evident over long periods of time. For those dysarthric individuals with progressive disease, the awareness that the present level of intelligibility may be difficult to maintain is sure to add to the stress already perceived.

Other stresses related to aging and to the immediate health needs of the individual complicate the matrix. The individual with dysarthria may also assimilate stress indirectly from that experienced by family or caregivers. Finally, getting to the session and participating in speech therapy may be stressful for some individuals. Most adults are new to the clinical speech pathology setting, and they may perceive it as childlike, boring, tedious, frustrating, and never-ending.

The speech–language pathologist treating a dysarthric individual should consider the potential psychological, social, and emotional impact of the speech disorder. Traditionally, speech–language pathologists have focused on identifying the speech process components of the problem, designing remedial programs to improve the specific areas of the disorder, or recommending assistive communicative devices. It is not axiomatic that improving communication skills will result in an immediate resolution of the entire communication problem. Despite improved communication skills, dysarthric individuals may continue to perceive themselves as disabled and, subsequently, may withdraw from communication opportunities. It is difficult to shed a coat of disability once it has been worn. Further, improved skills may not result in perfect intelligibility, regardless of how much effort has been expended by the clinician and client. The individual with dysarthria may insist on obtaining an unrealistic goal of producing 100% intelligible speech. Or the individual may continue to react to other physical, mental, or health problems that do not improve. Communication partners may have withdrawn so much opportunity for interaction, that the social bonds that encourage communication are weakened. People cannot always renew relationships or activities where they left off months, or even years, ago.

Compliance to Therapy

Speech–language pathologists may wonder why some dysarthric clients are not highly motivated to improve speech intelligibility. The clinician may wonder why a person whose communication world is limited would not take advantage of every possible opportunity to learn how to speak clearly or to learn how to use an assistive device. They wonder why the punishment inherent in communication breakdown may seem to be more powerful than the positive reinforcement for communication that flows easily. Basically, the speech–language pathologist is asking, "Why doesn't every dysarthric individual follow my suggestions?" This is called *compliance* and has been an area of great interest in the medical arena for many years (Gerber & Nekemkis, 1986).

Dysarthric clients vary in the commitment to speech therapy despite its golden goals. Commitment is dependent upon a person's positive and negative experiences with a task and on the bond between these two factors (Lemkau, Bryant, & Brickman, 1982). Some individuals come to the therapy situation with a compliant, committed personal attitude. Others may be cautious of accepting help from a stranger. Some individuals expect the clinician to accept all the responsibility for improvement, but others enter the therapy situation convinced that nothing can be done to improve their speech. It is hoped that few are noncompliant because they do not understand the nature of the speech problem or the procedures being used to treat it. Previous positive and negative experiences with speech therapy can also affect commitment to therapy. Unfortunately, little is known about the nature of dysarthric individuals' commitment to speech therapy or the factors that contribute to an unsuccessful experience and noncompliance. Understanding these factors could lead to obtaining a stronger commitment from the dysarthric client to achieving therapy goals.

Thus, it becomes critical for the clinician to clearly explore treatment goals with the dysarthric patient. This includes addressing the patient's perceptions of therapy and what the patient perceives as important for effective carryover of speech intelligibility strategies or use of an assistive device to their everyday life. Further, this exploration needs to be repeated over time so that adjustments in goal setting and strategies can be made to affect optimum generalization. This process of discussion and mutual goal setting empowers dysarthric patients to assume more responsibility for how they will achieve better communication and should be aimed at attaining a strong commitment from the patient to achieve the treatment goals.

Probe Questions

The questions in Table 5.2 were designed to help the speech–language pathologist explore and understand the psychological, social, and emotional impact of dysarthria on the individual during the therapy process. The questions are probe questions that should be followed later with more in-depth queries appropriate for a given client. These questions were not designed for scoring or for comparing one client with another. These questions may be repeated during the course of therapy to examine changing perceptions and the impact of therapy on the individual and on significant others.

Exploring the Psychosocial Impact of Dysarthria: The Family

Although the stroke, trauma, or progressive neurological disease that results in the dysarthria is incurred by the individual, in actuality, it is the family that acquires the problem. The family equilibrium is disrupted in many ways. The reactions of the family are likely to change from the point of identification or occurrence—such as shortly after the initial diagnosis of Parkinson's disease or from the onset of the stroke—to when rehabilitation is initiated, transpires, or is terminated. Reactions of patient and family are also likely to differ if the course is acute but stabilized, as in stroke, versus if the underlying etiology is a

Table 5.2
Probe Questions for the Client

Definition of the Problem

1. What concerns you about your speech now?
2. What kinds of sounds or words give you the most difficulty?
3. What other areas of talking give you difficulty, such as loudness or rate?
4. In what situations do you feel you have the most difficulty talking?

Impact of the Problem

1. How do you feel when you have difficulty being understood?
2. How do others react when you have difficulty being understood?
3. Do you ever avoid a situation or a person because of your speech difficulty? If yes,
    a. What is this situation (person)?
    b. Why do you think this happens?
    c. How do you feel when this happens?
4. How has your speech problem affected your interaction with your family?
5. How has your speech problem affected your social life (e.g., employment, etc.)?
6. Do you think you have less opportunity to talk now than previously? If yes,
    a. Why?
    b. How can you change this?

Motivation to Improve

1. Why would you like to improve your speech?
2. What would you like to improve?
3. What have you done on your own to improve your speech?
4. What techniques do you find help you to talk better?
5. Have you attended speech therapy sessions before this? If so,
    a. Where were they held?
    b. What were your goals?
    c. What were the results?
    d. How did you feel about the progress you made?
6. How will your family work to help you improve your communication?
7. How will we know when speech therapy is successful?
8. What would you like my role to be in helping you communicate more effectively?
9. What other questions do you have about what we will do together in therapy?

progressive disease. Bray (1987) provided a schema for understanding the reaction of family members to chronic illness. He cautioned that families vary in their reactions to chronic illness and observed that numerous, often amorphous, factors complicate their feelings and behaviors. The typical course of reactions exhibited by families include fear, denial, bargaining, depression, mourning, and rapprochement.

Bray (1987) described *fear* as the first response of the family. Often, family members are shocked by the occurrence or identification of the chronic illness. They may coalesce into a unified group to fight the problem. This may be manifested through criticizing, as family members attack or unreasonably question care or rehabilitation efforts. Another natural response is to flee. Although few family members would outright deny care to a chronically ill person, some may more insidiously withdraw emotional support and interaction from the affected individual. Another fear is based on not understanding or misunderstanding the course of a chronic illness; family members may automatically assume the worst possible consequences. There is also an egocentric type of fear in which family members imagine that they will experience the same chronic illness sometime in the future.

Denial is a second response exhibited by some or all family members. Bray (1987) described this as a defensive posture. Initially, denial may help to cushion the impact of the disorder on the family, but, eventually, it will result in providing less than optimal care and rehabilitation possibilities (Power, 1985).

A third response is referred to as *bargaining*. Bray stated that some families attempt to trade their "compliance and oversolicitness" for the patient's recovery. Bargaining can be summed up as an "if we, then you" situation. Although family involvement, concern, and commitment are necessary factors in the meaningful rehabilitation of the dysarthric individual, no guarantees of outcome can be made. Speech identical to that produced before the stroke, trauma, or disease occurred is an unreasonable expectation in spite of the best efforts of the clinician, patient, and family.

Depression constitutes the fourth possible reaction by the family. Depression in family members may be manifested by a lack of affect, a sense of giving up, and a pervasive sadness that invades all aspects of their lives. The depression felt by the dysarthric individual or by the family members may spread to persons outside the family. A vicious cycle can occur—others may limit or cut off interaction opportunities with the dysarthric individual or the family, thus reducing the social interaction needed for achieving an environment free of depression.

Mourning is defined as the quiescent phase (Bray, 1987). During this stage the family begins to accept the actual disability and feels sorrow for the loss that has occurred—or in the case of progressive disease, for the loss that will occur eventually. This letting-go may result in withdrawal from the dysarthric individual, as a new family system is being created.

The final stage in reaction to chronic illness as described by Bray is *rapprochement*. This stage usually occurs after rehabilitation efforts have been completed. The family now establishes its new equilibrium, often with family members accepting new roles. During this stage, the chronically ill person either is being reintegrated into former roles, or a role commensurate with his or her abilities and desires. At this point, the chronically impaired person may become a marginal member of the family.

The family equilibrium also is broken at a more fundamental, personal level. Each time the dysarthric individual tries to communicate and experiences difficulty, the reciprocal nature of the communication is compromised. Like society at large, most family members lack experience in communicating with persons who have sustained a speech or language impairment. They may exhibit the same negative attitudes that society holds toward the disabled, and in fact may be more intolerant, embarrassed, and frustrated than others outside the family unit as they attempt to interact with a person whose speech is difficult to understand. Family members may let down their social guard and exhibit their frustration in more open—if not hostile—ways than do persons outside the family, particularly in the confines of the home. Some family members may be overly solicitous and anticipate what the dysarthric individual may want to say, thereby denying the dysarthric person the opportunities to use his or her residual or improving speech and language skills. Other family members may place an unrealistic burden for improvement on the dysarthric speaker. Still others may believe that if only the clinician and patient work hard enough, "normal" speech will be recovered. Finally, some family members may fluctuate in their reactions to the dysarthric person. At times they may be sensitive, encouraging communicators, but at other times, they may provide few opportunities for any interaction at all.

Thus, the family is a complex factor in the life of the dysarthric individual and, hence, in the rehabilitation process. Nevertheless, speech–language clinicians should consider Luterman's (1984) advice to "come to realize that the people we deal with are part of a system and that we cannot treat one element [the person with the communication disorder] without some attention to the entire system [the family]" (p. 160).

Family as a System

The concept that a family is a system has become well accepted in the family theory, counseling, and speech–language pathology areas (e.g., Evans et al. 1991; Lubinski, 1994; Maitz, 1991). The components of the system include individual, marital dyads, parental relationships, sibling relationships, and relationships with other significant family members. Jones (1988) states that the family can be viewed as an interdependent, interacting system of roles in a state of dynamic equilibrium. Family roles are developed through verbal and nonverbal communication over time. Each member of the family brings individual characteristics, expectations, resources, and limitations to any family situation. Individuals and the family, itself, influence each other and in turn are influenced by societal rules and expectations. Thus, the family cannot be understood without any of its parts, yet the parts individually do not constitute the family. It is the interaction of family members and their evolution over time that creates a system.

Therefore, it can be seen that when a family member becomes dysarthric, there is an impact on the family system. Initially, the underlying condition of stroke, trauma, or progressive neurological disease creates a crisis for the individual and the family. Eventually, the resulting dysarthria produces chronic stress for the family system. Hill (1949) proposed a model for understanding family systems under stress and called this paradigm the ABCX model. The A variable constitutes the stressor event and the demands placed on the family system. The B variable describes the resources brought to the stressful situation by the individual family members. The family's definition of the problem is the C variable. The interaction of the A, B, and C variables creates the X variable, or the actual crisis.

This model has been expanded upon by McCubbin, Boss, Wilson, and Lester (1980) in the double ABCX model. The revised model, shown in Figure 5.1, provides a way of understanding how a family reacts to multiple stressors, over a period of time, and not just at the time of the crisis.

The primary crisis, the onset of stroke, trauma, or the identification of a progressive neurological disease is not static in time within the family. The family comes to the crisis with other demands on it (A variable). For example, there may be a variety of preexisting demands on the family prior to the event that resulted in dysarthria. These demands may include social, occupational, and financial problems within the family, itself, or between family members and individuals or groups outside the family. These demands do not disappear when the individual becomes dysarthric. The family with previous financial concerns may find that problem exacerbated and contributing to the present crises. A history of alcoholism or family estrangement or abuse will affect the present crisis. Thus, clinicians working with dysarthric individuals and their families

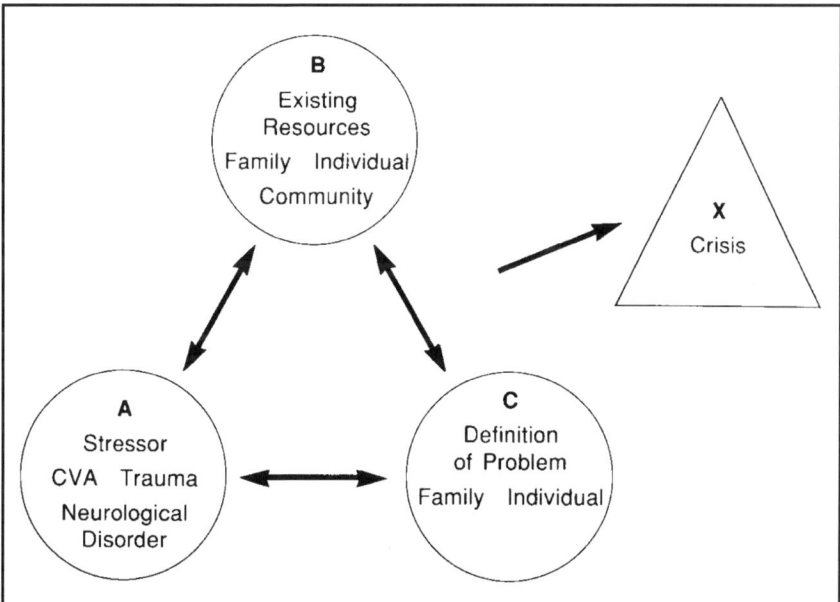

Figure 5.1. ABCX model of family stress. Adapted from "Generic Features of Families Under Stress," by R. Hill, 1949, *Social Casework, 49*, pp. 139–150, and "Family Stress Process: A Double ABC Model of Adjustment and Adoptation," by H. McCubbin and J. Patterson, 1983. In H. McCubbin, J. Patterson, and M. Sussman (Eds.), *Advancements and Developments in Family Stress Theory and Research*, New York: Hayworth Press.

must explore the demands on the family that existed before the individual became dysarthric and that potentially affect the present condition.

The family brings not only a history of other small and large demands but also a resource infrastructure (B variable) that has helped the family members to cope with previous stresses and problems. Some families have positive, functional styles that help them cope well with both everyday and major problems. Friedman (1986) stated that a family most likely to use its resources is one that has a broad repertoire of resources. Similarly, Imber-Black (1986) described families as perceptual problem-solving mechanisms. Families may not even be aware of the resources or strengths they are bringing to the problem situation.

Several researchers have described the resources and support that families may bring to any problem (e.g., Berkman, Oxman, & Seman, 1992; Imber-Black, 1986; Watkins, 1991). One set includes religious, cultural, and racial identity. These have helped to shape the family in particular ways over a long period of time. A second source of strength is the family's "inner language." Family members have special and idiosyncratic ways of communicating with each other that help to define them as a family. A third source of strength includes individual and family commitment, loyalties, and sense of connection. Individuals within a family, and the family as a whole, may be dedicated to its members and the survival of the family system in different ways.

The family's capacity to interact with the outside world also may be an important resource for the family. This determines how individual family members and the family as a whole interface with groups or systems outside themselves. Some families are inner-directed in that they seldom, if ever, seek assistance from anyone outside the family. This type of family is seen as a free-standing entity capable of providing its own assistance. Other families, in contrast, are open; they seek outside stimulation and assistance as needed. Probably, many families fall somewhere on this continuum between the closed, self-sufficient family and the open, society-integrating family. A family that hesitates to interface with groups outside its own boundaries may be more hesitant to accept rehabilitative and counseling efforts than a family that interacts easily outside its own unit.

Socioeconomic and educational status and access to medical and rehabilitation facilities serve as resources for families. Some families are inherently more knowledgeable about service availability and funding and are more aggressive in attaining them. However, Waaland and

Raines (1991) stated that "far too often, families find service lacking and expend their limited time advocating for appropriate services" (p. 25).

The family's adaptability may be added to this list of resources. Baird and Doherty (1986) defined *adaptability* as "flexibility in responding to demands imposed by stressors" (p. 371). A crucial element in a family's adaptability is its ability to shift family roles easily. The family's natural response to the crisis facing it is to maintain relative homeostasis; therefore, individual family members may need to assume different roles even though this may add extra demands.

Cohesion is a strength that a family may bring to a problem situation. Similar to Imber-Black's concept of commitment, loyalty, and sense of connection and inner language, cohesion emanates from the family's "tightly woven communication" (Baird & Doherty, 1986, p. 372). Cohesive families have clear roles, exhibit open communication, and provide support when it is needed.

Resources may also stem from outside the family. Informal family support systems include the extended family, friends, and community and religious groups. Social agencies and self-help groups offer support outside the familiar family system. As stated previously, some families may be more open than others to using the resources generated by these groups.

How families define an actual stressor is the third variable in Hill's ABCX model. Individuals may perceive the dysarthria-causing event and the resulting speech disorder in different ways. The definition of stress partly emanates from our societal definition of what is identified as a problem. It also originates from the perception of the individual. Such factors as the suddenness of onset, the degree of severity, the time it takes to adjust to the changes brought about by the problem, and the potential for solving of the problem all contribute to the individual's definition of the problem (Jones, 1988). One family member may view the dysarthria as an inevitable problem associated with advancing age, another may see it as a problem during each interaction, and still another may perceive it as remedial with time and therapy.

Speech–language pathologists need to explore how both family members and the dysarthric individual describe and view the problem. This exploration must take place over time, because the definition of the problem may change as the dysarthric person becomes more intelligible or family members gain more experience in communicating with the dysarthric person. Further, perception of the problem may change as other physical and emotional problems evolve. For example, the communication problem may be of secondary importance until the patient becomes more independent in ambulation. Finally, perception may be dependent upon the context within which the individual is communicating. What may be considered intelligible speech on a one-to-one basis in the home with a familiar family member may be perceived as unintelligible speech by unfamiliar caregivers in a nursing home setting.

Probe Questions for Family Members

The set of questions in Table 5.3 is based on Hill's ABCX model. The first set of questions explores the demands created by the dysarthria, the second searches for possible resources the family may bring to the situation, and the third focuses on how the family defines the problem. A combination of all three components should indicate the stress the family may be experiencing and consequently the loci of counseling needs.

Institutionalization of the Dysarthric Individual

The decision to institutionalize a family member is a difficult one. Contrary to the belief of some, most persons are not callously dumped in this setting (Committee on Aging, 1974). Often, the decision comes after a crisis or a burdensome, unsuccessful period of attempting to care for the individual at home. An older spouse may not be able to meet the physical needs of a neurologically impaired wife or husband. Some dysarthric individuals may need maximum assistance with activities of daily living that an older, perhaps frail, spouse cannot provide. There may be no spouse or family member to care for the dysarthric person at home. In-home services may be too expensive, too intrusive, or not easily and consistently available.

In other cases, the lifestyle of adult children may preclude providing full-time care for a parent. Adult daughters tend to be the primary caregivers for their parents, and their move into the workforce complicates the issue (Bernard & Thompson, 1970). Usually, the person who resides in a nursing home cannot live independently and needs maximum assistance in daily living (Rauth, 1968). How the loss of speech intelligibility contributes to the decision to institutionalize a dysarthric person is an unknown factor.

Table 5.3
Probe Questions for Family Members*

Demands

1. What significant events were occurring in your family prior to the onset of your (dad's, mom's, husband's, wife's, etc.) chronic illness or communication difficulties?
2. How have these events changed since the onset of the physical and communication problems?
3. Who has primary care or responsibility for your (dad's, etc.) physical needs?
4. How does this care affect (you, him, her, them)?
5. How has the chronic illness or communication difficulty affected your (dad's, etc.) social life?
6. How has the chronic illness or communication difficulty affected your/the primary caregiver's (your mom's, etc.) social life?
7. What physical stress or strains do you/the primary caregiver (your dad, etc.) have because of the physical problem?
8. What financial problems is your family incurring related to the physical or communication problem?
9. How has your/the primary caregiver's (your mom's, etc.) daily life changed since the onset of the problem?
10. What physical or psychological changes have you noted in you/the primary caregiver (your dad, etc.) since the inception of the problem?
11. How did the family change immediately after the onset of the problem? How has it changed over time?

Resources

1. How would you describe your family's strengths?
2. How has your family solved difficult problems in the past?
3. How willing is your (dad, etc.) to seek help from friends? counselors? religious institutions? social services? others?
4. During difficult times, is your family likely to call a family conference and discuss problems? Who is likely to be the leader or take-charge person in these situations?
5. Who will be the primary communication partners of your (mom, etc.)? Will this individual be available to come to therapy sessions on occasion?

Definition of the Problem

1. What do you perceive as the major problem facing your family at the present time?
2. Why is this problem so critical?

(continues)

Table 5.3 *Continued.*

Definition of the Problem *(continued)*

3. What do you think can be done about this problem?
4. Should the communication problem not be mentioned, then ask the following: How does your (mom's, etc.) communication problem compare to the problem you just mentioned?
5. Do other members of your family perceive your (dad's, etc.) problems in the same way as you do? If not, how are their views different?

*It is suggested that the interviewer use appropriate names or relationship markers rather than the generic terms, such as resident, client, or family members. For example, use "Mrs. Smith" or "your mother."

There are over 16,000 nursing homes in the United States serving 1.7 million elderly and chronically ill individuals (U.S. Department of Commerce, 1992). Although it is usually estimated that only about 5% of the elderly are institutionalized (Kastenbaum and Candy, 1973), many more will spend some time in a long-term care setting. In general, the nursing home resident population consists of very old, white females. The average nursing home resident is 82 years old, has at least four chronic disabilities, and will reside there at least one year. Most of these individuals will die in this setting. The number of individuals with dysarthria in nursing homes is not well documented but is likely to be significant inasmuch as dysarthria is associated with aphasia following stroke, progressive neurological diseases, head trauma, and can be evident during late-stage dementia (e.g., Bayles & Kaszniak, 1987; Cambell-Taylor, 1995; Hudson, 1981; Square & Martin, 1994).

Effects of Institutionalization

Any individual who enters a nursing home undergoes a drastic change in lifestyle. The individual must adhere to a regimented lifestyle in which there are few opportunities for self-determination and choice. Goffman (1961) and Bennett (1963) described this all-encompassing nature of institutional totality. In most nursing homes, the physical environment is designed for the efficient functioning of the staff in the provision of long-term custodial care. The staff of the facility controls or manages the daily life and possessions of the residents. The social environment is limited, particularly in the number and type of social roles the individual may assume. The primary social role for the individual with dysarthria is that of resident—one who receives care. There may be little regard for the person's privacy and personal possessions.

Many residents react to this drastic change in independence and lifestyle with feelings of fear, hostility, rejection, despair, loss, anxiety, dependency, and isolation (e.g., Ainsworth, 1977; Kahana, 1973; Lieberman, 1969). Some react negatively to their caregivers and become verbally and physically abusive; others withdraw from available social activities and passively receive care; still others attempt to instill guilt in family members who come to visit. Other individuals accept institutional life and interact positively with other residents, staff, and family. These individuals demonstrate exceptional adaptability. In general, most people will become accustomed to institutional life, though few regard it as a desired living experience.

Communication-Impaired Environment

Nursing homes have been described by Lubinski (1981, 1988, 1994, 1995) as an example of a communication-impaired or communication-deprived environment. This concept adds another dimension to Goffman and Bennett's definition of institutional totality. Table 5.4 lists 10 characteristics of a communication-impaired environment. These characteristics serve to limit the communication opportunities and how individuals perceive themselves as meaningful contributors to the life occurring in that setting. These characteristics must be weighed carefully considering the fact that, as a group, elders in nursing homes desire to communicate and feel that it is important to their well-being to do so (Lubinski, Morrison, & Rigrodski, 1981). It should be noted that although this concept is applied primarily to institutional life, community-based living arrangements may also restrict communication opportunities.

In addition to the restrictive physical and psychosocial environment of the nursing home setting, the residents themselves contribute to the impoverished communication atmosphere of long-term care settings. Residents make little effort to get to know each other, perceive others as incapable of communication, and are highly selective about whom they choose as communication partners. In an interview study of

Table 5.4
Characteristics of a Communication-Impaired Environment

In a communication-impaired environment you will find some combination of:
1. A lack of sensitivity to the value of interpersonal communication as the cornerstone of effective functioning and self-realization.
2. Restrictive rules that inhibit where, when, why, and to whom communication can occur.
3. A lack of desired communication partners of choice.
4. Few reasons to talk that emanate from internal needs or activities of choice.
5. Individuals who perceive that their communication contributes little to the environment.
6. A lack of places where private, personal conversations might occur.
7. Limited accessibility to activities and communication partners of choice.
8. A sensory confusing and limiting environment.
9. A lack of stimulating socialization opportunities.
10. A nonsupportive environment for caregivers.

communication in a nursing home, elderly residents stated that they did not talk to "communication-impaired" residents because they perceived such residents as being incapable of communication (Lubinski et al., 1981). It is not known how amenable nursing home residents are to communicating specifically with other residents who have dysarthria, either those who are difficult to understand or those who use an assistive communication device. It can be hypothesized, however, that the dysarthric individual, along with other severely communicatively impaired persons, is likely to be rejected as a communication partner. This, in turn, places more burden on staff and family to be available as communication partners for dysarthric individuals in long-term care settings.

Unfortunately, nursing home staff know little about communicating with elders in general, or those with dysarthria, in particular. Koury and Lubinski (1991) found that nursing assistants had limited knowledge of the communication problems of the elderly and could generate few strategies for communicating with communicatively impaired older persons. Thus, when confronted with an individual with reduced speech intelligibility, nursing assistants are likely to lack the skills for facilitating communication. As a result, they may avoid interaction with the dysarthric person. Therefore, in this setting, communication becomes a by-product of daily life rather than a priority of care.

Positive Communication Environment

Despite the bleak portrayal of nursing home life, improvements can be made that will result in a better quality of life for the residents and in greater job satisfaction for staff members. Major improvements would entail a drastic conceptual change in the design and management of nursing homes, as well as in the everyday interaction that occurs there. Ideally, nursing homes would mirror independent life in the community as nearly as possible. Maxwell Jones (1976) described this ideal institutional setting as a "therapeutic community." In a therapeutic milieu, residents and staff work cooperatively and share responsibility for daily life. Social interaction between residents and staff, and among the residents themselves, is viewed as the means of promoting self-actualization and self-determination. This concept emanates from the principle that people, even the institutionalized elderly, can and should be active participants in their own care and not simply passive respondents. Excellent reviews of the concept of the therapeutic community are contained in Rosenstock, Goldman, and Rothenberg (1969); Rossi and Filstead (1973); and Gottesman (1973).

Full implementation of a therapeutic milieu in all nursing homes may be unrealistic. Although there is increased governmental pressure to improve nursing homes, much of the emphasis is on factors such as cleanliness, dietary considerations, nursing care, and availability of rehabilitation and leisure activities. Although these are important aspects of nursing home life, they do not address the socialization that occurs between the residents and staff and among the residents themselves. Opportunities for choice and self-actualization are amorphous and difficult to evaluate. Thus, usually, nursing homes are not evaluated on the amount of socialization that occurs or on the quality of the communication that exists.

Staff, families, and residents may be unaware of what quality life in a nursing home entails. During the institutionalization process, families are likely to focus on the apparent cleanliness and nursing care in the setting. Staff accustomed to the usual scheme of interaction in the nursing home are likely to maintain the status quo. Residents are even less likely to make major changes. So much time in the nursing home is spent on meeting the physical demands of the residents and documenting caregiving that the cycle of dehumanization and depersonalization becomes entrenched and is considered the norm for that setting.

The communication disorders specialist can become involved in creating a more positive communication environment in nursing homes. This should benefit all residents, but especially those with communication difficulties such as dysarthria.

A positive communication environment is one in which residents and staff have maximum opportunity to interact with each other in a variety of meaningful activities. It is based on the following premises: (a) elderly and chronically ill residents want to talk and feel that it is important to their well-being to communicate; (b) staff are the primary communication partners of the residents and thus play a crucial role in the residents' communication life; (c) it is possible to change the physical environment to make it more conducive to communication; and (d) people need to be able to engage in activities that foster communication and to be allowed access to their choice of communication partners in order for optimum communication to occur.

The first step in creating this positive communication environment is to help administrators and staff understand the vital importance of communication to the daily lives and functioning of their residents. Communication should be as high a priority of care as a clean environment and adequate nursing. Staff, in particular the nursing assistants, should receive in-service training focusing on skills for initiating and facilitating conversations with residents and emphasizing their important role in communicating with residents (Koury & Lubinski, 1991). Nursing assistants need to know how assistive devices work and how valuable these devices can be to dysarthric residents. Also, they need to know how to manage the physical environment to promote visual and auditory aspects of communication. Finally, and most important, they need to become sensitive to their role in communicating with residents. Many staff persons are not aware of how vital their role is in communicating with residents or how their own verbal and nonverbal communication is received and interpreted by residents. Communication occurs between people who perceive themselves as similar, who have similar interests, and who work interdependently. Chipping away at what Goffman (1961) calls the staff–inmate split could be one of the most valuable ways to enhance communication in the nursing home environment.

Communication disorders specialists can work with the staff to identify the physical aspects of the environment that can be made more conducive to communication. Proper management of lighting and sound control can be incorporated easily by most nursing homes.

For example, adding lights in areas where conversations occur facilitates interaction as does attenuating the volume on a television set so that the residents can hear one another. Also, providing physical access to social activities in the institution can stimulate communication. Speech–language pathologists should work with activity directors in nursing homes to aid them in designing programs that are both meaningful and stimulating to the age and physical abilities of the residents. For further information, the reader is referred to Lubinski (1981, 1988, 1991, 1995) who, in a series of articles and book chapters, has outlined the concept of a positive communication environment, as well as identification and intervention strategies.

Stress of Dysarthria Therapy

The major focus of this chapter thus far has been on the impact of dysarthria on the individual and the significant others in the dysarthric person's environment. There is an additional person to be considered: the speech–language pathologist. The thrust of dysarthria therapy is to help the individual regain as much communicative competence as possible. Therapy, if successful, can result in the client's overall improved quality of life. When this is possible, both client and clinician feel successful. The joy of seeing a client communicate effectively can be an immense reward for the speech–language pathologist even if the client does not directly express his or her gratitude. Positive comments from family, caregivers, and other professionals can be added incentive for both client and clinician.

Progress in therapy with dysarthric clients is likely to be slow, limited, and prolonged. For those clients with degenerative diseases, the progressive loss of intelligibility, along with the loss of physical and mental abilities that can accompany the disease, may cause strain for client and clinician. Clients may expect progress even when it is not realistic, may reject assistive communicative devices, or may exert a less than optimum effort to use the communication skills that remain. The speech–language pathologist may be frustrated, if not angry, at a client's lack of compliance and minimal motivation. Further, families and significant others in the environment may pay little attention to therapy, reduce communicative opportunities for the dysarthric individual, and even sabotage therapy efforts in subtle ways. For example, placing a communication board out of the reach of a client may extinguish the client's motivation to use it.

Indeed, the help offered by the speech–language pathologist may be simultaneously intense, complicated, demanding, and tedious for the client. The speech–language pathologist who has a caseload of individuals who need this type of therapy may incur stress and, eventually, burnout.

It is only fairly recently that the profession of speech–language pathology has become aware that speech–language pathologists may react physically and emotionally to the work that they do. Miller and Potter (1982) and Potter and Rudensey (1984) were among the first to describe the personal impact of the speech–language pathologist's professional work. Miller and Potter found that 43% of speech–language pathologists were experiencing moderate to severe burnout. Although this work does not focus specifically on the speech–language pathologist working with the dysarthric client, many implications can be derived from the existing theories and empirical research on stress and the helping professions.

Helping Relationship

Speech–language therapy, in which one individual helps another to communicate, is one of the most intimate forms of helping relationships. The relationship between the client and clinician is a complex one. The clinician brings to the situation clinical knowledge, competence, and experience combined with a variety of important personal qualities. Numerous authors have delineated the following characteristics of a helping relationship: empathy, warmth, genuineness, concreteness, immediacy, self-understanding, and open communication (e.g., Murgatroyd, 1985; Rogers, 1951). The client, in turn, also brings certain factors to the relationship: a personal history, the communication handicap, the need and motivation to improve, other complicating physical and mental problems, and a social environment, which can be supportive or not. The client may be in the therapy situation by choice or because others have deemed it necessary. In addition, the client and clinician will form a working relationship over time, making their relationship dynamic, rather than static.

The helping relationship in dysarthria therapy focuses on assisting the individual to improve or maintain speaking abilities or to use compensatory strategies to communicate. Therapy also may focus on motivating the client and working with significant others to improve their strategies for communicating with the dysarthric individual. Thus, the helping relationship incorporates a series of decisions: judgments involving appropriate assessment methods, candidacy for therapy, therapeutic techniques, motivation, and counseling.

Stress

This process of dysarthria therapy may be a stressful one for the speech–language pathologist. Stress is a person's "physical, mental or emotional reaction to tension, conflict and pressure" (Greenberg & Valletutti, 1980, p. 2). The sources of stress may arise from the clinician's personal outlook, the client, significant others, and the work environment (Farmer, Monahan, & Hekeler, 1984). These factors are intertwined as they impact on the clinician.

The very nature of the helping relationship may be a source of stress for the clinician working with a dysarthric individual. Clinicians who are idealistic or perfectionistic may find this type of therapy stressful. Normal speech may not be attainable. Regression may occur. Therapy gains can evaporate even after months of success. Clinicians may expect the dysarthric client to maintain high levels of motivation and involvement in the therapy even though the client is facing multiple other problems. The clinician may experience role overload, wherein the clinician has too many tasks to perform, often without enough preparation time (Greenberg & Valletutti, 1980). Clinicians also bring to the therapy situation their own constellation of personal problems from other areas of their lives.

Stress may arise from the client or from significant others in the client's life. Clients may lack motivation, be noncompliant, fluctuate in their motivation and performance, become ill, and impose unrealistic expectations on the therapy process. Further, their own personal problems may hamper the helping process and indirectly cause stress for the clinician.

Stress can also stem from the work environment. Greenberg and Valletutti (1980) described such sources of stress as role ambiguity, role conflict, inequities in pay, and inadequate job status. Maslach (1982) added conflict between co-workers, poor relationships with supervisors, and even the goals of the work setting. The agency's definition of success in therapy may be contrary to how the clinician or client defines success. It may be very difficult for a clinician to continue therapy for a dysarthric client when third-party insurers expect rapid progress in functional communication. Although a client may need therapy to maintain existing skills, a large number of, if not most, governmental and private sources of therapy funding do not support maintenance therapy.

Burnout

The result of chronic stress incurred in a helping relationship is burnout. Maslach (1982) defined burnout as a "syndrome of emotional exhaustion, depersonalization and reduced personal accomplishment that occurs among individuals who do 'people work'" (p. 3). She states that burnout is a unique form of stress because it stems from the "social interaction between helper and recipient" (p. 3). Corey (1982) lists nine causes of helper burnout: repetition of therapy tasks, minimal reward for maximal expenditure of energy, unrealistic expectations, minimal evident progress, lack of collegial support, conflict between organization administration and clinician, few opportunities for independent decision making, few opportunities for self-improvement, and unresolved personal problems. A speech–language pathologist providing dysarthria therapy is likely to incur some, if not all, of these causes of burnout.

The results of burnout also are numerous. The effects of burnout include "physical depletion and chronic fatigue, feelings of hopelessness and helplessness, and development of a negative self-concept and negative attitudes toward work, life and other people" (Pines, 1982, p. 455). One of the most devastating effects of burnout is that the clinician stops caring about the client; provides only the most basic, nonchallenging therapy; and views the client and significant others in a cynical fashion. Eventually, the clinician internalizes a negative concept about the helping relationship and broadcasts this attitude to other clients, caregivers, and families.

Coping with Stress and Burnout

The first step in coping with stress and burnout is identification. A variety of tools are available for clinicians to use to help identify and measure their burnout, including those developed by Pines (1982) and Maslach and Jackson (1982). These tools stress identifying the sources of stress within the individual, the client–clinician relationship, and the work environment. They also focus on identification of stress effects and behaviors. For example, the physical effects of stress can include headaches, colds, gastrointestinal disorders, hypertension, and numerous other physical problems. Emotional stress effects can include feelings of hopelessness, frustration, powerlessness, and loneliness. Finally, the identification tools can help clinicians to delineate specific stress behaviors in their lives. These may include eating and sleeping disorders, withdrawing, engaging in medication and alcohol abuse, and other negative activities.

A number of positive actions can be taken to prevent or ameliorate stress and burnout among helping professionals. These include reducing the staff–client ratio, making client selection more flexible, changing job tasks, and taking time out (Pines, 1982). Maslach (1982) stated that a critical factor in helping to deal with burnout is the formal or informal support given by colleagues. She states that peers can provide help, insight, a basis for personal comparison, recognition, and a means of escape. Maslach added that colleagues can help ease the burden through positive humor. Other techniques that help reduce burnout include improving communication skills with colleagues, administrators, clients, and significant others.

Finally, for some clinicians a period of timeout will be crucial. This can be done through taking planned vacations, changing client types, and refocusing job tasks.

Some clinicians may be helped by assuming a new role within the organization, participating in a research project, or attending a professional workshop or continuing education course. See Farmer et al. (1984) for a number of suggested stress reducing techniques. Henderson and Bryan (1984) cautioned those in helping relationships to keep the client's problems in perspective, to encourage self-help, and to use humor to help clients over rough spots. Their final comment may be the most important one they make: "All helpers make mistakes when working with people with disabilities. They should learn from their mistakes and try not to repeat them" (p. 139).

Probe Questions for Speech–Language Pathologists

The questions in Table 5.5 can be used by speech–language pathologists to examine stress in their professional lives. This is not an exhaustive

Table 5.5
Probe Questions for Speech–Language Pathologists

Sources of Stress

1. What factors in my job do I find difficult?
2. How can I change these factors?
3. What kind and amount of personal and professional satisfaction do I receive from working with clients? families? other staff?
4. Are there opportunities for advancement?
5. What factors in my personal or family life are stressful?
6. Are my financial sources sufficient?
7. Is the institution I work in flexible and open to suggestions and change?

Effects of Stress

1. Does stress affect my physical well-being? How so? What are the symptoms?
2. Does stress affect my self-esteem and psychological well-being? How? What are the symptoms?
3. Does stress affect my everyday performance in therapy? diagnostics? family counseling? interactions with other staff? with my own family and friends?

Management of Stress

1. What do I do to cope with the causes and effects of stress?
2. Do I have a strong, meaningful support system? How do I use it?
3. Are there peers in my work environment with whom I can express my feelings?
4. Is professional help available to guide me through difficult stressful periods? Will I seek professional help and follow through with it?
5. Do I plan for time out? vacations? personal time? recreation? physical exercise?

---

diagnostic tool, but may help identify stress and, therefore, serve to initiate further self-evaluation or professional guidance.

Case Studies

The following case studies illustrate many of the concepts developed in this chapter. They will serve as the concluding remarks for the chapter. Although the names of the principals have been changed, the stories are true. The essence of these case studies is that the clients' needs are more complex than their dysarthria.

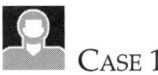 CASE 1

Colonel Dick Canter was a 58-year-old retired Army Reserve officer who suffered a stroke with resultant mild aphasia and moderately dysarthric speech. Although his language skills improved quickly to nearly normal status, his speech remained dysarthric. Divorced 10 years prior to sustaining the stroke, Dick had lived alone in Washington, D.C. Two adult daughters resided in Dick's hometown of Buffalo, New York, and one son lived in California. Over the years, Dick had maintained little contact with his children, communicating with them only occasionally.

Following the stroke, Trisha, Dick's oldest daughter, assumed power of attorney for her father's affairs and became the primary decision maker in his life. She closed his apartment, sold most of his furnishings, and entered her father in a nursing home near her home. While in the nursing home, Dick attended physical and speech therapy session, making excellent progress in physical therapy. His speech remained moderately dysarthric, however, and Trisha blamed that on the fact that her father had been a heavy drinker rather than on the fact that he had suffered a stroke (demands).

Speech therapy sessions held twice weekly focused on improving Dick's speech intelligibility in sentences and conversation, and emphasized self-monitoring of rate and articulatory clarity. During these sessions, Dick spoke of how unhappy he was living in the nursing home. He perceived himself as a youthful vigorous man in the company of a "bunch of old ladies." In reality, despite mild hypertension, he was physically fit and in good health. It was difficult for the speech clinician to focus treatment on improving speech intelligibility when Dick's primary concern (definition of the problem) was his need to live independently.

The social worker in the nursing home was sympathetic to Dick's situation but felt powerless to help him make changes in his living environment. Dick's daughter was intent upon keeping her father in the controlled setting of the nursing home. Even though Trisha agreed that her father might be motivated to improve his speech if he lived independently, she was afraid that if he left the nursing home he would begin to drink again. The speech clinician began to explore with Trisha the alternative living possibilities in the community, and it was during their discussions that Trisha revealed her long-held feelings about her father's drinking and his dominance over the family. At that time, Trisha herself had several problems unrelated to her father's situation; her life was complicated by a pending divorce, a chronically ill preschooler, and her own financial need to return to work (multiple demands on caregiver). For Trisha, it was easier to keep her father in the nursing home than to have him live elsewhere, regardless of his frustration and anger with that living arrangement (demands).

Eventually, Trisha agreed to move her father to a senior citizens' health-related facility. Although this facility was less restrictive than the nursing home, Dick continued to perceive himself as "living with a bunch of old ladies." Moreover, during his stay in the nursing home, he had established a personal relationship with a nurse there, and now he wanted a place where he could entertain her. During his weekly sessions with his speech clinician, he continued to focus on his need to live independently. His speech intelligibility improved somewhat, but he was preoccupied with changing his living environment, and that, rather than improvement of his speech, was his top priority. He told the clinician that in the setting in which he lived, there was "no one like me, no one with whom I can communicate and, therefore, no real need for me to improve my speech" (effects of institutionalization).

During the next year, the speech clinician maintained close contact with Trisha, gently encouraging her to consider allowing her father to live alone in an apartment for a trial period. Dick was highly motivated to try this. Finally, when 2 years had passed since Dick had sustained the stroke and he had had no alcohol during that time, Trisha agreed to look for a furnished apartment where her father could live for a 1-month trial period. She found a place, and this venture turned out to be successful. Eventually he moved to a small apartment close to shopping facilities and a bus line.

After he was settled in the apartment, Dick's motivation to improve his speech increased and therapy was resumed. At the present time, his speech, although not totally free of articulatory distortions, is very intelligible. He cares for all except his financial needs. Trisha continues to help in that area (resources). Shortly after moving to his present home, Dick flew to California to visit his son, whom he had not seen for several years. He reported that the visit resulted in a reunion with his son (resources).

There is no doubt that Dick used his speech clinician as a primary communication partner during the therapy process. This was difficult for the clinician, because improving speech intelligibility was a secondary rather than a primary goal for Dick, and this was evident in every therapy session (clinician stress).

The clinician questioned her own role in the therapeutic situation—a role that extended far beyond that of a speech clinician. It was obvious that Dick and his daughter were using the clinician to work through their own personal difficulties. The clinician was faced with several alternatives: to terminate the therapy, to refer the family to a counselor, to focus therapy on speech production only, or to help the family work through its problems while continuing to work on Dick's speech production. Because both Dick and his daughter refused to seek counseling outside of the speech therapy sessions, that was not a viable option. The clinician felt that the last alternative would be the most productive, and, considering the positive outcome, it is apparent that the clinician chose the correct alternative. In fact, Trisha stated that she had not believed that her father could live independently; it was the speech clinician's encouragement that convinced her to let him try.

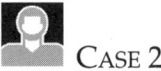 CASE 2

Helene Pierre is a 73-year-old woman who resides alone in a small apartment in an assisted living community in an area where three of her five children live. Two of her daughters visit several times per week (resources). The widow of a physician, she had been diagnosed with polio 43 years previously (demands). Although there was no dysarthria following the polio, for approximately 1 year, her speech intelligibility had begun to deteriorate as part of a postpolio syndrome (demands). Three months after hospitalization for a broken leg, followed by intensive physical therapy, a speech evaluation was suggested. Perceptual evaluation of Mrs. Pierre's speech revealed a slightly slower than normal rate, reduced prosody, and overarticulation of consonants. In general, her speech intelligibility was excellent, regardless of whether or not the context was known to the listener.

Mrs. Pierre, however, deliberately and drastically limited her communication with other residents and staff. She described herself as a woman used to managing a large home, family, and personal staff. She was used to participating in a number of civic activities and frequently had served as a hostess for social gatherings. Now she perceived that her speech was not understood by others, and she stated "I don't sound proper" (definition of the problem).

Mrs. Pierre's primary communication partners were the aides who helped her twice daily and her daughters who visited her once each week. She participated in none of the variety of programs available in her building and avoided participation in conversation at mealtimes with her tablemates. After a recent visit by a hometown friend, Mrs. Pierre described their conversations as "torturous and fatiguing" (demands).

In addition to breath control, phrasing, and self-monitoring, therapy focused on discussing communication opportunities with Mrs. Pierre. Part of each session was devoted to discussing the conversational demands of her existing and potential communication contexts, her views of how others perceived her speech, the communicative strengths she brought to each conversation, and how she evaluated her own speech (see Vogel, Miller, & Garcia, this volume, for further discussion of a top-down approach to treatment of dysarthria). Role-playing was the most effective technique employed to help Mrs. Pierre approach her communication opportunities more willingly. Scenarios focused on conversations with the aides, her daughters, and interactions with other residents. Alternating roles helped Mrs. Pierre to become aware of her speech patterns and to demonstrate her speech intelligibility. During the final therapy session, Mrs. Pierre stated, "I realize now that I really want to talk and that I need to talk as much as possible to maintain my present abilities and appreciate the life I have." Her comments demonstrated that, for her, there were two observable and functional outcomes of therapy—improvement in her speech intelligibility and her increased willingness to communicate.

References

Ainsworth, T. (1977). *Quality assurance in long-term care*. Germantown, MD: Aspen.

Antonak, R., & Livneh, H. (1995). Psychosocial adaptation to disability and its investigation among persons with multiple sclerosis. *Social Science Medicine, 40*, 1099–1108.

Baird, M., & Doherty, W. (1986). Family resources in coping with serious illness. In M. Karpel (Ed.), *Family resources: The hidden partner in family therapy* (pp. 359–383). New York: Guilford Press.

Bayles, K., & Kaszniak, A. (1987). *Communication and cognition in normal aging and dementia*. Boston: Little, Brown.

Bennett, R. (1963). The meaning of institutional life. *The Gerontologist, 3*, 117–124.

Berkman, L., Oxman, T., & Seman, T. (1992). In R. Wallace & R. Woolson (Eds.), *The epidemiologic study of the elderly* (pp. 196–212). New York: Oxford University Press.

Bernard, J., & Thompson, L. (1970). *Sociology of nurses and their patients in modern society*. St. Louis, MO: Mosby.

Bray, G. (1987). Family adaptation to chronic illness. In B. Caplan (Ed.), *Rehabilitation psychology desk reference* (pp. 171–184). Rockville, MD: Aspen.

Cambell-Taylor, I. (1995). Motor speech changes. In R. Lubinski (Ed.), *Dementia and communication* (pp. 70–83). San Diego: Singular.

Caplan, G., & Schecter, J. (1987). Denial and depression in disabling diseases. In B. Caplan (Ed.), *Rehabilitation psychology desk reference* (pp. 133–170). Rockville, MD: Aspen.

Committee on Aging. (1974). *Nursing home care in the U.S.: Failure in public policy*. Washington, DC: U.S. Government Printing Office.

Corey, G. (1982). *I never knew I had a chance*. Monterey, CA: Brooks, Cole.

Dunn, M. (1987). Social skills and rehabilitation. In B. Caplan (Ed.), *Rehabilitation psychology desk reference* (pp. 345–364). Rockville, MD: Aspen.

Evans, R., Bishop, D., Haselkorn, J., Hendricks, R., Baldwin, D., & Connis, R. (1991). From crisis to recovery: The family's role in stroke rehabilitation. *NeuroRehabilitation, 1,* 69–78.

Farmer, R., Monahan, L., & Hekeler, R. (1984). *Stress management for human services.* Beverly Hills, CA: Sage.

Friedman, E. (1986). Resources for healing and survival of families. In M. Karpel (Ed.), *Family resources: The hidden partner in family therapy* (pp. 65–92). New York: Guilford Press.

Gerber, K., & Nekemkis, A. (1986). *Compliance: The dilemma of the chronically ill.* New York: Springer.

Goffman, E. (1961). *Asylums.* Garden City, NY: Anchor Books.

Goodstein, R. (1983). Cerebrovascular accident and the hospitalized elderly: A multidimensional clinical problem {Overview}. *American Journal of Psychiatry, 140,* 141–147.

Gottesman, L. (1973). Milieu treatment of the aged in institutions. *The Gerontologist, 13,* 23–26.

Greenberg, S., & Valletutti, P. (1980). *Stress in the helping professions.* Baltimore: Brookes.

Henderson, G., & Bryan, W. (1984). *Psychosocial aspects of disability.* Springfield, IL: Thomas.

Hill, R. (1949). Generic features of families under stress. *Social Casework, 49,* 139–150.

Hudson, A. (1981). Amyotrophic lateral sclerosis associated with dementia, Parkinsonism, and other neurological disorders: A review. *Brain, 104,* 217–247.

Imber-Black, E. (1986). Toward a resource model in systematic family therapy. In M. Karpel (Ed.), *Family resources: The hidden partner in family therapy* (pp. 148–174). New York: Guilford Press.

Jones, K. (1988). *The impact of C.V.A. on the family system.* Unpublished doctoral dissertation, State University of New York at Buffalo, New York.

Jones, M. (1976). *Maturation of the therapeutic community.* New York: Human Sciences Press.

Kahana, E. (1973). The humane treatment of old people in institutions. *The Gerontologist*, 13, 282–289.

Kastenbaum, R., & Candy, S. (1973). The four percent fallacy: A methodological and empirical critique of extended care facility statistics. *International Journal of Aging and Human Development*, 4, 15–21.

Koury, L. N., & Lubinski, R. (1991). Effective in-service training of a staff working with communication-impaired patients. In R. Lubinski (Ed.), *Dementia and communication* (pp. 279–291). Hamilton, Ontario: B. C. Decker.

Lemkau, J., Bryant, F., & Brickman, P. (1982). Client commitment to the helping relationship. In T. Willis (Ed.), *Basic processes in helping relationships*. New York: Academic Press.

Lieberman, M. (1969). Institutionalization of the aged: Effects on behavior. *Journal of Gerontology*, 24, 330–339.

Livneh, H., & Antonak, R. (1994). Psychosocial reactions to disability: A review and critique of the literature. *Critical Reviews in Physical and Rehabilitation Medicine*, 6, 1–100.

Lubinski, R. (1981). Language and hearing programs in home health care and nursing homes. In D. Beasley & G. Davis (Eds.), *Aging: Communication processes and disorders* (pp. 339–356). New York: Grune & Stratton.

Lubinski, R. (1988). A model for intervention: Communication skills, effectiveness and opportunity. In B. Shadden (Ed.), *Communication behavior and aging* (pp. 294–308). Baltimore: Williams & Wilkins.

Lubinski, R. (1994). Family and environmental considerations in aphasia. In R. Chapey (Ed.), *Language intervention in adult aphasia* (3rd ed.). Baltimore: Williams & Wilkins.

Lubinski, R. (1995). Environmental considerations of elderly patients. In R. Lubinski (Ed.), *Dementia and communication* (pp. 257–278). San Diego, CA: Singular.

Lubinski, R., Morrison, E., & Rigrodski, S. (1981). Perception of spoken communication by elderly and chronically ill patients in an institutional setting. *Journal of Speech and Hearing Disorders*, 46, 405–412.

Luterman, D. (1984). *Counseling the communicatively disordered and their families*. Austin, TX: PRO-ED.

Maitz, E. (1991). Family systems theory applied to head injury. In J. Williams & T. Kay (Eds.), *Head injury* (pp. 65–80). Baltimore: Brookes.

Maslach, C. (1982). *Burnout: The cost of caring*. Englewood Cliffs, NJ: Prentice Hall.

Maslach, C., & Jackson, S. (1982). Burnout in health professions: A social psychological analysis. In G. Sanders & J. Suls (Eds.), *Social psychology of health and illness* (pp. 227–254). Hillsdale, NJ: Erlbaum.

McCubbin, H., Boss, P., Wilson, L., & Lester, G. (1980). Developing family invulnerability to stress. In J. Trost (Ed.), *The family in change*. Vasters, Sweden: International Library.

McCubbin, H., & Patterson, J. (1983). Family stress process: A double ABC model of adjustment and adaptation. In H. McCubbin, J. Patterson, & M. Sussman (Eds.), *Advancements and developments in family stress theory and research*. New York: Hayworth Press.

Miller, M., & Potter, R. (1982). Professional burnout among speech–language pathologists. *ASHA, 24*, 177–180.

Murgatroyd, S. (1985). *Counseling and helping*. London: British Psychological Society and Methuen.

Pines, A. (1982). Helpers and motivation and the burnout syndrome. In T. Willis (Ed.), *Basic processes in helping relationships*. New York: Academic Press.

Potter, R., & Rudensey, K. (1984). Coping with burnout. *Asha, 26*, 35–38.

Power, P. (1985). Family coping behaviors in chronic illness: A rehabilitation perspective. *Rehabilitation Literature, 46*, 78–83.

Rauth, T. (1968). *Nursing homes*. Springfield, IL: Thomas.

Rogers, C. (1951). *Client centered therapy*. Boston: Houghton Mifflin.

Rosenstock, R., Goldman, M., & Rothenberg, R. (1969). Rehabilitation of the long-term patient: An action research program in milieu therapy. *Journal of Chronic Disabilities, 27*, 493–503.

Rossi, J., & Filstead, W. (Eds.). (1973). *The therapeutic community*. New York: Behavioral Publications.

Safilios-Rothchild, C. (1970). *The sociology and social psychology of disability and rehabilitation*. New York: Random House.

Square, P., & Martin, R. (1994). The nature and treatment of neuromotor speech disorders in aphasia. In R. Chapey (Ed.), *Language intervention strategies in adult aphasia* (pp. 467–502). Baltimore: Williams & Wilkins.

Sussman, M. (1977). Dependent disabled and dependent poor: Similarity of conceptual issues and research needs. In J. Stubbins (Ed.), *Social and psychological aspects of disability* (pp. 247–260). Baltimore: University Park Press.

U.S. Department of Commerce. (1992). *Statistical abstracts of the United States*. Washington, DC: Author.

Waaland, P., & Raines, S. (1991). Families coping with childhood neurological disability: Clinical assessment and treatment. *NeuroRehabilitation, 1*, 19–28.

Wahrborg, P. (1991). *Assessment and management of emotional reactions to brain damage and aphasia*. San Diego, CA: Singular.

Watkins, C. (1991). Hassles of caring. *Nursing the Elderly, 3*, 25–27.

Chapter 6

Phonological Encoding and Speech Programming: The Disorders of Paraphasias and Apraxia of Speech

Robert S. Pierce

Two of the processes involved in speaking what is on one's mind are (a) the encoding of the message one wants to convey into a series of phonological segments, and (b) the progamming/planning of movements that articulate those segments. These processes can be impaired following neurological insult, creating the general disorders of paraphasias and apraxia of speech, respectively. In this chapter, Pierce discusses these two processes and their disorders, emphasizing issues relating to characteristics, diagnoses, and treatment.

1. *What causes the different types of paraphasias?*

2. *How can you distinguish the paraphasic pattern associated with a mild Wernicke's aphasia from that of a conduction aphasia?*

3. *How can one confidently diagnose apraxia of speech?*

4. *What are some of the basic principles of treatment for apraxia of speech? What kind of generalization and maintenance patterns result from this treatment?*

�֍   ✶   ✶

It is reasonably well established that the expression of language through the production of speech is accomplished by a number of processes. Of course, these processes can break down causing language and speech production disorders. However, drawing clear distinctions among these disorders has been controversial. This chapter discusses two of these processes and their disorders. One is the process of phonological encoding, a part of the language production system. Disorders within this system lead to paraphasic intrusions. The other is the programming of speech movements, a part of the speech production system. An impairment to this system causes apraxia of speech. It is essential to distinguish between these two disorders, if for no other reason than because the treatment approaches for each disorder are different. This chapter begins with a discussion of phonological encoding and the origin of paraphasias. After a brief discussion of speech production systems, it then discusses apraxia of speech, including issues relating to its characteristics, diagnosis, and treatment. The chapter concludes with a discussion of treatment for paraphasias.

Phonological Encoding and Paraphasias

This section reviews *phonological encoding;* that is, the process of converting linguistic intent into phonological output that drives the articulatory system. The process begins with activation of the phonological lexicon based on some input and ends with a syllabified order of phonemes that inputs into the articulatory processes. These articulatory processes subsequently make appropriate allophonic accommodations over the phonemic strings, such as aspirating voiceless stops in certain phonetic contexts and lengthening vowels in front of voiced stops. These accommodations occur even when the phoneme segments are incorrect and, accordingly, are not of interest in this section. Somewhere during this phonological encoding, paraphasic errors occur.

Figure 6.1 displays the events that occur during phonological encoding. As can be observed, the phonological lexicon can be activated by a number of input sources. During the expression of internal thought, activation comes from a person's semantic representation. Some authors suggest that conceptual knowledge, in the form of compilations of semantic features, contains a linking address that locates the appropriate entry in the phonological lexicon for a particular concept (Butterworth, 1992; Kohn & Smith, 1994b). Other authors argue that there is an intermediate stage, frequently referred to as a lemma (Dell, Schwartz, Martin, Saffran, & Gagnon, 1997; Levelt, 1989). A *lemma* is a nonphonological representation of a word whose activation is guided

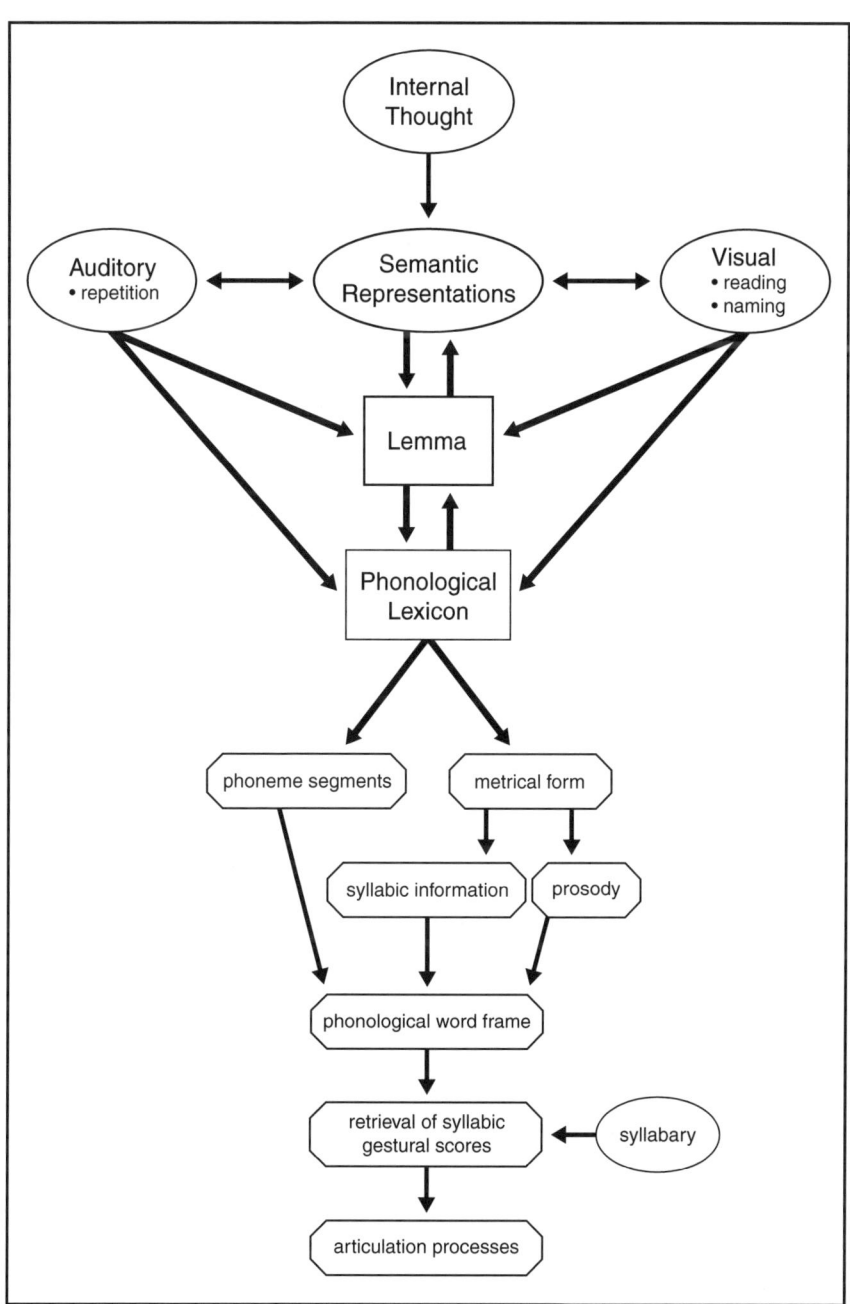

Figure 6.1. Model of phonological encoding.

by semantic, pragmatic, and syntactic considerations. Activation of the lemma then leads to activation of the phonological information. This stage is incorporated into Figure 6.1.

Activation of phonological representations can also come from auditory inputs (repetition) either through the semantic system or independently (as in echolalia and transcortical sensory aphasia where repetition occurs in the absence of comprehension). Independent, non-semantic, activation can either go directly to the lemma when repetition is based on word activation, or to the phonological lexicon when imitation is based on converting sounds to phonemes (as in repeating nonwords). Visual inputs during reading and naming can also activate the phonological lexicon. Again, this can occur either via the semantic system or independently (as in hyperlexia, demented patients' ability to read aloud with limited comprehension, the ability to name without semantic awareness [see Brennen, David, Fluchaire, & Pellat, 1996], and the ability to read aloud nonwords). In addition, activation could occur based on combined inputs from several sources (Hillis & Caramazza, 1995), such as when phonemic cuing helps patients retrieve words.

Although Figure 6.1 shows only one phonological lexicon, some authors argue that there is more than one (Orpwood & Warrington, 1995; but see also Coleman, 1998); however, this controversy will not be considered in this chapter. Other authors argue that different aspects of semantic meaning become activated at different times (Goodglass, Wingfield, & Ward, 1999). Early semantic activation may be sufficient to activate a specific word node in the lemma, which, in turn, activates both phonological information and additional semantic information.

The planning frame over which activation of the phonological lexicon occurs can range from the smallest unit to be spoken (i.e., a *morpheme*) to a clause (Buckingham, 1992; Dell & O'Seaghdha, 1992; Levelt, 1989), although words outside this frame can be concurrently active within the lexicon (see later discussion).

Activation of the phonological lexicon releases two types of information. One is metrical information, which consists of information about the syllables in the word (e.g., the number of syllables) and the prosody/stress pattern (Butterworth, 1992; Levelt, 1989; Wheeldon & Levelt, 1995). The second type of information consists of the phoneme segments associated with the activated lexical entries. Some theorists argue that the information activated at this stage consists of under-specified featural knowledge that is constructed into phonemic segments at a later stage (Beland, Caplan, & Nespoulous, 1990; Caplan & Waters, 1992; Kohn & Smith, 1995). However, others disagree (Buckingham, 1992; Dell, 1988) and, for the sake of simplicity, this chapter will consider the units activated at this stage to be intact phonemes. Other theorists state that this activated information is stored in a phonological buffer (Shattuck-Hufnagel, 1979, 1983). However, it is probably best to simply view this information (metrical form and phoneme segments) as being in a state of activation, which makes it more available for use in later processing stages as compared to information that is not activated. The activated phoneme segments are probably tagged for word position (Dell, 1986, 1988; Dell & O'Seaghdha, 1992; Shattuck-Hufnagel, 1992). That is, the word *cat* will activate a word-initial /k/ and a word-final /t/ in addition to the vowel. If activation of a lexical entry fails to release metrical and/or segmental information, information may become active based on some sort of default setting or by a random phoneme generator (Butterworth, 1979, 1992), or through the process of phonological reconstruction (Kohn & Smith, 1994b).

At some point, activated information within the phonological lexicon is called upon to be spoken, either when a certain level of activation is reached or a specified amount of time has passed. The process appears to begin with the metrical information (stress and syllabic information) combining to form a new syllabified frame that relates to phonological words rather than lexical words (Levelt, 1992; Levelt & Wheeldon, 1994). That is, lexical boundaries disappear and phonological words are developed based on a concatenation of the individual lexical items. For example, *demand it* (as in voters demand it) becomes *demandit* (with syllables *de-man-dit*); *gave it to him* becomes *ga-vi-tim*; and *neglect it* becomes *ne-glec-tit*. Similarly, the speech error *peel like flaying* (for *feel like playing*) may reflect an interchange of initial phonemes in adjacent phonological words, assuming that *feel like* had become *feelike* during the encoding process (Levelt, 1992).

This new phonological word frame then drives the selection or mapping of phoneme segments from the lexicon onto the frame. The order in which this mapping occurs has been a matter of controversy. Shattuck-Hufnagel (1987) felt that the word onsets were mapped last. Dell (1986, 1988) claimed that the different parts of the syllable (onset, nucleus, coda) were mapped in parallel. However, more recent work indicates that mapping occurs sequentially from left to right, both within a syllable (Kohn & Smith, 1995; Meyer, 1991) and from one syllable to the next (Kohn & Smith, 1995; Meyer, 1990; Wheeldon & Levelt, 1995). This mapping respects word position information, in that a word-initial position slot in the phonological word frame will select a phoneme from the available set of activated word-initial phonemes in the lexicon (Dell, 1988; Shattuck-Hufnagel, 1992). Mechanisms relating to this mapping process have been called a *scan copier* (Shattuck-Hufnagel, 1979, 1983) and a *phonological assembly subsystem* (PASS) (Butterworth, 1992). As phonemes are selected and mapped onto the phonological word frame, they may be removed from further use by either their activation levels returning to a resting level (Dell, 1988; Harley, 1993) or by being tagged as used by a check-off monitor (Shattuck-Hufnagel, 1979, 1983). The planning frame over which these phonological words are constructed and filled may be smaller than the planning frame that guides activation of information within the phonological lexicon. Dell and O'Seaghdha (1992) state that this planning frame may be more related to the prosodic structure of an utterance than the syntactic and may have an upper limit of the phrase.

Although information contained in filled phonological word frames could be sent directly to the articulatory processes for programming and execution, Levelt and Wheeldon (1994) argue that there is an intermediary step during which syllable gestural scores are retrieved from a mental syllabary. These syllable gestural scores contain the specifics of which articulatory gestures are needed to produce these syllables, not specifics as to how these gestures are to be made. These scores exist for syllables that are well practiced or learned. Articulatory gestures would still need to be computed anew for low frequency and new syllables.

Finally, the syllable gestural information is forwarded to the articulatory processes, which can act over several syllable scores at one time. These processes provide the allophonic accommodations and coarticulatory characteristics that are seen in the final speech output.

What Is Active in the Phonological Lexicon?

Because the phoneme segments that are mapped onto the phonological word frames are thought to come from the pool of activated segments in the phonological lexicon, it is important to consider what might be active within the lexicon at any given time. These activated entries can come from several different sources.

1. Because the planning frame governing lexical activation can range up to a clause, phonological information from all the units within the clause can be active at one time. This allows for slips-of-the-tongue in which phonemes are interchanged across words within the clause (e.g., *queer old dean* for *dear old queen*).

2. Spreading activation (connectionist) theories claim that, during the normal course of events, additional information becomes activated relating to the phonological and/or semantic components of the target words (Dell, 1986, 1988; Dell & O'Seaghdha, 1991, 1992; Dell et al., 1997; Harley, 1993). The semantic features highlighted in the semantic representation can activate (prime) other entries within the lemma that are consistent with those semantic features. For example, the semantic features that address the lexical entry of *cat* could also prime entries such as *dog* and *cow* because they share semantic features. As stated earlier, activation of a lemma activates the phoneme segments associated with that entry (tagged for word position). Activation can then spread backward from these phoneme segments to activate other lexical entries in the lemma that share those segments. For example, *cat* consists of the vowel, the word-initial /k/, and the word-final /t/. The word-initial /k/ could prime lexical entries such as *cap,* and the word-final segments could activate entries such as *mat* and *rat*. Further spreading activation could occur as these other entries' prime additional entries. For example, *dog* could be primed, based on the sharing of semantic features, and then prime *log* based on the sharing of phoneme segments (this is referred to as a mediated entry because of the presence of an intermediary step). The extent to which these other entries are activated, or primed, and remain active relates to the strength of the connections between entries (known as weights) and the function of a decay factor. For example, mixed entries (such as *rat* for *cat*) will have the most activation because priming occurs based on both semantic and phonological associations. Mediated entries have the least activation because priming goes through an intermediary step. For example, *dog* may have 20% of the activation that the target *cat* has and then spreads 20% of that to *log*. So, *log* has 4% (20% of 20%) of the activation of *cat*. Priming based only on semantic or phonological similarity will have levels in between mixed and mediated entries (Dell & O'Seaghdha, 1992; Harley, 1993). Weights may also vary based on the degree of the semantic and/or phonological relationship. Spreading activation, in particular the notions of weights and decay functions,

has a marked impact on the theories of paraphasia generation (Dell et al., 1997).

3. Reduced inhibition of inappropriate spreading activation and/or reduced clearing of used or unwanted information (e.g., a malfunctioning check-off monitor or an impaired ability of activation to return to resting levels) can lead to lexical entries remaining active long after they should be. This could lead to perseverations if those entries are selected again (Butterworth, 1992; Kohn, 1989).

4. Contextual or environmental contaminants could impose on lexical activation (Levelt, 1992; Shattuck-Hufnagel, 1992). These might be words that the person is hearing or reading, or perhaps extraneous thoughts that occur while phonological encoding is progressing. Some of these contaminants may be associated with the target words. For example, the proposition *climb the tree* may stimulate the concept of *playing*, which could mix with the original proposition and come out as *plimb the tree* (Shattuck-Hufnagel, 1992).

5. A person may have multiple plans as to what to say (something we have probably all experienced). For example, difficulty deciding whether to say *close* or *near* may produce *clear*, or choosing between *recognize* and *reflect* may lead to the production of *recoflect* (Meyer, 1992).

Where Do Paraphasias Come From?

The term *paraphasia* refers to a substitution. It can be a substitution of a whole word, an individual phoneme, or a combination. Typically, these substitutions are involuntary and should be distinguished from volitional substitutions that anomic patients (and normals) demonstrate when they cannot think of the word that they want. The following are descriptions of the different types of paraphasias and how they might be generated. These descriptions rely on the model of phonological encoding discussed earlier and shown in Figure 6.1.

Phonemic Paraphasias. *Phonemic paraphasias* are substitutions of individual phonemes. They can arise from a mild problem with the phonological information that is released when an entry in the phonological lexicon is activated (Kohn & Smith, 1994b). Some of the phonemes released with that activation may be incorrect. Phonemic paraphasias can also occur with problems in mapping phonemes from the phonological lexicon to the syllables in the phonological word frame (Kohn

& Smith, 1995). These phonemic errors can result in either another real word (*coke → coat*) or a nonword (*neologism*) that closely resembles the target word (*beef → peef*). The source of the erroneously mapped phonemes could be any of the entries that are concomitantly active in the phonological lexicon (as discussed previously). For example, one patient produced the sequence *his hat is on the . . . shop . . . she . . . top . . . shef . . . shelf*. Presumably, the *sh* phoneme from *shelf* was inaccurately mapped onto the word-initial position in *top*. Another patient (Darley, Aronson, & Brown, 1975), when asked to repeat a sentence containing *roast beef*, produced *road peach . . . peef . . . beef*. A phonemic paraphasia transformed *roast* to *road*. The patient then substituted the word *peach* for *beef*. In an attempt to correct this error, she apparently correctly activated *beef*, combining it with the previous production of *peach* (whose activation had not dissipated). It is not clear whether the word-final /f/ combined with the word *peach* or whether the word-initial /p/ combined with the word *beef* to get the neologism *peef*. Another patient produced the utterance *pamples you can hold* when referring to her new glasses. Her neologistic distortion of *temples* could have resulted from a mapping problem or from the release of an inaccurate group of phonemes when the lexical entry for *temples* was activated. Although phonemic paraphasias occur in patients with both Wernicke's and conduction aphasia, they are the prominent symptom in conduction aphasia (Buckingham, 1992).

Verbal Paraphasias. *Verbal paraphasias* are whole word substitutions that do not bear a semantic or phonological resemblance to the target word (e.g., *cat → house*). Kohn and Smith (1994b) hypothesize that they arise from an impairment to the phonological addresses contained in the semantic representation. If these addresses are markedly impaired, then they are unable to guide selection of a lexical entry, so the selection occurs randomly (or based on activation from sources other than the semantic representation).

Apparent verbal paraphasias can also occur when (a) phonemic paraphasias change the correct target word into an unrelated real word (*cup → pup*), or (b) an incorrect semantically related error is subjected to further phonemic errors (*cat → dog → log*) (Dell et al., 1997).

Formal (Phonic Verbal) Paraphasias. Whole word substitutions that share some phonemes with the target (e.g., *harp → hanger, latch → limp,* *record player* → *roll pickle*) are called *formal* (*phonic verbal*) *paraphasias*. Kohn and Smith (1994b) state that they arise from a less severe impairment to the phonological addresses in the semantic representation. When partially intact, these addresses can activate entries in the phonological lexicon that are phonologically related to the target (phonological neighbors).

Spreading activation theory accounts for formal paraphasias differently (Gagnon, Schwartz, Martin, Dell, & Saffran, 1997; Martin & Saffran, 1992). As depicted in Figure 6.2, during naming, activation spreads from the semantic nodes (activated by the concept depicted in the picture) to the lexical entries (lemmas). Activation occurs to the target entry in the lemma as well as to semantically related entries. Subsequently, activation spreads backward to the semantic nodes and forward to the phonological nodes associated with the lexical entries. Activation then again spreads back to the lexical entries, this time activating ones that are phonologically related to the target entry based on the phonological nodes from which the spreading arises. Assuming an abnormally rapid rate of decay of the activation levels, then the phonologically related lexical entry (which was activated most recently) has an advantage over the target and semantically related entries (which were activated earlier in the process and decayed rapidly). Accordingly, the phonologically related entry is likely to be selected for production, producing a formal paraphasia. Martin, Dell, Saffran, and Schwartz (1994) further demonstrated, through the use of computer simulations, that abnormally rapid decay rates caused an increase in formal paraphasias. Furthermore, their simulations showed that more normal decay rates lead to a reduction in the incidence of phonic verbal paraphasias. These simulation results mirrored the performance of N.C., a patient with deep dysphasia (similar to Wernicke's aphasia), who demonstrated a high incidence of formal paraphasias early post onset and then a reduction in these errors with recovery. The authors hypothesized, therefore, that N.C.'s errors were partially caused by an abnormally rapid rate of decay of activation levels throughout the phonological encoding system, which became less rapid with recovery.

In contrast to Martin and Saffran (1992), Harley and MacAndrew (1992) reported that increasing the decay rate for lexical entries did not cause a change in error patterns (particularly an increase in formal paraphasias). However, as pointed out by Martin, Saffran, and Dell (1996), the

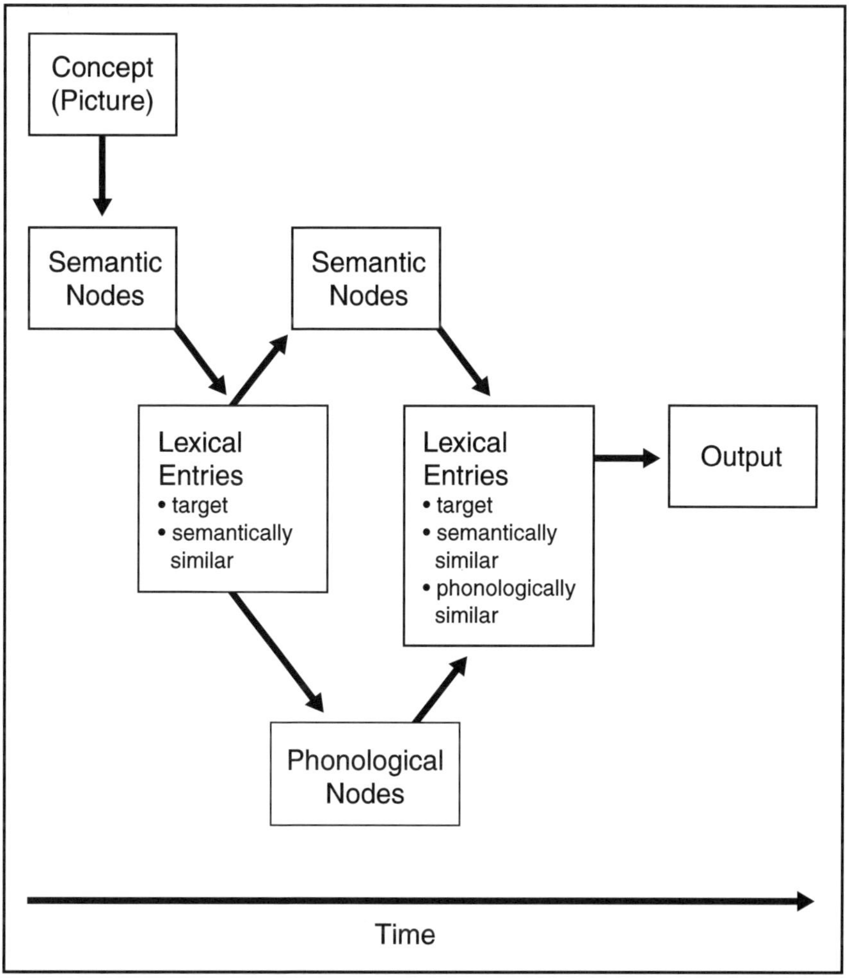

Figure 6.2. Representation of the spreading activation that could account for phonic verbal paraphasias. *Note.* Adapted from Figure 2 in "A Computational Account of Deep Dysphasia: Evidence from a Single Case Study," by N. Martin and E. Saffran, 1992, *Brain and Language, 43*, p. 257.

lexical entries in Harley and MacAndrew's simulations could maintain their activation based on input from the phonological and semantic nodes that were not decaying rapidly. The change in error patterns arises when all levels (semantic, lexical, and phonological) decay rapidly, as simulated by Martin et al. (1994).

Apparent formal paraphasias can also occur when a correctly selected word is subjected to a phonemic paraphasia (*dog* → *log*) (Dell et al., 1997).

Semantic Paraphasias. *Semantic paraphasias* are whole word substitutions that share semantic features with the target (*dog* → *cat*). They could arise from impaired semantic representations. Partial semantic representations could be activated that subsequently address incorrect lexical entries. Because the same semantic representations may be used for comprehension and production, aphasic patients with this type of semantic paraphasia will probably show comprehension problems as well. However, semantic paraphasias can arise when the semantic representations appear to be intact (Caramazza & Hillis, 1990). The semantic information can prime several related lexical entries, with the wrong one being selected for production. In this case, comprehension would be intact.

N.C.'s semantic paraphasias during repetition were again accounted for within the theory of spreading activation (Martin et al., 1994, 1996). During repetition, the spread of activation flows differently than during naming (see Figure 6.3). Phonological nodes are activated first, then lexical. Activation spreads back to the phonological and forward to the semantic nodes, and then back to the lexical entries activating semantic competitors for the first time. Given a rapid rate of decay of activation levels, the semantic competitors are at an advantage for production because they are activated most recently. Computer simulations and N.C.'s recovery pattern (showing a decrease in semantic paraphasias during repetition) are consistent with this model.

Semantic paraphasias can also occur whenever the semantic nodes within the spreading activation model are more active than at other times. This could occur based on intrinsic characteristics of the target word and its competitors, such as words with high imageability ratings that are thought to contain richer semantic networks (Martin et al., 1996). Other semantically related words could intrude into the planning unit for phonological encoding for a variety of reasons, as discussed earlier (e.g., contextual or environmental contaminants).

Neologisms. Nonword errors are *neologisms*. They can occur with an impairment to the information released from the phonological lexicon (Kohn & Smith, 1994b). In cases of severe impairment, neologisms will

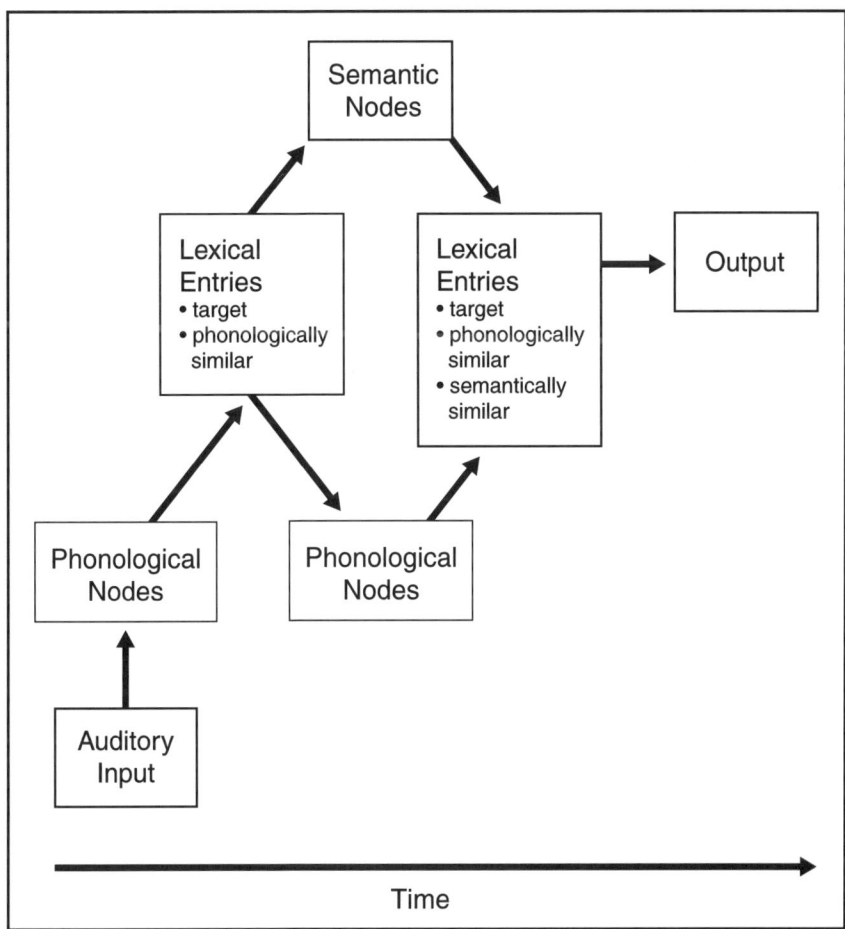

Figure 6.3. Representation of the spreading activation that could account for semantic paraphasias. *Note.* Adapted from Figure 7 in "Origins of Paraphasias in Deep Dysphasia: Testing the Consequences of a Decay Impairment to an Interactive Spreading Activation Model of Lexical Retrieval," by N. Martin, G. Dell, E. Saffran, and M. Schwartz, 1994, *Brain and Language, 47*, p. 637.

show little resemblance, if any, to the target words because the phonemes released from the lexicon will be mostly incorrect ones. In addition, faulty information about syllable structure can also be released such that the spoken words may have extra syllables (e.g., *umbrella* → *umbrellorena*). In cases of milder impairment, neologisms will be closer to the target, sharing a greater number of correct phonemes, and will have fewer extra syllables (the *temples* → *pamples* error mentioned above is a good example). Neologisms also result from phonemic paraphasias that occur during the mapping process.

In very severe cases, there may be a complete failure to release phonological information from the lexicon. Accordingly, there is no target from which neologisms can diverge. These instances are referred to as anomia-driven, no target, or abstruse neologisms. Butterworth (1979, 1992) suggests that a random string of phonemes is generated. Kohn and Smith (1994b) argue that these neologisms result from the process of phonemic reconstruction that occurs during the mapping process (respecting phonotactic rules, of course).

Combination Errors. *Combination errors* can occur whenever two or more of these processes go wrong on the same word. For example, one patient with Wernicke's aphasia produced *telebone* for *umbrella*. Presumably the phonemic paraphasia /f/ → /b/ was overlaid on the word substitution *umbrella* → *telephone*, suggesting that the target word was active within the phonological lexicon planning frame when the mapping process occurred. No doubt the experienced clinician can think of many such examples.

Evolution of Paraphasias

Kohn and Smith (1994a) state that the evolution of the impairment to the phonological addresses within the semantic representation will allow for aborted attempts to become verbal paraphasias and subsequently formal paraphasias. Improvement in the release of information from the phonological lexicon will be reflected in neologisms that evolve from being totally different from the targets (assuming one can be identified) and containing extra syllables, to ones that are closer to the target, sharing more phonemes and syllables. An indication that this evolution in the quality of neologisms may not occur is the presence of consistent patterns of phonemic perseveration (Kohn, Smith, & Alexander, 1996). This poor prognosis may also relate to the persistence of poor single word comprehension. Phonemic paraphasias stemming from mapping difficulties evolve from severely distorted productions created by multiple mapping errors, to fewer mapping errors, that create words more similar to the targets (and thus more identifiable by the listener). In general, therefore, evolution of symptoms involves the production of fewer errors and errors that are closer to their intended targets. This allows for more successful communication as the listener is better able to discern the communication message, particularly within the context of the situation.

Comparing Milder Levels of Two Disorders

Patients with conduction aphasia demonstrate the primary symptom of phonemic paraphasia, presumably relating to problems with the phonemic mapping process. Patients with Wernicke's aphasia demonstrate most or all of the different types of paraphasias, presumably because of problems in semantic, lemma, and/or phonological lexicon activation. It has traditionally been espoused that the symptomatology of Wernicke's aphasia evolves to resemble that of conduction aphasia. However, the experienced clinician recognizes that mild Wernicke's aphasia is not equivalent to conduction aphasia. This difference has been highlighted recently by Kohn and Smith (1994a). They compared two patients who had quantitatively similar levels of severity (relatively mild). One was thought to demonstrate conduction aphasia resulting from problems with the mapping process; the other was thought to have a mild Wernicke's aphasia with problems associated with the release of inaccurate information from the phonological lexicon. Both patients made more errors with increasing word length. Both also produced neologisms and phonemic paraphasias. However, the conduction aphasic (CA) patient produced more word fragments, always involving the initial portions of the words and typically relating to the target. This can occur because mapping progresses one syllable at a time, and the patient can stop after a syllable to self-correct errors or the process can abort. The Wernicke's aphasic (WA) patient produced fewer word fragments (most of them were not target related) because the planning frame for phonological encoding is at minimum the morpheme. Whatever phonological information that was released for that morpheme would be mapped in its entirety. The CA patient produced more errors as the word unfolded. If phoneme mapping is impaired, then the phonological representations may fade as mapping progresses, thus leading to more errors toward the end of the word than at the beginning. The WA patient produced errors that were more evenly distributed within the words, presumably related to faulty activation of the stored lexical information (see also Kohn & Smith, 1995). The CA patient's nonword errors were closer to the target than were the nonword errors of the WA patient. That is, the CA patient produced more target phonemes and fewer nontarget phonemes than did the WA patient. The WA patient added syllables and consonants within syllables, whereas the CA patient seldom did either of these (because lexical information was intact). The CA patient was more successful in oral reading than in repetition of sentences (similar results were reported by Canter, Trost, & Burns, 1985; Caplan, 1987; Nespoulous, Joanette, Ska, Caplan, & Lecours, 1987). Possibly the printed word provides a more permanent activation of the lexical entry than does the fleeting stimulus associated with repetition that can fade before production is completed (see also Friedrich, Glenn, & Marin, 1984; Martin et al., 1996). The WA patient did equally well in both conditions.

Anatomy of Paraphasias

Wernicke's aphasia results from damage to Wernicke's area in the posterior superior temporal gyrus (often extending into the middle temporal gyrus). Patients whose lesions involve more than half of Wernicke's area have a much poorer prognosis for recovery than do patients whose lesions involve less than half of Wernicke's area (Kohn et al., 1996; Naeser, 1994; Palumbo, Alexander, & Naeser, 1992). Conduction aphasia results from damage to the lower parietal lobe, particularly the supramarginal gyrus, white matter just deep to it, and/or portions of the insula (Anderson et al., 1999; Palumbo et al., 1992). Those conduction aphasic patients who initially demonstrate auditory comprehension deficits appear to have parietal lobe lesions that also extend into part (less than half) of Wernicke's area or the temporal isthmus (Palumbo et al., 1992). Pairing these lesion patterns with the types of paraphasias evidenced by these two aphasic syndromes, placed within a broader distributed network model of word retrieval (Tranel, Damasio, & Damasio, 1997), it is conceivable that damage to Wernicke's area disrupts the phonological lexicon while damage to the lower parietal lobe impairs the phoneme mapping process (see also Coleman, 1998).

From Planning to Production

Typically, the verbal production of messages uses three stages: planning, programming, and execution. A linguistic intent or message is developed using the processes described previously. The output of these processes serves as the input to the programming system in order to initiate the spoken representation of these messages. The manner in which the transformation from planning to programming occurs remains poorly understood (Kent, Adams, & Turner, 1996). However, one conceptualization is that the planning stage generates phonological goals relating to perceptually acceptable acoustic outputs (Abbs, 1986). Particular movements or actions of specific muscles are not dictated by these goals. Rather, it is the role of the programming system to convert these goals into appropriate movement patterns.

The programming system generates the complex, multiple-movement sequences that are needed for speech production (Duffy, 1995; Square & Martin, 1994). Specifically, the programming system determines and organizes multiple-movement gestures across different muscle groups or articulators (e.g., jaw, larynx, tongue, lips, and palate; Abbs, 1986; Gracco, 1995; Gracco & Lofquist, 1994; Keller, 1987). For example, the programming system organizes jaw, laryngeal, and lip activity during bilabial productions, or palate, lips, jaw, and tongue activity during the production of nasals. This is a primary distinction between the programming system and the execution system, which acts on individual muscles or small muscle groups that carry out simpler movements within a specific articulator (Keller, 1987; Kuehn, Lemme, & Baumgartner, 1989).

The specific motor commands developed by the programming system do not have to be identical each time the same utterance is produced. There are many configurations of the vocal tract that can produce the same perceptually acceptable acoustic goal. This notion of motor equivalence relates to the capacity of the motor system to obtain the same end product (acoustic representation) despite considerable variation in the movements that contribute to that output (various vocal tract shapes) (Hughes & Abbs, 1976). Toward this end, the programming system receives sensory information from many different sources, including the somato-sensory areas of the cerebral cortex, the basal ganglia, and the cerebellum (in addition to visual and auditory feedback) (Kuehn et al., 1989; Square & Martin, 1994). It can use this sensory information to modify its motor commands either before the movements are initiated or during their execution. Movements can be modified prior to initiation in order to accommodate the specifics of the vocal tract configuration present at that time. Movements can be modified during their execution to accommodate unexpected conditions or perturbations. For example, limiting the movement of the jaw during bilabial closure leads to greater movement of the lip to achieve the closure (Abbs, 1986; Folkins & Abbs, 1976). This sensory information can interact with central preprogrammed motor commands for well-learned movements executed under typical and predictable conditions (Gracco, 1995; Gracco & Lofquist, 1994). Its role may be enhanced for less well-learned movements or when production conditions are less typical or predictable (Borden, 1979).

Disruptions in the programming system result in apraxia of speech that is characterized by difficulty in planning/organizing interarticulatory movements for the production of speech. Breakdowns in the execution of these motor commands by one or more muscle groups cause dysarthria and usually are associated with some degree of weakness, slowness, incoordination, or alteration of muscle tone (Duffy, 1995), symptoms that typically are absent in apraxia of speech (although the two disorders can co-occur). Programming problems can occur for speech movements exclusively. Thus, patients can be apraxic for speech movements but not for nonspeech movements (i.e., no oral apraxia). In contrast, execution problems typically affect both speech and nonspeech movements because they both rely on the same system of upper and lower motor neurons.

Apraxia of Speech

The past decade or so has witnessed an essentially new era of how we think about apraxia of speech. This evolution has evolved around two considerations. One is the recognition that, because patients seldom have a pure apraxia of speech without a concomitant aphasia, the speech behavior that was being studied may have reflected impairments at levels other than motor planning/programming. Most notably, apraxia of speech frequently occurs in patients who also have Broca's aphasia. Accordingly, it becomes difficult to tease out which aspects of their errors are caused by their aphasic-based linguistic difficulties (e.g., phonological encoding problems) or by their apraxia (see Marquardt & Cannito, 1996). What is no longer permissible is to test an individual who has Broca's aphasia and apraxia of speech and automatically assume that the errors he or she makes are caused by the apraxia. Researchers must show that their subjects demonstrate apraxia in conjunction with either a nonexistent or a very mild aphasia.

The second consideration relates to the level of analyses that is used to study speech errors. Perceptual analyses using broad phonetic transcriptions risk glossing over important variations in speech sound productions. They tend to force perceived errors into phonemic categories that imply a sound substitution has occurred. They minimize the ability to identify distorted productions. For example, when trying to say *bat,* an apraxic individual may have difficulty programming the inter-articulatory movements needed to produce an appropriate voice onset time for the voiced sound /b/. If sufficiently disturbed, the voice onset time (VOT) may fall into the range that is perceived as a voiceless sound, so the listener may perceive *pat*. However, suggesting that this individual incorrectly substituted (retrieved) the /p/ phoneme for the /b/ phoneme would inaccurately characterize the events that occurred. The correct phoneme was retrieved but distorted in its production. For example, Wambaugh, West, and Doyle (1997) presented a case study where VOTs for stops and affricates that were devoiced (and perceived as substitutions) were distinctly different from the VOTs produced during correct voiceless stops and affricates. This suggests the errors were distortions and not substitutions. Although not perfect, narrow phonetic transcriptions are better able to identify distortions that were either not noted previously or were misconstrued as substitutions.

A third consideration that deserves more systematic attention relates to the severity of the apraxia. A hallmark of studies with apraxic speakers is the identification of increased variability in performance (e.g., Seddoh et al., 1996). For example, the duration of between-word intervals varies considerably across apraxic speakers (Strand & McNeil, 1996). Does this variation relate systematically to the severity of the apraxia? Similarly, Odell, McNeil, Rosenbek, and Hunter (1991) reported that some apraxic speakers evidenced open junctures between syllables in words but others did not. Is this related to severity or to idiosyncratic strategies employed by certain individuals? Hough and Klich (1998) reported that certain speech planning/programming errors were noticeably more impaired in an individual with more severe apraxia than in one with a less severe impairment. Although it is intuitive that disrupted aspects of speech programming should vary as a function of severity, it may be that certain behaviors reflect individual speakers' approaches to dealing with their problem. More systematic research in this area could be informative.

Because of these considerations (particularly the first two), early databases on apraxia of speech are viewed as suspect. The field is literally beginning to rebuild its database, adhering to more stringent subject selection criteria and experimental methods. For reviews of the older literature and some considerations of how the new differs from the old, the reader is referred to Duffy (1995); McNeil, Robin, and Schmidt (1997); Pierce (1991); and Square and Martin (1994).

Description

Unlike phonemic paraphasias that reflect the inaccurate selection and/or sequencing of phonemes, apraxia of speech impairs the ability to plan/program the articulatory movements that are needed to produce those sounds (in the presence of relatively normal muscle strength and coordination). Apraxic speakers have difficulty producing both vowels and consonants. Traditional thought has been that apraxic speakers follow a general hierarchy based on motor complexity, producing fewer errors on vowels, more on consonants, and the most on consonant blends (Canter et al., 1985; Monoi, Fukusako, Itoh, & Sasanuma, 1983). However, studying a small group of subjects with pure apraxia and using narrow phonetic transcription, Odell et al. (1991) reported a relatively equal number of errors on vowels and consonants. Most of the vowel errors (64%) were distortions, of which 74% were sound prolongations. Only 10% were judged as substitutions. This contrasted with the errors made by the subjects with paraphasic difficulty, whose errors were judged as substitutions 65% of the time and distortions only 24%. Almost all of the apraxic speakers' vowel errors (93%) occurred next to consonants that were produced in error.

Longer vowel durations is a frequent finding in recent studies of apraxia (Hough & Klich, 1998; Seddoh et al., 1996; Strand & McNeil, 1996). Strand and McNeil (1996) argued that these longer durations are not likely to be caused by reduced speed of movements, citing several studies that showed apraxic speakers to be able to achieve essentially normal velocities of movement. They feel it is more likely that the speakers were extending the steady state of the vowels in order to achieve specific articulatory configurations or to obtain afferent information for use in motor control. Interestingly, these vowel durations became much longer when the words were produced in sentences (e.g., "I cook stew slowly.") than when produced either in isolation or in series (e.g., *cook, cook, cook*) (Hough & Klich, 1998; Strand & McNeil, 1996). Apparently, increasing the overall articulatory demands of an utterance has an impact on performance for individual segments.

The ability to modify durations based on linguistic convention has also been studied. Similar to normals, the less severe apraxic speaker studied by Hough and Klich (1998) was able to shorten vowel duration before a voiceless final consonant compared to before a voiced final consonant, both when the words were produced in isolation and when embedded in a sentence. However, the more severely impaired speaker could do this only when the words were produced in isolation. Rogers (1997) reported that this shortening effect is exaggerated in apraxic speakers compared to those with aphasia or dysarthria. Hough and Klich (1998) and Strand and McNeil (1996) found that apraxic speakers could shorten vowel duration as words became longer (e.g., *sue, suing, suingly*), but that the magnitude of these reduced durations was less than those of the normal controls. These findings suggest that apraxic speakers are sensitive to these linguistic conventions, but they are impaired in their ability to produce them.

Apraxic speakers produce errors on consonants as well as vowels. Again, the traditional thought is that errors of substitution are the most common on imitative tasks (Canter et al., 1985; Monoi et al., 1983; Nespoulous et al., 1987). However, using pure apraxic speakers and narrow phonetic transcription, Odell, McNeil, Rosenbek, and Hunter (1990) found that the majority of errors (54%) were distortions. Most (66%) of these distortions were prolonged segments. Consonant clusters had more errors than did consonant singletons, and most of these errors were omissions. Of the substitutions, most (63%) were only one distinctive feature away from the target. Place was the feature most prone to error, with dental and palatal articulations being the most vulnerable. Alveolar articulations were the most likely replacements (similar to the results of Klich, Ireland, & Weidner, 1979). Manner was typically retained by the substituting phoneme, but liquids and fricatives were the manners most often in error. Voiced phonemes were more prone to error than were voiceless ones. Some results that differed from previous research were that errors occurred relatively equally across word position, with the most errors in medial position, and that the relatively same number of errors occurred in one-, two-, and three-syllable words.

McNeil, Odell, Miller, and Hunter (1995) reported that the location and type of error was relatively consistent across repeated trials of the same word for apraxic speakers, especially compared to individuals evidencing phonemic paraphasias.

Apraxic speakers demonstrate increased durations of vowels, consonants, and inter-segment transitions (Kent & Rosenbek, 1983; Seddoh et al., 1996). Some also demonstrate open junctures (pauses) between syllables (Kent & Rosenbek, 1982, 1983; Odell et al., 1991) and longer pauses between words (Strand & McNeil, 1996). One possible reason for the longer pauses between syllables and words (and perhaps the lengthened phoneme segments) is to provide time for them to program the next segment. It is thought that apraxic speakers reduce the unit over which they try to program articulatory movements. Rogers and Storkel (1999) provide evidence that apraxic speakers cannot program more than one syllable at a time. In addition, some apraxic speakers may have difficulty programming across segments within a syllable and separate these segments so that they can be programmed independently. The intrusion of a neutral schwa sound between consonants in a cluster (Canter et al., 1985) may be for this purpose. Reduced co-articulation (Hough & Klich, 1998; McNeil, Hashi, & Southwood, 1994; Southwood, Dagenais, Sutphin, & Garcia, 1997; Ziegler & van Cramon, 1985, 1986) may also reflect the programming of segments within a syllable in a sequential, rather than an integrated, manner. The extent to which a particular individual needs to reduce his or her programming unit to a segment or a syllable may depend on the severity of his or her apraxia. Hough and Klich (1998) found that their severely apraxic subject showed significantly reduced anticipatory lip rounding before the vowel /u/, but their less severely impaired subject did not.

Increased segment, transition, and pause durations may contribute to the perception of slow, labored speech that is characteristic of apraxic speakers. Finally, the reduction in programming units to segments, syllables, or even words makes it very difficult to maintain any kind of normal intonation pattern over a longer utterance. Accordingly, it is not surprising for apraxic speakers to show marked prosodic impairments.

Diagnosis

There are few tests specifically designed to diagnose apraxia of speech. Those that are published (*Apraxia Battery for Adults*, Dabul, 1979), referenced in a book (*Motor Speech Evaluation*, Wertz, LaPointe, & Rosenbek, 1984), or have been informally developed and put in the clinical files often have similar tasks. The most common of these are:

1. A spontaneous speech sample, including conversation and picture description
2. Oral reading of a standard paragraph
3. Vowel prolongation
4. Alternate motion rates (syllable diadochokinesis)
5. Repetition of monosyllabic words with identical sounds in the initial and final position of a word (e.g., mom, zoos)
6. One repetition of multisyllabic words
7. Repetition of multisyllabic words several times each
8. Repetition of words of increasing length (e.g., flat, flatter, flattering)
9. Repetition of sentences containing multisyllabic words
10. Counting forward and backward

These tasks are very useful for allowing an apraxia of speech to show itself. That is, apraxic speakers will usually have difficulty with these tasks. However, the clinician must be aware that poor performance on these tasks does not guarantee that the patient has apraxia of speech. Aphasic patients, particularly those with paraphasic difficulties, will also have difficulty with these tasks. Accordingly, an accurate diagnosis must be based on careful observation of the behaviors that are elicited by these tasks. Table 6.1 contains a list of behaviors included in the *Apraxia Battery for Adults* (Dabul, 1979). Dabul suggests that if five or more of the behaviors listed in Table 6.1 are present, apraxia of speech can be identified and that the more behaviors present, the greater the severity of the disorder. However, only two of these behaviors—intrusion of the schwa sound and abnormal prosody—can be confidently allocated exclusively to apraxia (versus aphasia; see also McNeil et al. 1997). Others (e.g., receptive-expressive gap) can be characteristic of patients with apraxia but also of those with paraphasic difficulties. Still others (e.g., highly inconsistent errors) are more characteristic of paraphasic than apraxic speakers.

Table 6.1
Inventory of Articulation Characteristics of Apraxia

The subject exhibits phonemic anticipatory errors (*gl*een glass for *gr*een glass)
The subject exhibits phonemic perseverative errors (boo*b* for boo*th*)
The subject exhibits phonemic transposition errors (A*rif*ca for A*fri*ca)
The subject exhibits phonemic voicing errors (*b*en for *p*en)
The subject exhibits phonemic vowel errors (m*o*an for m*a*n)
The subject exhibits visible and audible searching
The subject exhibits numerous and varied off-target attempts at the word
The subject's errors are highly inconsistent
The subject's errors increase as phonemic sequence increases
The subject exhibits fewer errors in automatic speech than in volitional speech
The subject exhibits marked difficulty initiating speech
The subject intrudes a schwa sound /ə/ between syllable or in consonant clusters
The subject exhibits abnormal prosodic features
The subject exhibits awareness of errors and inability to correct them
The subject exhibits a receptive-expressive gap

Note. From *Apraxia Battery for Adults* (p. 12), by B. Dabul, 1979, Austin, TX: PRO-ED. Copyright 1979 by PRO-ED, Inc. Reprinted with permission.

Therefore, an uncritical tallying of error behaviors cannot ensure the presence of apraxia of speech. In addition to the two behaviors identified above, if the clinician identifies audible and/or visual groping for articulatory positions and movements (as compared to juggling of sounds until the correct one is retrieved) and a pattern of perceived substitutions that are close to the targets and relatively consistent and predictable, then this would increase the probability that apraxia is contributing to the patient's errors.

Treatment

Much has been written about treating apraxia of speech. When the apraxia is severe, the goal for treatment is the production of speech sounds in isolation, syllables, and words. If the patient is successful in producing sounds simply by imitating the clinician's verbal productions, then imitation can be considered the preferred technique. The eight-step continuum suggested by Rosenbek, Lemme, Ahern, Harris, and Wertz (1973) leads the patient from the production of speech by imitation to more spontaneous use of speech in role-playing situations. Deal and Florance (1978) suggest that the difficulty experienced by some patients, particularly with the middle steps in the eight-step continuum, can be alleviated by using an accumulative measure for reaching criteria at the lower steps before progressing to higher steps. Presumably, this accumulative measure provides the patient with a greater number of correct and stable responses in the early stages before moving on. Dabul and Bollier (1976) also outline an imitative approach, although they emphasize nonmeaningful speech movements for improving the sequencing of speech movements. These authors suggest that individual consonants should be trained in isolation and that the vowel /a/ should be added to the trained consonant to form syllables. Finally, the syllables are combined into sequences and words. Dabul and Bollier recommend nonmeaningful stimuli, reasoning that apraxic speakers need to learn movement patterns that can be applied to difficult words by using a sound-by-sound procedure.

When imitative approaches are not successful, other techniques can be tried. One technique is to substitute another stimulus for an auditory one or to combine an auditory stimulus with another type of stimulus. For example, some patients can produce words more accurately when reading Collins, Cariski, Longstretch, and Rosenbek (1980), and Simmons (1980) reported a case of a blind apraxic speaker whose verbal production improved when auditory and tactile (Braille) stimuli were combined.

When treating severe apraxia, direct techniques may be needed. Wertz et al. (1984) suggest phonetic derivation; that is, observing the speech or nonspeech movements produced by the speaker and modifying them to form specific sounds. For example, humming can be used to generate voiced sounds, and placing the tongue behind the upper teeth and producing a clicking sound can lead to the production of /t/. A technique that is often coupled with derivation is phonetic placement, in which the clinician uses visual stimuli and describes and demonstrates how sounds are made in the mouth. In addition, the clinician manually manipulates the patient's articulators to achieve appropriate positions and movements. Square, Chumpelik, Morningstar, and Adams (1986) report success with a phonetic placement technique, the PROMPT system, used with adult apraxic patients. PROMPT stands for Prompts for Restructuring Oral Muscular Phonetic Targets and was developed by Chumpelik (1984) for use with developmentally apraxic children. It is a tactile-based program that employs a highly structured set of finger placements on the patient's face and neck to represent oral positions. These finger placements provide feedback to help the patient determine a target position toward which to move and, in addition, can cue aspects of production such as duration, continuance, and tongue tension. Chumpelik states that these placements can facilitate movements between phonemes in connected speech by chaining a series of prompts. The clinician can cue the position for each sound or for one sound that represents the primary target positions in a word. Square et al. (1986) report that their adult apraxic patients also improved their production of sounds in multisyllable words and short sentences with the use of PROMPT. Freed, Marshall, and Frazier (1997) report on a single severely apraxic patient who learned to produce a core vocabulary of 30 words over a 41-week period using PROMPT. Although no generalization to untrained target words occurred during the study, the patient's family reported that he also began producing another 10 to 12 untreated nontarget words in appropriate contexts.

Stevens and Glaser (1983) describe Multiple Input Phoneme Therapy for severely impaired patients who demonstrated an inability to imitate speech. In this program, the clinician uses whatever spontaneous output the patient provides (typically an involuntary utterance) and turns it into a voluntary utterance. The clinician "inputs" (verbally produces) the utterance, and the patient is allowed to imitate the clinician's input only upon request. After the patient imitates the clinician accurately, the clinician inputs additional words beginning with phonemes that were present in the original utterance. For example, if the patient involuntarily produces the word *one*, the clinician would produce words such as *wash, win, wet, walk, white, up, us, no, new, night,* and *nose*. Following successful completion of the Multiple Input Phoneme Therapy tasks, other tasks are used to strengthen the patient's volitional use of words and phrases (see Wertz et al., 1984, for examples of these tasks). Both PROMPT and Multiple Input Phoneme Therapy are discussed in Square-Storer (1989).

Melodic Intonation Therapy (MIT) is a procedure that has been recommended for use with patients who have good comprehension but very limited verbal output. It emphasizes the melodic pattern of a phrase or sentence; the patient is required to tap out the rhythm and intone or sing the words of the phrase or sentence. Subsequent steps in the program are used to shape these productions into natural speech. The procedure for MIT was outlined by Sparks and Holland (1976) and Sparks and Deck (1994). Several investigators have reported success with MIT after modifying the program (Dunham & Newhoff, 1979; Hyland & McNeil, 1987; Marshall & Holtzapple, 1976).

Unfortunately, functional speech is not an attainable goal for all patients, and for some it is necessary to consider nonverbal avenues of communication. These can range from gestural systems such as American Indian Sign (Amer-Ind; Skelly, 1979) and finger spelling to language boards and electronic communication devices. Some nonverbal techniques have been used with success and some have not. It is important to recognize that the value of these nonverbal systems depends on whether a patient can use them successfully after leaving the treatment session. Of course the nature and extent of a patient's medical condition, and the presence and severity of aphasia, will have an impact on this process. The interested reader is referred to Hux, Beukelman, and Garrett (1994); Rao (1994); and Yorkston and Waugh (1989) for information concerning the use of nonverbal communication systems with aphasic and apraxic individuals.

For treatment of moderate apraxia of speech, Wertz et al. (1984) discuss imitating contrasts. This involves imitating target consonants in a variety of vowel contexts (e.g., contrasting *pet* and *pat*) and imitating target consonants in contrast to other consonants (e.g., contrasting *sigh* with *tie*). The degree of similarity between the contrasting phonemes can be manipulated to increase or decrease the difficulty of the task. Wertz et al. also discuss the use of contrastive stress drills. In these exercises, the patient produces target sentences several times, varying the location of the primary stress in the sentence by either imitation or answering questions.

A series of single case studies has been presented recently by Wambaugh and her colleagues that evaluates the effect of traditional treatment on patients with chronic aphasia and moderate or severe apraxia of speech. Wambaugh, Kalinyak-Fliszar, West, and Doyle (1998) treated three patients using minimal contrast pairs (comparing the target sound with the sound most frequently substituted for it) supported by cuing based on integral stimulation, modeling with the use of silent junctures, and articulatory placement cues. With the exception of /ç/ in word-final position, the three subjects showed significant improvement in the targeted sounds in both words that were treated and not treated. However, generalization to untreated sounds was minimal. Generalization to other stimuli (phrases and oral reading tasks) was variable; however, no treatment effort was devoted to promoting this generalization. Maintenance of these gains at a 6-week follow-up was quite good, although a slight decrement in performance was noted.

A different case study (Wambaugh, Martinez, McNeil, & Rogers, 1999) of an individual who had severe apraxia of speech demonstrated considerably more difficulty maintaining his gains. He tended to overgeneralize newly trained sounds to words containing previously trained sounds (reducing their accuracy during the maintenance stage). By subsequently training both the new and the previous sounds together, the patient's prior level of accuracy was reestablished.

In contrast to treating individual sounds, Wambaugh, West, and Doyle (1998) treated one subject on the production of three groups of sounds (stops, fricatives, and glides/liquids). The subject was able to produce all of the target sounds correctly in single words. Treatment involved producing short sentences that contained more than one sound from the targeted class (e.g., *Sue fills the vase.*). Improvement was seen for all three sound groups on both trained and untrained words. Maintenance was good; however, generalization across sounds groups was minimal.

Pairing speech with another activity such as gestures (Rosenbek, Collins, & Wertz, 1976), tapping, using a pacing board (Helm, 1979), or finger counting (Simmons, 1978) has been reported as successful for some patients with moderate apraxia of speech. However, pairing verbal and gesture training with a severely apraxic patient improved his ability to produce target sounds during repetition but not oral reading (Raymer & Thompson, 1991). As patients begin to increase the accuracy of their verbal productions, the paired activity can be phased out. In addition, instructing moderately apraxic patients to prolong their speech and reduce their rate has led to improvement (Southwood, 1987). Dworkin, Abkarian, and Johns (1988) reported that an apraxic patient's speech improved when a hierarchy of nonspeech and articulatory tasks was paced using a metronome.

Wertz et al. (1984) provide several suggestions for treating the mildly apraxic patient. These include introducing a faster rate of speech, imposing increasingly longer delays, and providing a decreasing amount of assistance from the clinician. Tasks can be made more difficult by requiring the production of infrequently occurring words and by introducing unfamiliar topics. The responses required can range from answering simple questions and discussing familiar topics to participating in conversation and discussing unfamiliar topics. Oral reading tasks are also useful for treating the mildly apraxic patient. Finally, strengthening the patient's ability to self-monitor and correct errors is essential.

Case Study

 APRAXIA OF SPEECH

M.W. was a 65-year-old male who, in May 1984, suffered a left hemisphere stroke that resulted in a mild right hemiparesis and aphasia. Due to recurring medical complications, M.W. received only 2 or 3 months of speech–language therapy during the first year post onset. In September 1985, approximately 16 months post stroke, he began speech–language therapy at the Kent State University Speech and Hearing Clinic.

Results of an initial evaluation with the *Boston Diagnostic Aphasia Examination* (BDAE; Goodglass & Kaplan, 1983) revealed that M.W. was performing at the 80th percentile on the auditory and graphic subtests and at the 20th percentile on the verbal tasks. Oral apraxia was identified. His speech was limited to production of the syllable /ma/. M.W. also displayed a mild to moderate Broca's aphasia; he had difficulty in thought organization and a mild deficit in auditory and visual comprehension. His primary communication deficit was a severe apraxia of speech.

Oral motor tasks were introduced to increase agility of the oral musculature. Speech tasks included verbal imitation of vowels to initiate voicing and the use of integral (auditory plus visual) stimulation for consonant production in CV combinations beginning with the bilabial stops. Writing (of functional words and phrases) and gestures (specifically Amer-Ind) were incorporated into the therapeutic regimen as functional means of communication and as aids to increasing verbal output.

M.W.'s communicative ability was reevaluated in January 1986. The *Communicative Abilities in Daily Living* (CADL; Holland, 1980) was administered. Communication was primarily through writing, pointing, and the production of one-word verbal responses. Humor, reading, writing, sequential relationships, and calculation all were within the normal range of performance.

Treatment tasks focused on increasing the accuracy and consistency of production of bilabials at the word and phrase level, and on increasing nasal and fricative production in CV and CVC combinations using imitation with and without integral stimulation. Self-cuing strategies that were successful in initiating functional speech production included writing and preposturing of the articulators. M.W. was encouraged to use these cues to initiate spontaneous speech. He also was encouraged to transfer his written functional phrases to speech. The clinician asked M.W. questions or instructed the patient to request or provide information.

Reevaluation of the patient's communication skills with the *Minnesota Test for the Differential Diagnosis of Aphasia* (Schnell, 1965) at 24 months post onset in May 1986 revealed that M.W. produced intelligible one- and two-word utterances. Treatment tasks at this time focused on continuing to increase articulatory accuracy of words and phrases through integral stimulation with particular emphasis on fricatives. A task aimed at prolonging vowels was implemented to improve sound and syllable transitions. Stress and intonation drills, with accompanying visual cuing on words to be stressed, were introduced to attempt to improve his verbal communication.

Administration of the BDAE in December 1986, at 31 months post onset, revealed that M.W. produced three- and four-word utterances with labored, halting production and exaggerated articulatory postures. Blends, affricates, and some fricatives were consistently misarticulated (primarily distortions). An imitation task with visual cues was used to expand M.W.'s functional utterances. Placement cues, integral stimulation, and imitation alone were used to increase articulatory accuracy of affricates and fricatives in CV combinations and words.

Informal evaluation of M.W.'s apraxia in October 1987 (41 months post onset) yielded labored productions of five-word verbal utterances with frequent problems related to initiation and oral posturing. Therapy focused on increasing the accuracy of /ʂ/ and affricates in words and simple sentences through imitation. A task aimed at improving the rhythmic production of utterances was introduced to elicit a more automatic manner of production while speaking. The task used an "MIT-like" approach, using hand tapping during the production of six- and seven-word utterances.

At the termination of treatment, M.W. still had difficulty with speech initiation and accuracy of some sounds. Speech naturalness was reduced with a halting quality. However, he was communicating verbally with both family and non–family members.

Treatment for Paraphasias

In contrast to the wealth of information that exists for treating apraxia of speech, there is far less information concerning the treatment of paraphasic errors. This is understandable in that treatment for apraxia is direct and lends itself to the formulation of specific programs and procedures. Treating paraphasias is more indirect, and there are few, if any, procedures specific to the disorder.

Paraphasias come from breakdowns in the retrieval of phonological information and the mapping of that information into syllabic slots. These errors are subsequently produced with minimal articulatory disruption. Paraphasias typically occur in patients with Wernicke's and conduction aphasia. Those patients with better auditory comprehension skills often recognize their errors and may attempt to self-correct them. Particularly for patients with conduction aphasia, these attempts may lead them closer to the target, and eventual success is not uncommon.

Improving auditory comprehension is an important focus of treatment for paraphasic speakers. As comprehension improves, it seems that the phonological encoding system improves. Errors become less frequent and less severe. Productions become closer to the target and are more easily identifiable by the listener. In addition, improved comprehension facilitates the self-monitoring of errors, which can lead to successful self-correction.

Although imitation is often used successfully in treating apraxia of speech, this approach is not the best for treating paraphasic errors. Patients with paraphasic errors often produce more errors on imitation than on spontaneous speech tasks. In fact, the repetition impairment typically is viewed as the hallmark of conduction aphasia. Imitation also reduces patients' ability to self-correct errors. Because imitation plays such a small role in normal daily communication, it makes more sense during treatment sessions to emphasize patients' strengths (spontaneous speech) rather than weaknesses (imitation). This is not to say that patients should not repeat their responses several times, especially if it contains an error. This type of repetition is beneficial for most patients, although potentially frustrating as well. What should be minimized is asking patients to imitate something that has been presented only through the auditory channel. It is better for the response to be elicited in some other manner, such as oral reading, answering questions, completing sentences, naming, describing pictures, and discussion. The severity of the aphasia will dictate the type and level of tasks that are appropriate. For example, Boyle (1989) reported a decrease in the number of phonemic paraphasias in a patient following a treatment program of structured oral reading tasks. Similar results were presented for a patient with conduction aphasia using sentence-level oral reading tasks with imposed delays (Sullivan, Fisher, & Marshall, 1986).

Because apraxia of speech is considered a speech motor control disorder that can occur along with various linguistic deficits, it is generally treated independently of the other deficits. In contrast, paraphasias are typically an integral part of a larger language disorder characterized by deficits in comprehension, word retrieval, thought formulation, and writing. Therefore, treatment focuses on language impairment, and the paraphasia problem is handled indirectly. Because it is difficult to predict which words will be subjected to paraphasic error, treatment tasks should reflect variables that influence other aspects of the patient's performance. For example, variables that influence the accuracy of word retrieval, sentence formulation, or thought organization ability should guide the construction of the task. It is not uncommon for the visual input modality to be less impaired than the auditory input modality in patients with paraphasic errors. The clinician can capitalize on this difference by using visual along with auditory cues during auditory input tasks. As a paraphasia occurs, the patient can attempt to correct the error, then move on. A technique for reducing paraphasic intrusions in some patients involves instructing the patient to think of or write the first letter of a word or the entire word to be produced. As other language skills improve, the number of paraphasias should decrease and the patient's ability to self-correct should increase.

It is important that successful communication be emphasized more and that phonemic accuracy be emphasized less. Patients should be encouraged to value the successful communication of a message even though it might contain a paraphasic error. Similarly, listeners should be counseled to appreciate the meaning of a patient's verbal message and not to demand phonemic accuracy. The listener can learn to use context to facilitate his or her comprehension of the speaker's message. For additional insights into treating paraphasic speakers, the reader is referred to Marshall (1994) and Simmons-Mackie (1997).

Case Study

Paraphasia

V.H. suffered a stroke in January 1997 and was first seen by this author on February 4, 1997, through the auspices of home health care. V.H. demonstrated a severe conduction aphasia. She demonstrated extensive phonemic paraphasias that caused both real and nonreal word substitutions. She scored 4/60 on the *Boston Naming Test* (BNT; Kaplan, Goodglass, & Weintraub, 1983). Word imitation for common words was 40% accurate. Oral reading of common words was 60% accurate. She scored 8/43 and 10/44 on spoken and written modified versions of the *Peabody Picture Vocabulary Test–Revised* (PPVT–R; Dunn & Dunn, 1981), respectively. She scored 5/10 on the sentence reading subtest (VI) of the *Reading Comprehension Battery for Aphasia* (RCBA; LaPointe & Horner, 1979). When asked to verbally describe the *Cookie Theft Card*, V.H. could not provide any units of content (nouns, verbs, etc.) successfully. Her family indicated that they could understand less than 20% of what V.H. tried to convey verbally.

Treatment was conducted twice per week with plenty of homework involving reading comprehension and writing tasks. Treatment sessions emphasized traditional tasks of naming, oral reading, responding to simple questions, describing pictured activities, and reading comprehension. In addition, because sessions were held in V.H.'s home, many treatment activities involved items within her apartment and aspects of her favorite activities (e.g., shopping, cooking, sewing, quilting). The difficulty level of the stimuli used in these tasks was increased as V.H.'s performance improved. Throughout all of these tasks, attention was devoted to the paraphasic intrusions. When errors occurred, V.H. was alerted to the error (although most of the time she was able to accurately self-monitor these errors), allowed the opportunity to try the word again, and cued as needed (with a verbal model and written word cues). If she was not able to produce the word correctly after a couple of attempts, we moved on to the next item.

By July, V.H. had made good progress in all aspects of treatment. Her score on the BNT was 21. She scored 16 and 20 on the auditory and reading versions of the modified PPVT–R, respectively. She scored 8/10 on the sentence subtest of the RCBA and 4/10 on the short paragraph subtest (which she couldn't attempt during the evaluation). When describing the *Cookie Theft Card*, she produced 4 units of content that were accurate and free of paraphasic intrusion. Functionally, V.H. was relatively successful reading the *TV Guide*, some basic recipes, and short bits from the newspaper. She was able to converse about familiar topics (where she went for dinner, what activities her family was involved with, what she watched on TV). She began asking questions in addition to answering them. Although her utterances were not free of paraphasic errors, content was much higher and words that were in error were more identifiable. She was able to convey her ideas successfully approximately 50% of the time. V.H. was much more accurate at self-monitoring her paraphasic errors, and her ability to correct them increased to about 40%. Her family stated that they could converse more with V.H. and greatly appreciated this ability to interact with her. Unfortunately, V.H. had another massive stroke and treatment was never resumed.

Acknowledgment

The author acknowledges the assistance of Dr. Monica Strauss on portions of this chapter.

References

Abbs, J. (1986). Invariance and variability in speech production: A distinction between linguistic intent and its neuromotor implementation. In J. Perkell & D. Klatt (Eds.), *Invariance and variability in speech processes* (pp. 202–225). Hillsdale, NJ: Erlbaum.

Anderson, J., Gilmore, R., Roper, S., Crosson, B., Bauer, R., Nadeau, S., Beversdorf, D., Cibula, J., Rogish III, M., Kortencamp, S., Hughes, J., Gonzalez-Rothi, L., & Heilman, K. (1999). Conduction aphasia and the arcuate fasciculus: A reexamination of the Wernicke-Geschwind model. *Brain and Language, 70,* 1–12.

Beland, R., Caplan, D., & Nespoulous, J. (1990). The role of abstract phonological representations in word production: Evidence from phonemic paraphasias. *Journal of Neurolinguistics, 5,* 125–164.

Borden, G. (1979). An interpretation of research on feedback interruption in speech. *Brain and Language, 7,* 307–319.

Boyle, M. (1989). Reducing phonemic paraphasias in the connected speech of a conduction aphasic subject. In T. Prescott (Ed.), *Clinical aphasiology* (pp. 379–394). Austin, TX: PRO-ED.

Brennen, T., David, D., Fluchaire, I., & Pellat, J. (1996). Naming faces and objects without comprehension: A case study. *Cognitive Neuropsychology, 13,* 93–110.

Buckingham, H. (1992). Phonological deficits in conduction aphasia. In S. Kohn (Ed.), *Conduction aphasia* (pp. 77–116). Hillsdale, NJ: Erlbaum.

Butterworth, B. (1979). Hesitation and the production of verbal paraphasias and neologisms in jargon aphasia. *Brain and Language, 18,* 133–161.

Butterworth, B. (1992). Disorders of phonological encoding. *Cognition, 42,* 261–286.

Canter, G., Trost, J., & Burns, M. (1985). Contrasting speech patterns in apraxia of speech and phonemic paraphasias. *Brain and Language, 24,* 204–222.

Caplan, D. (1987). Phonological representation in word production. In E. Keller & M. Gopnik (Eds.), *Motor and sensory processes of language* (pp. 111–124). Hillsdale, NJ: Erlbaum.

Caplan, D., & Waters, G. (1992). Issues arising regarding the nature and consequences of reproduction conduction aphasia. In S. Kohn (Ed.), *Conduction aphasia* (pp. 117–149). Hillsdale, NJ: Erlbaum.

Caramazza, A., & Hillis, A. (1990). Where do semantic errors come from? *Cortex, 26,* 95–122.

Chumpelik, D. (1984). The prompt system of therapy: Theoretical framework and applications for developmental apraxia of speech. *Seminars in Speech and Language, 5,* 139–156.

Coleman, J. (1998). Cognitive reality and the phonological lexicon: A review. *Journal of Neurolinguistics, 11,* 295–320.

Collins, M., Cariski, D., Longstretch, D., & Rosenbek, J. (1980). Patterns of articulatory behavior in selected motor speech programming disorders. In R. Brookshire (Ed.), *Clinical aphasiology* (pp. 196–208). Minneapolis, MN: BRK.

Dabul, B. (1979). *Apraxia Battery for Adults.* Austin, TX: PRO-ED.

Dabul, B., & Bollier, B. (1976). Therapeutic approaches to apraxia. *Journal of Speech and Hearing Disorders, 41,* 268–276.

Darley, F., Aronson, A., & Brown, J. (1975). *Audio seminars in speech pathology: Motor speech disorders.* Philadelphia: Saunders.

Deal, J., & Florance, C. (1978). Modification of the eight-step continuum for treatment of apraxia of speech in adults. *Journal of Speech and Hearing Research, 43,* 89–95.

Dell, G. (1986). A spreading activation theory of retrieval in sentence production. *Psychological Review, 93,* 283–321.

Dell, G. (1988). The retrieval of phonological forms in production: Tests of predictions from a connectionist model. *Journal of Memory and Language, 27,* 124–142.

Dell, G., & O'Seaghdha, P. (1991). Mediated and convergent lexical priming in language production: A comment on Levelt et al. (1991). *Psychological Review, 98,* 604–614.

Dell, G., & O'Seaghdha, P. (1992). Stages of lexical access in language production. *Cognition, 42,* 287–314.

Dell, G., Schwartz, M., Martin, N., Saffran, E., & Gagnon, D. (1997). Lexical access in aphasic and nonaphasic speakers. *Psychological Review, 104,* 801–838.

Duffy, J. (1995). *Motor speech disorders: Substrates, differential diagnosis, and management.* St. Louis, MO: Mosby.

Dunham, M., & Newhoff, M. (1979). Melodic intonation therapy: Rewriting the song. In R. Brookshire (Ed.), *Clinical aphasiology* (pp. 286–294). Minneapolis: BRK Publishers.

Dunn, L., & Dunn, L. (1981). *Peabody Picture Vocabulary Test–Revised.* Circle Pines, MN: American Guidance Service.

Dworkin, J., Abkarian, G., & Johns, D. (1988). Apraxia of speech: The effectiveness of a treatment regimen. *Journal of Speech and Hearing Disorders, 53,* 280–294.

Folkins, J., & Abbs, J. (1976). Additional observations on responses to resistive loading of the jaw. *Journal of Speech and Hearing Research, 19,* 820–831.

Freed, D., Marshall, R., & Frazier, K. (1997). Long-term effectiveness of PROMPT treatment in a severely apractic-aphasic speaker. *Aphasiology, 11,* 365–372.

Friedrich, F., Glenn, C., & Marin, O. (1984). Interruption of phonological coding in conduction aphasia. *Brain and Language, 22,* 266–291.

Gagnon, D., Schwartz, M., Martin, N., Dell, G., & Saffran, E. (1997). The origins of formal paraphasias in aphasics' picture naming. *Brain and Language, 59,* 450–472.

Goodglass, H., & Kaplan, E. (1983). *Boston Diagnostic Aphasia Examination.* Baltimore: Williams & Wilkins.

Goodglass, J., Wingfield, A., & Ward, S. (1999). Decision latencies for phonological and semantic information in object identification. *Brain and Language, 66,* 294–305.

Gracco, V. (1995). Central and peripheral components in the control of speech movements. In F. Bell-Berti & L. Rafhael (Eds.), *Producing speech: Contemporary issues* (pp. 417–431). New York: AIP Press.

Gracco, V., & Lofquist, A. (1994). Speech motor coordination and control: Evidence from lip, jaw, and laryngeal movements. *Journal of Neuroscience, 14,* 6585–6597.

Harley, T. (1993). Phonological activation of semantic competitors during lexical access in speech production. *Language and Cognitive Processes, 8,* 291–309.

Harley, T., & MacAndrew, S. (1992). Modeling paraphasias in normal and aphasic speech. In *Proceedings of the 14th Annual Conference of the Cognitive Science Society* (pp. 378–383). Hillsdale, NJ: Erlbaum.

Helm, N. (1979). Management of palilalia with a pacing board. *Journal of Speech and Hearing Disorders, 44,* 350–353.

Hillis, A., & Caramazza, A. (1995). Converging evidence for the interaction of semantic and sublexical phonological information in accessing lexical representations for spoken output. *Cognitive Neuropsychology, 12,* 187–227.

Holland, A. (1980). *Communicative abilities in daily living.* Austin, TX: PRO-ED.

Hough, M., & Klich, R. (1998). Lip EMG activity during vowel production in apraxia of speech: Phrase context and word length effects. *Journal of Speech, Language, and Hearing Research, 41,* 786–801.

Hughes, O., & Abbs, J. (1976). Labial-mandibular coordination in the production of speech: Implications for the operation of motor equivalence. *Phonetica, 44,* 199–221.

Hux, K., Beukelman, D., & Garrett, K. (1994). Augmentative and alternative communication for persons with aphasia. In R. Chapey (Ed.), *Language intervention strategies in adult aphasia* (3rd ed., pp. 338–358). Baltimore: Williams & Wilkins.

Hyland, J., & McNeil, M. (1987). The effects of an intoning therapy on the speech of a developmentally apraxic adult. In R. Brookshire (Ed.), *Clinical aphasiology* (pp. 288–299). Minneapolis: BRK.

Kaplan, E., Goodglass, H., & Weintraub, S. (1983). *The Boston Naming Test.* Philadelphia: Lea & Febiger

Keller, E. (1987). The cortical representation of motor processes of speech. In E. Keller & M. Gopnik (Eds.), *Motor and sensory processes of language* (pp. 125–162). Hillsdale, NJ: Erlbaum.

Kent, R., Adams, S., & Turner, G. (1996). Models of speech production. In N. Lass (Ed.), *Principles of experimental phonetics* (pp. 3–45). St. Louis, MO: Mosby.

Kent, R., & Rosenbek, J. (1982). Prosodic disturbance and neurological lesion. *Brain and Language, 15,* 259–291.

Kent, R., & Rosenbek, J. (1983). Acoustic patterns of apraxia of speech. *Journal of Speech and Hearing Research, 26,* 231–248.

Klich, R., Ireland, J., & Weidner, W. (1979). Articulatory and phonological aspects of consonant substitutions in apraxia of speech. *Cortex, 15,* 451–470.

Kohn, S. (1989). The nature of the phonemic string deficit in conduction aphasia. *Aphasiology, 3,* 209–240.

Kohn S., & Smith, K. (1994a). Distinctions between two phonological output deficits. *Applied Psycholinguistics, 15,* 75–95.

Kohn, S., & Smith, K. (1994b). Evolution of impaired access to the phonological lexicon. *Journal of Neurolinguistics, 8,* 267–288.

Kohn, S., & Smith, K. (1995). Serial effects of phonemic planning during word production. *Aphasiology, 9,* 209–222.

Kohn, S., Smith, K., & Alexander, M. (1996). Differential recovery from impairment to the phonological lexicon. *Brain and Language, 52,* 129–149.

Kuehn, D., Lemme, M., & Baumgartner, J. (1989). *Neural bases of speech, hearing, and language.* Boston: College-Hill.

LaPointe, L., & Horner, J. (1979). *Reading Comprehension Battery for Aphasia.* Austin, TX: PRO-ED.

Levelt, W. (1989). *Speaking: From intention to articulation.* Cambridge, MA: MIT Press.

Levelt, W. (1992). Accessing words in speech production: Stages, processes and representations. *Cognition, 42,* 1–22.

Levelt, W., & Wheeldon, L. (1994). Do speakers have access to a mental syllabary? *Cognition, 50,* 239–269.

Marquardt, T., & Cannito, M. (1996). Treatment of verbal apraxia in Broca's aphasia. In G. Wallace (Ed.), *Adult aphasia rehabilitation* (pp. 205–228). Boston: Butterworth-Heinemann.

Marshall, R. (1994). Management of fluent aphasic clients. In R. Chapey (Ed.), *Language intervention strategies in adult aphasia* (3rd ed., pp. 389–406). Baltimore: Williams & Wilkins.

Marshall, R., & Holtzapple, P. (1976). Melodic intonation therapy: Variations on a theme. In R. Brookshire (Ed.), *Clinical aphasiology* (pp. 115–141). Minneapolis, MN: BRK.

Martin, N., Dell, G., Saffran, E., & Schwartz, M. (1994). Origins of paraphasias in deep dysphasia: Testing the consequences of a decay impairment to an interactive spreading activation model of lexical retrieval. *Brain and Language, 47,* 609–660.

Martin, N., & Saffran, E. (1992). A computational account of deep dysphasia: Evidence from a single case study. *Brain and Language, 43,* 240–274.

Martin, N., Saffran, E., & Dell, G. (1996). Recovery in deep dysphasia: Evidence for a relation between auditory-verbal STM capacity and lexical errors in repetition. *Brain and Language, 52,* 83–113.

McNeil, M., Hashi, M., & Southwood, H. (1994). Acoustically derived perceptual evidence for coarticulatory errors in apraxic and conduction aphasic speech production. *Clinical Aphasiology, 22,* 203–218.

McNeil, M., Odell, K., Miller, S., & Hunter, L. (1995). Consistency, variability, and target approximation for successive speech repetitions among apraxic, conduction aphasic, and ataxic dysarthric speakers. *Clinical Aphasiology, 23,* 39–55.

McNeil, M., Robin, D., & Schmidt, R. (1997). Apraxia of speech: Definition, differentiation, and treatment. In M. McNeil (Ed.), *Clinical management of sensorimotor speech disorders* (pp. 311–344). New York: Thieme.

Meyer, A. (1990). The time course of phonological encoding in language production: The encoding of successive syllables of a word. *Journal of Memory and Language, 29,* 524–545.

Meyer, A. (1991). The time course of phonological encoding in language production: Phonological encoding inside a syllable. *Journal of Memory and Language, 30,* 69–89.

Meyer, A. (1992). Investigation of phonological encoding through speech error analyses: Achievements, limitations, and alternatives. *Cognition, 42,* 181–211.

Monoi, H., Fukusako, Y., Itoh, M., & Sasanuma, S. (1983). Speech sound errors in patients with conduction and Broca's aphasia. *Brain and Language, 20,* 175–194.

Naeser, M. (1994). Neuroimaging and recovery of auditory comprehension and spontaneous speech in aphasia with some implications for treatment in severe aphasia. In A. Kerterz (Ed.), *Localization and neuroimaging in neuropsychology* (pp. 245–296). New York: Academic Press.

Nespoulous, J., Joanette, Y., Ska, B., Caplan, D., & Lecours, A. (1987). Production deficits in Broca's and conduction aphasia: Repetition versus reading. In E. Keller & M. Gopnik (Eds.), *Motor and sensory processes of language* (pp. 53–82). Hillsdale, NJ: Erlbaum.

Odell, K., McNeil, M., Rosenbek, J., & Hunter, L. (1990). Perceptual characteristics of consonant productions by apraxic speakers. *Journal of Speech and Hearing Disorders, 55,* 345–359.

Odell, K., McNeil, M., Rosenbek, J., & Hunter, L. (1991). Perceptual characteristics of vowel and prosody production in apraxic, aphasic, and dysarthric speakers. *Journal of Speech and Hearing Research, 34,* 67–80.

Orpwood, L., & Warrington, E. (1995). Word specific impairments in naming and spelling but not reading. *Cortex, 31,* 239–265.

Palumbo, C., Alexander, M., & Naeser, M. (1992). CT scan lesion sites associated with conduction aphasia. In S. Kohn (Ed.), *Conduction aphasia* (pp. 51–76). Hillsdale, NJ: Erlbaum.

Pierce, R. (1991). Apraxia of speech versus phonemic paraphasia: Theoretical, diagnostic, and treatment considerations. In D. Vogel & M. Cannito (Eds.), *Treating disordered speech motor control* (pp. 185–216). Austin, TX: PRO-ED.

Rao, P. (1994). Use of Amer-Ind code by persons with aphasia. In R. Chapey (Ed.), *Language intervention strategies in adult aphasia* (3rd ed., pp. 359–367). Baltimore: Williams & Wilkins.

Raymer, A., & Thompson, C. (1991). Effects of verbal plus gestural treatment in a patient with aphasia and severe apraxia of speech. In T. Prescott (Ed.), *Clinical aphasiology* (pp. 285–298). Austin, TX: PRO-ED.

Rogers, M. (1997). The vowel lengthening exaggeration effect in speakers with aprasia of speech: Compensation, artifact, or primary deficit? *Aphasiology, 11*, 433–446.

Rogers, M., & Storkel, H. (1999). Planning speech one syllable at a time: The reduced buffer capacity hypothesis in apraxia of speech. *Aphasiology, 13*, 793–806.

Rosenbek, J., Collins, M., & Wertz, R. (1976). Intersystemic reorganization in the treatment of apraxia of speech. In R. Brookshire (Ed.), *Clinical aphasiology* (pp. 255–260). Minneapolis, MN: BRK.

Rosenbek, J., Lemme, M., Ahern, M., Harris, E., & Wertz, R. (1973). A treatment for apraxia of speech in adults. *Journal of Speech and Hearing Disorders, 38*, 462–472.

Schnell, H. (1965). *Minnesota Test for Differential Diagnosis of Aphasia*. Minneapolis: University of Minnesota Press.

Seddoh, S., Robin, D., Sim, H., Hageman, C., Moon, J., & Folkins, J. (1996). Speech timing in apraxia of speech versus conduction aphasia. *Journal of Speech and Hearing Research, 39*, 590–603.

Shattuck-Hufnagel, S. (1979). Speech errors as evidence for a serial ordering mechanism in sentence production. In W. Cooper & C. Walker (Eds.), *Sentence processing* (pp. 295–340). Hillsdale, NJ: Erlbaum.

Shattuck-Hufnagel, S. (1983). Sublexical units and suprasegmental structure in speech production planning. In P. MacNeilage (Ed.), *The production of speech* (pp. 109–136). New York: Springer-Verlag.

Shattuck-Hufnagel, S. (1987). The role of word-onset consonants in speech production planning: New evidence from speech error patterns. In E. Keller & M. Gopnik (Eds.), *Motor and sensory processes of language* (pp. 17–52). Hillsdale, NJ: Erlbaum.

Shattuck-Hufnagel, S. (1992). The role of word structure in segmental serial ordering. *Cognition, 42*, 213–259.

Simmons, N. (1978). Finger counting as an intersystemic reorganizer in apraxia of speech. In R. Brookshire (Ed.), *Clinical aphasiology* (pp. 174–179). Minneapolis, MN: BRK.

Simmons, N. (1980). Choice of stimulus modes in treating apraxia of speech: A case study. In R. Brookshire (Ed.), *Clinical aphasiology* (pp. 302–307). Minneapolis, MN: BRK.

Simmons-Mackie, N. (1997). Conduction aphasia. In L. LaPointe (Ed.), *Aphasia and related neurogenic language disorders* (2nd ed., pp. 63–90). New York: Thieme.

Skelly, M. (1979). *Amer-Ind gestural code*. New York: Elsevier.

Southwood, M. (1987). The use of prolonged speech in the treatment of apraxia of speech. In R. Brookshire (Ed.), *Clinical aphasiology* (pp. 277–287). Minneapolis, MN: BRK.

Southwood, M., Dagenais, P., Sutphin S., & Garcia, J. (1997). Coarticulation in apraxia of speech: A perceptual, acoustic, and electropalatographic study. *Clinical Linguistics & Phonetics, 11*, 179–204.

Sparks, R., & Deck, J. (1994). Melodic intonation therapy. In R. Chapey (Ed.), *Language intervention strategies in adult aphasia* (3rd ed., pp. 368–379). Baltimore: Williams & Wilkins.

Sparks, R., & Holland, A. (1976). Method: Melodic intonation therapy. *Journal of Speech and Hearing Disorders, 41*, 287–297.

Square, P., Chumpelik, D., Morningstar, E., & Adams, S. (1986). Efficacy of the PROMPT system of therapy for the treatment of acquired apraxia of speech: A follow-up investigation. In R. Brookshire (Ed.), *Clinical aphasiology* (pp. 221–226). Minneapolis, MN: BRK.

Square, P., & Martin, R. (1994). The nature and treatment of neuromotor speech disorders in aphasia. In R. Chapey (Ed.), *Language intervention strategies in adult aphasia* (3rd ed., pp. 467–499). Baltimore: Williams & Wilkins.

Square-Storer, P. (Ed.). (1989). *Acquired apraxia of speech in aphasic adults.* New York: Taylor and Francis.

Stevens, E., & Glaser, L. (1983). Multiple input phoneme therapy: An approach to severe apraxia and expressive aphasia. In R. Brookshire (Ed.), *Clinical aphasiology* (pp. 148–155). Minneapolis, MN: BRK.

Strand, E., & McNeil, M. (1996). Effects of length and linguistic complexity on temporal acoustic measures in apraxia of speech. *Journal of Speech and Hearing Research, 39,* 1018–1033.

Sullivan, M., Fisher, B., & Marshall, R. (1986). Treating the repetition deficit in conduction aphasia. In R. Brookshire (Ed.), *Clinical aphasiology* (pp. 172–180). Minneapolis, MN: BRK.

Tranel, D., Damasio, H., & Damasio, A. (1997). On the neurology of naming. In H. Goodglass & A. Wingfield (Eds.), *Anomia: Neuroanatomical and cognitive correlates* (pp. 65–90). New York: Academic Press.

Wambaugh, J., Kalinyak-Fliszar, M., West, J., & Doyle, P. (1998). Effects of treatment for sound errors in apraxia of speech and aphasia. *Journal of Speech, Language, and Hearing Research, 41,* 725–743.

Wambaugh, J., Martinez, A., McNeil, M., & Rogers, M. (1999). Sound production treatment for apraxia of speech: Overgeneralization and maintenance effects. *Aphasiology, 13,* 821–838.

Wambaugh, J., West, J., & Doyle, P. (1997). A VOT analysis of apraxic/aphasic voicing errors. *Aphasiology, 11,* 521–532.

Wambaugh, J., West, J., & Doyle, P. (1998). Treatment for apraxia of speech: Effects of targeting sound groups. *Aphasiology, 12,* 731–744.

Wertz, R., LaPointe, L., & Rosenbek, J. (1984). *Apraxia of speech in adults: The disorder and its management.* New York: Grune & Stratton.

Wheeldon, L., & Levelt, W. (1995). Monitoring the time course of phonological encoding. *Journal of Memory and Language, 34,* 311–334.

Yorkston, K., & Waugh, P. (1989). Use of augmentative communication devices with apractic individuals. In P. Square-Storer (Ed.), *Acquired apraxia of speech in aphasic adults* (pp. 267–283). New York: Taylor and Francis.

Ziegler, W., & van Cramon, D. (1985). Anticipatory coarticulation in a patient with apraxia of speech. *Brain and Language, 26,* 117–130.

Ziegler, W., & van Cramon, D. (1986). Disturbed coarticulation in apraxia of speech. *Brain and Language, 29,* 34–47.

Chapter 7

Nature and Management of Acquired Neurogenic Dysfluency

Michael P. Cannito, Jon Deal, and Anthony DiLollo

Cannito, Deal, and DiLollo review existing literature, much of it case studies, on the problem of acquired neurogenic dysfluency. This disorder, although itself heterogeneous, is diagnostically differentiated from developmental stuttering, acquired psychogenic stuttering, and nonfluent aphasia. Potential sites of lesion are considered, and a comprehensive framework for treatment is advanced.

1. *Describe diagnostic considerations for dysfluency in terms of differentiation from other superficially similar disorders and in terms of subcategories within this generic diagnostic label. Why is this differentiation significant for treatment?*

2. *What site(s) of lesion have been posited as underlying the phenomenon of acquired neurogenic dysfluency?*

3. *Outline treatment approaches for acquired neurogenic dysfluency. What kinds of considerations might figure in the selection of one approach as opposed to another?*

❊ ❊ ❊

In the context of this chapter, *neurogenic dysfluency* refers to an onset of dysfluency in adult life that follows, or is associated in some way with, nervous system damage. There are three categories of acquired, adult onset dysfluency. First, the dysfluency may be a form of *occult stuttering*. Van Riper (1971) called this type of dysfluency *interiorized stuttering* and implied that under conditions of great stress, the dysfluency (stuttering) can no longer be hidden. The point is that adult onset of dysfluency may simply be the sudden appearance of stuttering that for years had been hidden or interiorized. This dysfluency is not a new problem; it is simply the sudden appearance of an old problem. If occult, or interiorized, stuttering can be ruled out, there are two other possible etiologies: The dysfluency may be of psychogenic or neurogenic origin.

When occult stuttering has been ruled out, and there has been no demonstrable neurological insult and there are no neurological signs, then the dysfluency may be considered to be of psychogenic origin. Freund (1966) has described this type of dysfluency as a hysterical conversion neurosis. *Psychogenic dysfluency* has been discussed in the literature by a number of authors (Baumgartner & Duffy, 1997; Deal, 1982; Deal & Doro, 1987; Dempsey & Granich, 1978; Helm-Estabrooks & Hotz, 1998; Shapiro, 1999; Wallen, 1961; Weiner, 1981). These reports suggest that dysfluency that is neither developmentally nor neurologically based, occurs in adulthood, is of sudden onset, and is temporally linked to some form of psychological trauma or cumulative psychological stress may be termed psychogenic dysfluency.

There is a third category, *neurogenic dysfluency*, that also occurs in adulthood, may have a rapid onset, and is temporally linked to a demonstrable neurological insult or at least to demonstrable neurological signs. This chapter is concerned with the dysfluency of neurologic origin. The remainder of the chapter will attempt to define the characteristics of neurogenic dysfluency, differentiate neurogenic from other types of dysfluency, identify etiologies of neurogenic dysfluency, differentiate different forms of neurogenic dysfluency, and suggest treatment strategies.

Terminology

There appears to be little consensus on what to call these dysfluencies that begin in adulthood. Terms such as *acquired stuttering, cortical stuttering, neurogenic stuttering*, and *stuttering associated with acquired neurological disorders* will be encountered in any review of the literature on adult onset dysfluency (Baumgartner & Duffy, 1997; Cullata & Goldberg, 1995; Helm-Estabrooks, 1999).

It should be noted that the wording in this chapter's title is "Neurogenic Dysfluency," not "Neurogenic Stuttering." *Dysfluency* is used instead of *stuttering* because there is some question as to the appropriateness of the term *stuttering* used in the context of neurogenic stuttering. Culatta and Leeper (1988) have made a rather eloquent case for not using the term *stuttering* in this context. Their basic premise is that all forms of dysfluency are not stuttering, and they urge that the term *stuttering* be reserved for "that well-defined and researched developmental dysfluency disorder, the causes of which remain unknown" (p. 487). Although much of the literature to be discussed uses the term *stuttering*, *dysfluency* will be substituted whenever possible. As Culatta and Leeper suggest, *dysfluency* may be the more appropriate term because there are differences between neurogenic dysfluency and developmental stuttering. *Dysfluency* may then be used as a descriptor without automatically, and perhaps subconsciously, drawing parallels to developmental stuttering.

By substituting *dysfluency* for *stuttering*, in an effort to avoid confusion with developmental stuttering, another confusion may arise. One of the etiologies associated with neurogenic dysfluency is stroke. Stroke may produce aphasia, and aphasia is often described along a fluent–nonfluent continuum. Thus, a distinction must be made between *dysfluency* and *nonfluency*. Although dysfluency and nonfluency sometimes are regarded as synonymous, they are not. There are persons who demonstrate a nonfluent aphasia and who also demonstrate dysfluency. There are also those individuals who are dysfluent but are not nonfluent. Albert, Goodglass, Helm, Rubens, and Alexander (1981) describe nonfluency as follows: "Nonfluent speech is slow, laboriously produced, with abnormal speech rhythm and melody, poor articulation, shortened phrase length, and preferential use of substantive words (such as nouns and main verbs) rather than grammatical words (such as conjunctions and auxiliary verbs). Nonfluent speech, often called telegraphic or agrammatic, is frequently associated with anteriorly located lesions and is usually a feature of the anterior dysphasias" (pp. 4–5). Dysfluency implies stuttering-like behaviors such as sound and syllable repetitions, stuttering-like blocks, sound prolongations, and other stuttering-like phenomena. Dysfluency does not include articulation disorders, telegraphic speech, or agrammatic speech. Nonfluency implies a linguistic deficit; dysfluency implies a nonlinguistic motor control problem.

Other aphasic symptomatology from which acquired neurogenic dysfluency should be differentiated includes the word-finding pauses and hesitations of anomia as well as reaproachment phenomena, wherein an aphasic patient repeatedly attempts pronunciation of a word, each time generating different phonological errors but progressively approximating the correct production. Although word-finding pauses and reaproachment behaviors are disruptive to the fluidly of speech, their underlying mechanisms are linguistic, and they are part and parcel of the primary aphasia (see Chapter 6 of this volume for discussion).

The Clinical Reality of Neurogenic Dysfluency

There is no question that neurogenic dysfluency occurs. Rather, the question is, Is the dysfluency a clinically distinct and separate disorder, or is it a manifestation of other well-defined clinical syndromes? The literature does not provide an answer that is unambiguous.

Neurogenic dysfluency can occur following a variety of neurological insults, including stroke, head trauma, brain tumor, and certain disease processes, such as Parkinson's disease, dementia, and AIDS. Considering the variety of etiologies, it is unlikely that neurogenic dysfluency is a unitary disorder. Yet there are enough descriptive reports and discussions in the literature to make the case that neurogenic dysfluency occurs as an isolated disorder, without concomitant aphasia, apraxia, or dysarthria. Reading the literature on neurogenic stuttering is like reading the literature on aphasia. Henry Head in 1926 described the literature on aphasia as "chaos." The same may be said of the more recent literature on neurogenic stuttering. Readers are confronted with concepts such as "stuttering in aphasia," "aphasic stuttering," "apraxic stuttering," "dysarthric stuttering," and "isolated stuttering." The conclusion to be drawn is that the dysfluency may be part of a larger clinical entity, or it may be an entity unto itself. A rose by any other name may smell as sweet, but neurogenic stuttering may not be neurogenic stuttering, may not be neurogenic stuttering, may not be neurogenic stuttering, and on and on.

Neurogenic Dysfluency and Aphasia

Luchsinger and Arnold (1965) and Schuell, Jenkins, and Jimenez-Pabon (1964) have pointed out that dysfluency may be present in the evolution of aphasia. This implies a transient phenomenon that is simply part of the natural history of aphasia and that there is nothing particularly unique or interesting about the dysfluency. Others have been more specific about dysfluency and its association with aphasia.

Arend, Handzel, and Weiss (1962), Helm and associates (Helm, Butler, & Benson, 1978; Helm, Butler, & Canter, 1980), and Mazzuchi, Moretti, Carpeggiani, Parma, and Paini (1981) have provided more information about the relationship of dysfluency and aphasia. The following conclusions may be drawn from their reports:

1. Aphasia and dysfluency occur simultaneously, and both persist.
2. Aphasia and dysfluency occur simultaneously, and both are transient.
3. Dysfluency precedes aphasia, but both are transient.
4. Dysfluency precedes aphasia, but the dysfluency is transient and the aphasia persists.
5. Aphasia precedes the dysfluency, but the aphasia is transient and the dysfluency persists.
6. Dysfluency may be an isolated phenomenon, present without aphasia.

There are case reports supporting each of the situations listed.

This state of affairs would not present clinicians with any particular difficulty if we could predict when the dysfluency would persist, if we could predict when the dysfluency would be transient, if we could specify the time domain for "transient," and if we could predict when the dysfluency would persist with or without aphasia. Unfortunately, at this point we are not able to predict the above with any comfortable level of certainty. An additional complication is the theory that the dysfluency is not neurogenic in origin at all; rather, the dysfluency is the result of an emotional reaction to the communication difficulties resulting from the aphasia. Although they do not completely rule this out, Helm et al. (1978) do us the favor of presenting case reports that weaken the theory. They also suggest that dysfluency may persist when the dysfluent patient has difficulty drawing three-dimensional figures, copying block designs, and producing and sustaining sequential motor tasks. Neither of their patients who experienced transient dysfluency had these difficulties, but six of their eight patients with persistent dysfluency did.

Dysfluency as a Component of Speech Motor Disorders

Dysfluency has been shown to be a component of aphasia. It may also be a component of certain motor speech disorders. As Rosenbek (1980) pointed out, van Riper states that "the integrity of a spoken word demands great precision in the timing of its components. When, for any reason, that timing is awry or askew, a temporally distorted word is produced, and when this happens, the speaker has evinced a core of stuttering behavior" (Van Riper, 1971, p. 401). Certainly various motor speech disorders result in the timing of speech production being "awry" and "askew." That being the case, it is no surprise that dysfluency has been a reported feature of speech motor disorders.

Apraxia of Speech

Various investigators note the marked prevalence of stuttering-like dysfluencies in association with articulatory programming problems of apraxia of speech (Johns & Darley, 1970; Trost, 1971; Yairi, Gintautas, & Avent, 1981) often accompanied by Broca's or motor aphasia. In their early observations on this subject, Johns and Darley (1970) noted that patients exhibiting apraxia of speech "as a group, do a creditable job of miming secondary stutterers, both acoustically and behaviorally" (p. 580) by exhibiting circumlocution; word substitution; false starts; anticipatory struggle; blocks; and part word, word, and phrasal repetitions. No other disorder, motor or otherwise, produces such a strong temptation to theorize about stuttering (let alone dysfluency) as does apraxia of speech. The temptation stems from the similarities between apraxia of speech and stuttering. This temptation was too strong for Rosenbek to resist, resulting in an article dealing with the relationship between the two disorders (Rosenbek, 1980).

The problem that arises is that it is tempting to regard stuttering as a form of apraxia of speech. Rosenbek was not able to support that thesis in 1980, and we will not attempt to support it now. We will simply refer clinicians to the literature on apraxia of speech, much of which can be found in the text by Wertz, Rosenbek, and LaPointe (1983).

Dysarthria

Certain forms of dysarthria are associated with dysfunction in neuromuscular substrates intimately involved with the timing of speech production. The hypokinetic dysarthria of Parkinson's disease or other extrapyramidal involvement (Darley, Aronson, & Brown, 1975) has been reported to produce dysfluency as a primary characteristic.

Canter (1971) included a patient with Parkinson's disease when he described characteristics of neurogenic stuttering, and Helm et al. (1980), Helm-Estabrooks (1986, 1999), and Shapiro (1999) also wrote of the dysfluencies associated with Parkinson's disease as neurogenic stuttering. Koller (1983) reported dysfluency associated with Parkinson's disease and other forms of extrapyramidal disease.

Palilalia

Palilalia is a form of motor speech perseveration. It has been described as multiple repetitions of a word, phrase, or sentence in a context of decreasing loudness and increasing rate (Critchley, 1927; LaPointe & Horner, 1981). In an acoustic study, however, Kent and LaPointe (1982) describe a palilalic patient whose reiterant utterances remained fairly uniform across a repetition train. These authors suggest that there may, therefore, be subtypes of palilalic disturbances. Palilalia has been reported in association with numerous neuropathologies, including postencephalitic Parkinson's disease, pseudobulbar palsy, Alzheimer's disease, multiple infarct dementia, and idiopathic cerebral calcinosis (Helm, 1979). Rosenbek (1984) differentiates palilalia from "neurogenic stuttering" on the basis of infrequent syllable repetition in the former but pervasive syllable repetitions in the latter. Helm-Estabrooks (1986) points out that stuttering "involves repetitions, blocks, and prolongation of phonemes" (p. 208), whereas palilalia operates at the whole word/phrase level. Palilalia represents a distinctive subcategory of acquired neurogenic dysfluency (Horner & Massey, 1983).

Neurogenic Dysfluency as a Clinical Entity

The literature contains documentation that dysfluency is a component of aphasia, apraxia of speech, and dysarthria. Other neurogenic speech and language disorders have dysfluency as a component. The communication problems stemming from head injury and right hemisphere strokes also may have dysfluency as a characteristic (Andrews, Quinn, & Sorby, 1972; Horner & Massey, 1983; Lebrun & Leleux, 1985; Quinn & Andrews, 1977; Schiller, 1947). Helm-Estabrooks (1999) also reported on a number of cases in which (acquired) dysfluency was the first sign of progressive neurological disease. This prompted her to emphasize the importance of the early identification of acquired dysfluency and to suggest that "adult onset of stuttering should be considered a potentially positive neurological sign" (p. 265). However, Baumgartner and Duffy (1997), in a review of the literature on neurogenic and psychogenic stuttering, state that acquired dysfluency has "been reported in people with no other communication disorder, or no other clinical or neuroimaging evidence of neurologic disease" (p. 76). Therefore, in the literature cited thus far, and in the literature yet to be discussed, there are sufficient case reports to support the concept of neurogenic dysfluency as a distinct clinical entity, albeit an uncommon one.

Some Evidence of a Neural Substrate for Fluency

Helm-Estabrooks (1999) has emphasized the highly heterogeneous nature of conditions that have been documented to lead to acquired neurogenic dysfluency. She states that damage to the cerebral cortex, basal ganglia, cerebellum, and brainstem have all been associated with the onset of acquired dysfluency. Such diverse lesion site data appear to indicate evidence of a diffusely represented neural substrate for fluency.

To find further evidence of a neural substrate for fluency, we can look to some of the functional brain imaging studies with developmental stutterers. The research group of Pool, Watson, Freeman, and their colleagues performed a series of single photon emission computerized tomography (SPECT) regional cerebral blood flow (rCBF) studies to investigate the neurological aspects of developmental stuttering (Pool, Devous, Freeman, Watson, & Finitzo, 1991; Watson, Pool,

Devous, Freeman, & Finitzo, 1992; Watson et al., 1994). These studies suggest that neurological areas implicated in developmental stuttering are widespread and may include inferior frontal cortex, superior and middle temporal cortex, and anterior cingulate cortex.

Ingham et al. (1996), however, performed a systematic replication of the Pool et al. (1991) study but used the more modern imaging technique of position emission tomography (PET). Subjects for this study were 10 adult males who were diagnosed with chronic developmental stuttering and 19 adult males who did not stutter. The groups were rigorously matched for age and body dominance. All subjects underwent three 40 s PET-acquisition scans and a full-brain MRI scan. MRI data was used to accurately identify regions of interest (ROIs) for each subject. Results indicated a lack of evidence for any functional or anatomical lesions in the brains of men who stutter.

Although the Ingham et al. (1996) resting study failed to replicate the findings by Pool et al. (1991), this same research group (Fox et al., 1996) and others (e.g., Wood, Stump, McKeehan, Sheldon, & Proctor, 1980; Wu et al., 1995) have found widespread brain differences between stutterers and nonstutterers during the performance of speech tasks (i.e., functional-activation studies). These findings suggest that the neural systems of stuttering include a diffuse overactivity of the cerebral and cerebellar motor systems, a right dominance of the cerebral motor system, a lack of normal self-monitoring of activations of left anterior superior temporal phonological circuits, and a deactivation of a verbal fluency circuit between the left frontal and left temporal cortex.

In reviewing brain imaging research on developmental stuttering, Watson and Freeman (1997) concluded that neuroimaging techniques have demonstrated evidence of multifocal anomalous brain functions for speech and language processing in stutterers. This led them to suggest a model of the neural basis of fluency that incorporated cognitive, linguistic, and speech motor components in a widely dispersed fluency generating system. Stuttering, then, could result from a breakdown in any one of these components, or a breakdown in the coordination between components.

DeNil (1999) has also suggested that there is evidence of a "neurophysiological basis of stuttering." He has proposed a diffusely represented fluency generating system, similar to that suggested by Watson and Freeman (1997), taking the position that acquired neurogenic dysfluency and developmental stuttering may represent differential breakdowns of the same system. Results of a PET study by DeNil, Kroll, Kapur, and Houle (2000) appear to present some support for such a model.

The suggestions by Watson and Freeman (1997) and DeNil (1999) of a diffusely represented fluency generating system also appear to be in line with some neurophysiological models of speech production that emphasize a widely distributed neural network subserving fluency. Among such models are those proposed by Fairbanks (1954), Dalton and Hardcastle (1989), and Perkins, Kent, and Curlee (1991). These models suggest that speech is produced by the coordinated interaction of a number of different subsystems that are diffusely represented in the brain. As such, breakdown at any of a number of points within this coordinated system could produce dysfluencies of varying types. Such models appear to fit nicely with the brain imaging data on developmental stuttering, as well as with the lesion data associated with acquired neurogenic dysfluency.

Differential Diagnosis of Acquired Neurogenic Dysfluency

When faced with a patient who presents with the putative diagnosis of acquired dysfluency, clinicians must be able to determine whether the dysfluency is a form of developmental stuttering, psychogenic dysfluency, or neurogenic dysfluency. Differentiating neurogenic dysfluency from developmental stuttering would seem to be a simple task. All we need to do is ask. If the patient denies stuttering as a child, we can assume that the present dysfluency is new and then determine whether it is neurogenic or psychogenic. Unfortunately, as every clinician knows, it is not that simple.

This is not to imply that patients are not truthful. Stuttering has been difficult for professionals to define; thus, it is too much to ask that the patients be even more adept at defining it. A great many people say that they stuttered when they were children but outgrew it. Conversely, a number of people (albeit a smaller number) seem dysfluent, but they would be offended to be called stutterers. Careful questioning of the patient, family, and others who know the patient may well resolve the issue.

To add to the difficulty, several cases have been reported in the literature (e.g., Helm-Estabrooks, 1999) in which childhood stuttering worsened or reappeared with the onset of neuropathology in adulthood. Should these cases be diagnosed and treated as neurogenic dysfluency, or should they be considered aspects of the individual's developmental stuttering? Helm-Estabrooks (1999) proposed a definition of "stuttering associated with acquired neurological disorders" (SAAND) that specifically included both *acquired* and *reacquired* disorders of fluency. At this time, there appears to be little direct research that either supports or challenges such a definition.

Due to the relatively small number of studies that have been published on neurogenic dysfluency, the literature is not as helpful as one would hope. However, some guidelines are available. Canter (1971) listed seven characteristics that he believed differentiated developmental stuttering and neurogenic dysfluency. Making slight modifications to Canter's guidelines, Helm-Estabrooks (1999) proposed a set of six speech behaviors that she believed could be used for the differential diagnosis of "neurogenic stuttering." The characteristics put forward (Helm-Estabrooks, 1999) as guidelines for differential diagnosis are the following:

1. Dysfluencies occur on grammatical words nearly as frequently as on substantive words.

2. The speaker may be annoyed but does not appear anxious.

3. Repetitions, prolongations, and blocks do not occur only on initial syllables of words and utterances.

4. Secondary symptoms such as facial grimmacing, eye blinking, or fist clenching are not associated with moments of disfluency.

5. There is no adaptation effect.

6. Stuttering occurs relatively consistently across various types of speech tasks. (p. 260)

The literature does not support each of these guidelines equally. Market, Montague, Buffalo, and Drummond (1990) collected a large amount of data on neurogenic dysfluency via a questionnaire survey of speech–pathologists throughout the United States. They reported general support for five of the guidelines (guidelines 1–5 as listed above; guideline 6 was not studied) suggested by Helm-Estabrooks (1999), as they found that these behaviors occurred in "relatively high percentage levels" in individuals with neurogenic dysfluency. However, a substantial minority of Market et al.'s (1990) respondents (over 30%) did not support items 2 and 4, suggesting some heterogeniety on these variables. Less than half of the respondents agreed with a lack of adaptation effect (item 5).

In a comprehensive review of the literature on neurogenic dysfluency, Ringo and Dietrich (1995) found support for only four of the guidelines being useful in the differential diagnosis of neurogenic dysfluency versus developmental stuttering. Both Market et al. (1990) and Ringo and Dietrich (1995) found support for the contention that neurogenic dysfluency is characterized by dysfluencies on function words as well as on content words. However, Ringo and Dietrich (1995) point out that many developmental stutterers also produce dysfluencies on function words, and that the case studies presented in the literature do not address the relative frequency of dysfluencies on function words as opposed to substantive words that would be required to support the guideline as stated by Helm-Estabrooks (1999).

Similarly, Ringo and Dietrich (1995) suggest that, despite their finding that a majority of individuals with neurogenic dysfluency will produce at least some non-word-initial dysfluencies, the observed patterns may not be that different from those seen with developmental stutterers, meaning that this aspect of neurogenic dysfluency may not be very useful in differential diagnosis. Ringo and Dietrich found general support for the remaining four guidelines suggested by Helm-Estabrooks, but point out that any conclusions drawn from the current data on neurogenic dysfluency must be considered with caution, as "observations and comparisons are restricted by the lack of detailed data collected in studies of neurogenic stuttering" (p. 118).

It is likely that clinicians will find exceptions to all of these guidelines. As discussed previously, the fact that neurogenic dysfluency is not a unitary disorder means that this population will likely be very heterogeneous in nature. It is important to remember that even though exceptions exist, these guidelines should be considered by clinicians when attempting to differentiate developmental stuttering and neurogenic dysfluency.

Neurogenic Dysfluency Versus Psychogenic Dysfluency

Assuming that developmental stuttering has been ruled out, differentiating between neurogenic and psychogenic dysfluency also would seem to be a simple task. If there are neurological signs and symptoms, or if there is a history of neurological dysfunction, the dysfluency would seem to be neurogenic in origin. If no neurological signs or symptoms are present, the dysfluency would seem to be psychogenic. Again, the clinical reality is not so simple.

Nowack and Stone (1987) reported two cases of acquired dysfluency that suggested neurogenic and psychogenic dysfluency are not mutually exclusive. One patient had an episode of viral meningitis but had no speech symptoms for at least 6 years afterward. She began to experience neurological changes at the same time she was experiencing a series of psychological stresses. She also began to exhibit dysfluencies. When the neurological and the psychological problems resolved, so did the dysfluencies. The second patient suffered a left hemisphere stroke, apparently with aphasia but no stuttering. Several years later, a right hemisphere stroke was followed by persistent stuttering. When she later underwent a series of psychological stresses, the dysfluency was exacerbated.

Attanasio (1987) reported a case of what he considered to be a psychogenic dysfluency; however, his patient also had a history of epilepsy. Similarly, Deal and Doro (1987) described what they felt was a case of episodic, hysterical stuttering; however, their patient had sustained a head trauma 30 years prior to the onset of the dysfluency. It is not always easy to rule out a neurological component.

Baumgartner and Duffy (1997), in a retrospective review of the literature on neurogenic and psychogenic dysfluency, found that 20 out of 69 cases of patients diagnosed with psychogenic dysfluency also had confirmed neurologic disease. Helm-Estabrooks (1999) and Helm-Estabrooks and Hotz (1998) have also reported on several cases where the differentiation between neurogenic and psychogenic dysfluency cannot be made by confirmation of neurologic disease alone.

Consequently, in an attempt to aid differential diagnosis, some researchers have tried to identify features of individuals with neurogenic dysfluency that differentiate them from individuals with psychogenic dysfluency. Deal (1982) proposed eight guidelines for differentiating psychogenic and neurogenic dysfluency:

1. The onset is sudden.

2. The onset is temporally linked to a significant episode(s) of psychological stress.

3. The pattern of dysfluency is primarily repetition of initial or stressed syllables.

4. Dysfluencies are not reduced by choral reading, masking noise, delayed auditory feedback (initially), singing, or different communicative situations.

5. There are no islands of fluency (initially).

6. The patient demonstrates no particular concern about the dysfluency.

7. There are usually no secondary symptoms.

8. The pattern of dysfluency is present during mimed speaking.

Although these guidelines provide a useful description of some of the differentiating characteristics of psychogenic dysfluency, they are not unequivocally supported in the literature. For example, Rentschler, Driver, and Callaway (1984) described a dysfluent patient whose clinical features did not support the lack of masking effect, the lack of concern about the dysfluency, or the apparent dysfluency during mimed reading. Other researchers also have reported anxiety, struggle, and secondary behaviors in selected cases (Lebrun, Leleux, Rousseau, & Devereux, 1983; Nowack & Stone, 1987).

More recently, Baumgartner and Duffy (1997) reviewed cases of psychogenic dysfluency from the literature and identified five features that differentiate psychogenic from neurogenic dysfluency:

1. The rapid and favorable response to behavioral therapy and associated management strategies

2. The presence of oral and nonoral struggle behaviors and other potential signs of anxiety

3. The presence of intermittent, situational, and stimulus-related (reading versus conversation) episodes of stuttering

4. The association of dysfluencies with unusual, pseudo-telegraphic, or agrammatical speech (in patients *without* aphasia)

5. An overall impression of "bizarreness" of the dysfluencies

Like the guidelines provided by Deal (1982), all of these features may not apply to 100% of cases of psychogenic dysfluency. Nevertheless, these are guidelines that clinicians may find helpful when attempting to determine whether dysfluency is of neurogenic or psychogenic origin.

Differentiating Types of Acquired Neurogenic Dysfluency

There is one statement about neurogenic dysfluency that may be difficult to contradict. That is, neurogenic dysfluency is not a unitary disorder. Helm-Estabrooks (1999) states that "neurogenic stuttering is associated with a variety of conditions affecting various areas of the brain, including the cerebral cortex, basal ganglia, cerebellum, and brain stem" (p. 256). Descriptions of neurogenic dysfluency are also not consistent. They vary in terms of the speech characteristics, the appearance with respect to the proposed neurological event(s) associated with the dysfluency, the persistence of the dysfluency, and the proposed neurological etiology. It is often difficult to find order in the literature. Helm-Estabrooks (1986) suggested three major diagnostic groups for neurogenic dysfluency: stroke-induced dysfluency, head trauma-induced dysfluency, and dysfluency with extrapyramidal disease.

Stroke-Induced Dysfluency

Lebrun, Leleux, et al. (1983) estimated that two thirds of the reported cases of neurogenic dysfluency were subsequent to stroke. Aphasia is a frequent sequella of stroke, and dysfluency is often associated with aphasia. Although frequently associated with left hemisphere lesions, dysfluency has been reported for patients with right hemisphere lesions and bilateral lesions as well.

Dysfluency and Vascular Lesions With and Without Aphasia

Single Left Hemisphere Vascular Episodes. Caplan (1972) investigated the dysfluencies of five patients with anomia and apraxia. He felt that the dysfluencies were prominent enough to be called stuttering. Caplan provided a great deal of information about the dysfluencies, but little about the etiology or the course of the dysfluencies. Since he did not elaborate, we have assumed that the five patients had suffered single episode, unilateral left hemisphere stroke, inasmuch as these strokes usually are the culprits when aphasia is present. If our assumption is correct, then Caplan's report is of five patients who had neurogenic dysfluency and aphasia following a single, left hemisphere stroke. Donnan (1979) reported two cases of patients with acquired neurogenic dysfluency, one of whom had only a single left-sided vascular episode. The patient initially presented as having complete expressive aphasia, but after 3 days she began to speak again, but with stuttering. After 2 weeks, the stuttering had largely resolved itself, and there was only slight word-finding difficulty.

Rosenfield (1972) described the sudden onset of stuttering in a 53-year-old female who suffered vascular headaches. Following one episode of headache, she began to stutter but without any aphasia, apraxia, or motor deficit. The stuttering gradually resolved over an 8-week period. Rosenfield's patient had no prior history of dysfluency. Rosenbek, Messert, Collins, and Wertz (1978) reported seven cases of acquired dysfluency. Four of these patients apparently had single, left hemisphere vascular episodes; one had a history of premorbid stuttering. Of the other cases reported, one had sustained a right hemisphere stroke, one had suffered multiple strokes, and one was reported to have possible generalized intellectual impairment. Fluency returned for only one of the four patients with a unilateral left hemisphere stroke. Mazzuchi et al. (1981) reported neurogenic dysfluency in 16 patients, 11 of whom had vascular events. Of these 11 patients, 3 had aphasia and dysfluency concurrently and both persisted, 2 had transient aphasia and persistence of the dysfluency, 3 had transient dysfluency and persistence of aphasia, and 3 had "isolated stuttering" without aphasia. Although in general the neurogenic dysfluency either disappeared or greatly decreased after weeks or months, several of the case descriptions indicate that the dysfluency persisted. Thus, it would seem that (a) isolated neurogenic dysfluency does occur from single left hemisphere vascular episodes, and (b) neurogenic dysfluency and aphasia often occur together and either, both, or neither may persist.

Dysfluency and Bilateral or Multiple Vascular Episodes. Arend et al. (1962) described two patients with acquired neurogenic dysfluency, one of whom had two vascular events within a 2-year period. Both events seemed to involve the left hemisphere. Right hemiparesis that resolved in a few months was present following the first event, but no aphasia or dysfluency was observed. The second event produced "motor and amnestic aphasia with paraphasia and stuttering." After 4 months, the aphasia resolved but the dysfluency persisted. One of two cases reported by Donnan (1979) suffered several vascular episodes involving the left hemisphere. After the first, she had only right arm and hand paraesthesia. The second episode, a few months later, produced right-sided paraesthesia and weakness and sudden onset of severe stuttering. She eventually underwent left carotid endarterectomy and upon recovery was fluent. She was still fluent months later when a right carotid endarterectomy was performed and at a follow-up examination 12 months later. One dysfluent patient discussed by Rosenbek et al. (1978) suffered multiple strokes. This person was reported to have a language disorder of an undetermined type (possibly aphasia), dysarthria, and stuttering. The dysfluency persisted at a 2-month follow-up session.

Helm et al. (1978) reported 10 patients with acquired neurogenic dysfluency, one of whom had sustained two left-sided vascular episodes. The patient with multiple episodes in the left hemisphere was aphasic following the first episode; the second episode produced aphasia and dysfluency. The aphasia persisted but the dysfluency was transient.

Bilateral Vascular Episodes. Five of the cases of dysfluency reported by Helm et al. (1978) were dysfluent following bilateral vascular episodes. For four of these patients, a right-sided vascular episode preceded the left-sided event. In three of these patients, dysfluency and aphasia were concurrent following the left (second) episode; dysfluency persisted in one patient. One patient suffered a left-sided episode first and was aphasic but not dysfluent. Following the subsequent right-sided episode, persistent stuttering was added to the aphasic component. Nowack and Stone (1987) report two cases of acquired dysfluency. One of the patients was a 55-year-old female who suffered a left hemisphere stroke and was apparently severely aphasic initially, but she recovered "good functional communicative ability." She suffered a second stroke involving the right hemisphere, with resultant persistent dysfluency. Carotid bypass surgery was attempted at that time but was unsuccessful. Several years later—14 years after the left hemisphere stroke and 6 years after the right hemisphere involvement—she experienced a series of psychological stresses that exacerbated the dysfluency. She was treated for the dysfluency problem. The authors report that after "several" sessions the dysfluency was decreased, but still present.

Dysfluency and Right-Sided Vascular Episodes. Dysfluency may also occur following right hemisphere vascular episodes, although that has not been reported frequently. Of the seven cases of dysfluency reported by Rosenbek et al. (1978), one had sustained a right hemisphere stroke. Other than the dysfluency, speech and language were reported to be normal. The dysfluency appeared 96 hours after the stroke and was treated 24 hours later; after an additional 96 hours and six therapy sessions, the dysfluency disappeared. Horner and Massey (1983) provide a detailed account of progressive dysfluency in a patient following a right hemisphere stroke. What makes this report especially interesting is that the dysfluency did not appear until 2 years after the occurrence of the stroke—for whatever reason, the dysfluency did not manifest itself initially. When it finally did appear, the dysfluency had features of both stuttering and palilalia; however, palilalia seems the more appropriate descriptive label. In any event, the point is that the disorder persisted.

Fleet and Heilman (1977) described the onset of left hemiplegia and dysfluency in a 42-year-old female who sustained a right hemisphere stroke. The patient was bilingual and had a familial history of stuttering. Although her father and her brother stuttered, she had not.

The dysfluency did not appear until several weeks following the stroke, and the onset was described as gradual. Subsequently her left hemiplegia decreased. Her dysfluency decreased also, but it did not resolve completely.

Summary: Dysfluency and Vascular Episodes. Based upon the literature cited, the following conclusions seem warranted:

1. Dysfluency occurs following vascular episodes.

2. Dysfluency often occurs with aphasia, but can occur in isolation. When dysfluency occurs in isolation, it tends to be a transient phenomenon.

3. Dysfluency can follow single left hemisphere lesions, bilateral lesions, multiple lesions within the same hemisphere, or right hemisphere lesions.

    a. Dysfluency associated with a single left hemisphere lesion tends to be transient.

    b. Dysfluency associated with bilateral lesions and with multiple unilateral lesions tends to persist.

    c. Dysfluency associated with right hemisphere lesions needs further study.

Helm-Estabrooks (1986) and Shapiro (1999) describe characteristics of stroke-induced dysfluency that may help the clinician identify this type. They state that stroke-induced dysfluency is usually sudden in onset. Also, it usually occurs on initial phonemes of substantive words during conversation, although some dysfluency on medial phonemes and on functor words may also occur for many patients. There is generally no adaptation effect with these patients. As discussed previously, these patients will often demonstrate co-occurring aphasia, but they may also display buccofacial apraxia and, rarely, secondary motor signs. Seizure disorder is not usually associated with stroke-induced dysfluency. Reduced performance in carrying a tune, tapping rhythms, block designs from a model, stick designs from memory, sequential hand positions, and three-dimensional drawing have also been reported for this patient group.

Head Trauma-Induced Dysfluency

Dysfluency has been reported as a sequella of head trauma (Baratz & Mesulam, 1981; Helm et al., 1978; Helm et al., 1980; Mazzuchi et al., 1981; Quinn & Andrews, 1977). Reviewing this literature, Helm-Estabrooks (1986) suggests features that differentiate head trauma-induced stuttering from stroke-induced stuttering. She states that with head trauma there is less sudden onset, less likelihood of aphasia, greater likelihood of seizure disorder, greater likelihood of adaptation effect, and greater likelihood of secondary behaviors. In addition, these patients may also demonstrate reduced performance in carrying a tune, tapping rhythms, block designs from a model, stick designs from memory, sequential hand positions, and three-dimensional drawing.

Dysfluency with Extrapyramidal Disease

As discussed previously, acquired dysfluency is often a characteristic associated with progressive extrapyramidal disease, particularly that of Parkinson's. From studies by Helm et al. (1980) and Koller (1983), Helm-Estabrooks (1986) and Shapiro (1999) have described some typical characteristics of this type of neurogenic dysfluency. They state that the onset of dysfluency in these patients is likely to be gradual and progressive, and that dysfluencies are usually produced on the initial phonemes of substantive words in conversation. The patient with extrapyramidal disease is also more likely to show an adaptation effect than will patients with stroke- or head trauma-induced dysfluency. In addition, the extrapyramidal disease patient will usually show no signs of aphasia, buccofacial apraxia, or secondary motor involvement. They may, however, demonstrate reduced performance in carrying a tune, tapping rhythms, and sequential hand positions.

Other Nonvascular Etiologies

Other disorders associated with dysfluency include dialysis dementia (Rosenbek, McNeil, Lemme, Prescott, & Alfrey, 1975), Alzheimer's disease (Quinn & Andrews, 1977), tumor (Helm et al., 1980), polysystemic central nervous system degeneration (Lebrun, Leleux, et al., 1983), and upper motor neuron disease (Lebrun, Retif, & Kaiser, 1983). The latter case was peculiar in that stuttering was the original presenting symptom, followed only subsequently by other pyramidal motor signs. This course mitigates against an explanation of psychogenic reactivity to neuropathology inasmuch as stuttering was the first salient symptom (Lebrun, Leleux, et al., 1983). Similarly, Quinn and Andrews (1977) and Helm-Estabrooks (1986, 1999) have reported cases in which dysfluent speech was the only initial presenting symptom of what turned out to be progressive neurological disease. Helm-Estabrooks stated that it is important for speech–language pathologists to consider adult onset of dysfluency as a potential sign of neurological disease and to encourage complete neurological and neuropsychological examinations of such patients.

Finally, dysfluency has been reported in association with drug usage (Duffy, 1994; Elliot & Thomas, 1985; McClean & McClean, 1988; Meghji, 1994; Nurnberg & Greenwald, 1981; Quader, 1977). Rentschler and colleagues (1984) report an interesting case of "stuttering" following lithium treatment for depression. This patient exhibited characteristics reminiscent of both acquired and developmental stuttering. Similarities to acquired stuttering included absence of adaptation effect, associated neuropsychological impairments (i.e., block design), and dysfluencies in all word positions and in function as well as content words. Similarities to developmental stuttering were speech anxiety, improvement with choral reading and masking noise, and secondary behaviors, including cheek puffing, head movement, and facial grimacing.

Assessment

In the preceeding sections, we have discussed some of the guidelines for the differential diagnosis of neurogenic dysfluency as opposed to both developmental stuttering and psychogenic dysfluency, and we have looked at some of the features of the major diagnostic groups of neurogenic dysfluency. In order to perform an adequate evaluation of a patient presenting with potential acquired neurogenic dysfluency, the guidelines and features previously discussed need to be addressed.

Helm-Estabrooks (1999, pp. 258–259) recommends beginning the evaluation with a detailed case history that, along with the regular identifying information, should include the following:

1. Onset of current speech problem and any treatment received

2. Handedness of individual and family members
3. Individual's past history and treatment of speech, language, or learning problems
4. Years of education and age when completed
5. Employment history
6. Family history (with dates) to include the following:
   a. Neurologic disease
   b. Head trauma
   c. Periods of unconsciousness
   d. Seizures
   e. Substance abuse
   f. Prescriptive and nonprescriptive medications
   g. Surgery and hospitalizations
   h. Psychiatric problems and treatment

Such a case history will provide information that will allow the clinician to begin to address issues such as differential diagnosis and the identification of diagnostic category.

However, evaluation of the specific speech patterns of the individual will be needed before the clinician can proceed with forming a diagnosis. Helm-Estabrooks (1999) suggests that this should begin with the administration of a standardized aphasia exam, such as the *Aphasia Diagnostic Profiles* (Helm-Estabrooks, 1992), in order to rule out aphasia as the basis of the patient's dysfluencies.

As is common in the assessment of developmental stuttering, it is recommended that multiple speech samples be collected from the patient under a variety of conditions (Helm-Estabrooks, 1986, 1999). These conditions should include conversation, oral reading, repetition of short phrases containing both functor and substantive words, and automatized speech, such as the days of the week. The oral reading should be of a standard passage, such as "The Grandfather Passage," and should be performed multiple times in succession in order to test for the adaptation effect. Analysis of the speech samples should include identification of the frequency, type (i.e., repetition, prolongation, or block) and duration of dysfluencies, the location of the dysfluencies (i.e., on initial or medial phonemes), and the grammatical location of the dysfluencies (i.e., on functor or substantive words).

Some additional neurobehavioral tasks are also suggested in the identification of diagnostic categories of neurogenic dysfluency (Helm-Estabrooks, 1986; Shapiro, 1999). The clinician should observe the patient during speech tasks to identify any secondary motor signs, such as fist clenching, facial grimmacing, and eye blinking. The patient should be asked to sing a familiar song, and the clinician should note if the patient can carry a tune. As noted earlier, other tasks—such as rhythmic tapping, sequential hand movements, block design (e.g., from the *Wechsler Adult Intelligence Scale*), and three-dimensional drawing (e.g., a block or a house)—have been found to be useful in differentiating the type of neurogenic dysfluency and should be included in any evaluation protocol.

Treatment

Approaches to treatment of acquired neurogenic dysfluency have been many and varied. All can be generally subcategorized under two broad headings: managing the underlying pathology and direct symptom modification.

Managing the Underlying Pathology

Again, two generic divisions can be made for approaches that seek to manage the neuropathologies associated with dysfluent speech. First are such treatments as pharmacotherapy, surgery, or prosthetic devices that have attempted to enhance the physiological substrate of speech. Second are the speech–language therapies that address the primary communication deficit (i.e., aphasia, apraxia of speech, or dysarthria). Pharmacotherapy for acquired neurogenic dysfluency has not been widespread. Baratz and Mesulam (1981) used anticonvulsant medication to treat dysfluency in a 42-year-old female who exhibited stuttering and aphasia in association with multifocal brain damage and seizure disorder following a closed head injury. Three hundred mg of phenytoin and 90 mg of phenobarbital daily were prescribed. Her stuttering resolved, and her word-finding abilities improved within a week. Recurrence of seizure-like phenomena were associated with the return of stuttering. Stabilization of the seizures was eventually achieved using 200 mg of phenytoin and 800 mg of carbamazepine daily. Schreiber and Pick (1997) used antidepressant medication to successfully treat neurogenic dysfluency in three males ages 26–30 years. They reported that treatment of the patients with paroxetine resulted in the complete disappearance of their dysfluencies. In two cases described by Nowack and Stone (1987), in which acquired stuttering was associated with bilateral cerebral disease and seizure disorder, pharmacotherapy in combination with speech therapy (i.e., relaxation and airflow) was also effective.

A purely surgical intervention for acquired neurogenic dysfluency has been limited to one case reported by Donnan (1979). Severe stuttering was associated with repeated transient ischemic episodes. Word-finding difficulties were also noted. Carotid angiography revealed bilateral carotid artery stenosis, with greater stricture on the left side. A left carotid endarterectomy was performed successfully. When the patient regained consciousness, the stuttering had resolved and remained so at the 2-month follow-up. Presumably restoration of cerebral blood flow restored speech–language function. Another procedure that has been reported by Bhatnagar and Andy (1989) and Andy and Bhatnagar (1992) involved the surgical implantation of a "chorionic stimulation electrode" in the thalamic nucleus of four patients, all of whom suffered from chronic pain and presented with neurogenic dysfluency. After implantation of the electrode, thalamic stimulation was found to alleviate the pain and considerably improve the fluency of each patient.

The use of a prosthetic or assistive device for neurogenic dysfluency was originally described by Helm (1979), who designed a pacing board for use with a palilalic patient with progressive Parkinson's disease. This device was approximately 13 by 2 inches and consisted of eight colored sections separated by raised wooden dividers running the length of the board. Helm reported that the patient was able to speak syllable by syllable without dysfluency "while tapping his finger from left to right, from segment to segment" (p. 352). The technique was based upon Luria's suggestion that automatic movements can be replaced by intentional movements to increase motor control in Parkinson's disease. Because patients with palilalia appear to have a movement termination deficit, Helm felt that the pacing board imposed an external "stop-go control" that the patient could no longer generate internally. It is noteworthy that the patient continued to use the pacing board for real communicative interactions after being transferred to another facility. Since that time pacing boards and similar devices (e.g., a wood-mounted toggle switch) have also been found to be clinically useful with more stuttering-like forms of neurogenic dysfluency (Helm-Estabrooks, 1986, 1999). It has also been reported that some patients are able to progress from the use of a pacing instrument to tapping the table, and then to tapping their thigh, thus eliminating the need for a device (Helm-Estabrooks, 1999).

Helm and Butler (1977) reported that use of external control stimuli can also be applied to dysfluent patients who require a more salient, ongoing stimulus. One patient exhibited persistent dysarthria accompanied by frequent blocks and occasional prolongation of initial and medial phonemes, following what appears to have been a series of transient cerebrovascular episodes. The patient was not aphasic, but some naming difficulty was noted. Use of a pacing board merely increased the speaking difficulty. In order to provide a more salient external stimulus, an electrolarynx was vibrated against the palm of her left hand during reading and conversation. Helm and Butler report that this technique reduced reading time by approximately 50%. The number of blocks dropped from 38 to 8. Similar effects were noted for the application of transcutaneous nerve stimulation to the bicipital groove of the left arm. When stimulation was removed, the dysfluencies returned. Attempts to use continuous auditory stimulation, such as masking noise, have not been as effective. Helm and Butler suggested that the effects of tactile stimulation on verbal output in acquired speech disorders warrant further investigation.

Another type of speech prosthesis that has proved useful in the management of some forms of neurogenic dysfluency is the portable delayed auditory feedback (DAF) unit. Such a unit is battery powered and small enough to be carried in a shirt pocket. It employs a throat-mounted microphone that delivers binaural audiosignals via molded ear pieces (e.g., Aberdeen Speech Aid, manufactured by Malden Care). Variable gain and delay intervals are usually included. Clinical use of the portable DAF unit as a permanent speech aid was originally reported by Hanson and Metter (1980), who found it to provide long-term improvement in rate and loudness in a patient with hypokinetic dysarthria, secondary to progressive supranuclear palsy. This patient, however, was not described as being dysfluent. Subsequently, Downie, Low, and Lindsay (1981) experimented with DAF units with 11 parkinsonian patients, 2 of whom benefited significantly from the device. Both patients were dysfluent, exhibiting hesitations and blocks "akin to stammering." Speech improvement was said to come and go as "abruptly as the apparatus was switched on or off" (p. 852). A 50-msec delay time was found to be most optimal. One patient, the more severe, became habituated to the device after a year of continuous use. The other continued to find it a valuable aid to communication at a 2-year follow-up. It should be recognized that the use of a portable DAF device as a permanent speech aid is quite different from the in-clinic use of DAF as an adjunct to a broader behavioral program of therapy (Hanson & Metter, 1980). It is possible that the use of delayed sidetone with such a short delay interval (in comparison with the 200–250 msec delay found most effective for developmental stutterers) might also constitute an external control stimulus akin to pacing. Thereby each echo would serve as a stop-go boundary for termination and initiation of the flow of speech.

Another set of therapeutic strategies that target the underlying disorder consists of the conventional speech–language therapies for the acquired neurogenic communicative disorders of aphasia, dysarthria, and apraxia of speech. The primary goal of traditional aphasia therapy is multimodality stimulation of the language system (Schuell et al., 1964). The primary goal of apraxia therapy is the retraining of speech motor programming functions (Rosenbek, 1985), whereas the primary goal of dysarthria therapy is compensated intelligibility (Rosenbek & LaPointe, 1985). Implicit in these approaches is the assumption that dysfluency is a direct result of the primary communicative deficit and, therefore, dysfluency will resolve as the primary deficit resolves. Example cases illustrating such parallel variation in fluency and aphasia have been reported in the literature; however, so have counter-examples of patients whose fluency did not improve (Andrews et al., 1972; Rosenbek et al., 1978). It does seem reasonable, at the present stage of knowledge, to initially target a primary deficit in cases for whom that deficit and the acquired dysfluency appear to be closely linked. This is particularly true when the primary deficit is the overriding contributor to disruption of communication. In addition, prior remediation of the primary disorder may make direct symptom modification of dysfluency less complicated at a later stage of therapy.

Direct Modification of Dysfluent Symptoms

Approaches that target direct symptom modification of dysfluency as the treatment goal are borrowed in their entirety from the extensive developmental stuttering literature. These "stuttering therapies" can also be divided into two general classes: fluency-shaping therapy and stuttering modification therapy (Guitar, 1998). Fluency-shaping involves establishing some form of fluency that is reinforced and modified to resemble normal speech, then generalized outside of the clinical setting to the patient's everyday environment. Fluency-shaping techniques have been applied to cases of acquired neurogenic dysfluency. Rosenbek et al. (1978) and Rosenbek (1984) describe a patient with intact language who stuttered following a right parietal lobe CVA. One day after onset, he was placed on a program of syllable timed speech. This involved a rate reduction to approximately 50 words per minute (wpm) by increasing both articulation time (i.e., phoneme prolongation) and pause time. Treatment also included a significant counseling component. The patient was fluent after six sessions and remained so at follow-up 1 month later. From their survey of speech–language pathologists, Market et al. (1990) reported that the majority of clinicians treating neurogenic dysfluency use the fluency-shaping techniques of slow rate, easy onset, or a combination of the two, with a reportedly high degree of success (82.2%). However, little additional information about these patients is provided, and questions regarding spontaneous recovery, especially given the known transient nature of some forms of neurogenic dysfluency, as well as issues such as amount of time in therapy, the amount of time lapsed between the onset of dysfluency and the initiation of therapy, and lack of data on patients who did not receive therapy, suggest caution in the interpretation of the high degree of success reported for these techniques.

Delayed auditory feedback (DAF) has also been used in the treatment of acquired neurogenic dysfluency. Marshall and Starch (1984) used DAF with a 32-year-old "acquired stutterer" to establish fluency at 4 years post onset of stuttering. To date, the most ambitious attempt at a treatment study involving DAF with neurogenic dysfluency was undertaken by Marshall and Neuburger (1987). These authors used single subject, multiple baseline designs with three severely dysfluent patients. Etiologies included closed head trauma, right parietal skull fracture with left temporal hematoma, and brainstem contusion. The patients were seen on an outpatient basis for 1-hour sessions, two to three times per week. Treatment followed conventional fluency therapy programs, in which an initial feedback delay of 250 msec was used to slow the speaking rate by requiring the patient to prolong each word to compensate for DAF; this delay interval was gradually reduced in 50-msec steps to zero. Frequency of stuttering events and reading rate were measured across baseline, treatment, and maintenance conditions for a variety of connected discourse tasks. The DAF treatment reduced dysfluencies in all three patients. Only one patient, however, sustained dysfluency reduction throughout the maintenance (i.e., treatment withdrawal) period. Generalization to nontreatment settings was not noted, but neither was any transfer training incorporated in the short-term experimental therapy. The authors conclude that "DAF has 'potential' as a treatment procedure in the management of acquired stuttering" (p. 363).

Stuttering modification therapy is based on interpretations of stuttering as learned avoidance and struggle behavior. Such therapies attempt to decrease avoidance behavior, improve negative attitudes toward speech, and reduce speech-related fear (Guitar, 1998). Stuttering modification therapy also has been applied to acquired neurogenic dysfluency. Nowack and Stone (1987) reported two cases of dysfluency associated with bilateral cerebral disease. As mentioned previously, neuropharmacological treatment was combined with a program of speech therapy that the authors regarded as broadly "anxiolytic." Both patients experienced marked speech anxiety. Treatment techniques included progressive relaxation and breathing exercises incorporating release of unphonated airflow in nonspeech tasks. The authors suggest that improvement in these cases followed alleviation of considerable psychological stress by speech therapy.

Electromyographic (EMG) biofeedback as an aid to relaxation during speech has been employed in the treatment of neurogenic stuttering (Helm-Estabrooks, 1986, 1999). Following a protocol originally developed for developmental stutterers, EMG treatment was used with a case of moderately severe "stuttering" secondary to a series of minor strokes. After a 4-month course of biweekly sessions, dysfluency was reduced to a mild level. Other forms of biofeedback therapy for more direct work on speaking variables also have been recommended (see Chapter 10 in this volume).

Combined approaches drawing upon various treatment strategies also have been employed. Rosenbek (1984) indicates that therapy using syllable-timed speech, which was successful with one neurogenic dysfluent patient, also had a strong counseling component oriented toward reassurance that fluent speech was still possible. Nowack and Stone (1987) combined pharmacotherapy with relaxation-breathing techniques. Given the strikingly heterogeneous nature of the disorder, an eclectic approach toward treating acquired neurogenic dysfluency would seem advisable. The available literature provides a fertile basis for clinical experimentation with a variety of potential combinations and permutations.

Summary

In an effort to bring order to the diverse array of treatment approaches that have been employed with acquired neurogenic dysfluency patients, a classification scheme is provided in Figure 7.1. Selection of a particular treatment strategy is not simple and may devolve into trial-and-error therapy in many cases. There remain no clear-cut guidelines. If medical management of the physiological substrate is indicated as part of an overall medical plan (e.g., for seizures or arterial circulation), one should attempt to monitor dysfluencies systematically before and after such intervention. There is at least some reason to be guardedly optimistic that physical intervention may decrease dysfluency. In most cases, however, it becomes the speech–language pathologist's responsibility to attempt to remediate the neurogenic patient's dysfluent speech.

The decision of whether to address the primary communicative deficit, or to attempt direct symptom modification of dysfluency, may be bolstered by a range of diagnostic information. Neurologic examination and brain-imaging studies may be useful in determining whether lesion loci are within the classic speech–language or motor control areas (Heuer, Sataloff, Mandel, & Travers, 1996). Chronic neurogenic dysfluency, not associated with the classic neurogenic communication disorders, tends to stem from bilateral subcortical involvement (Helm-Estabrooks, 1986). Traditional aphasia and motor speech evaluations

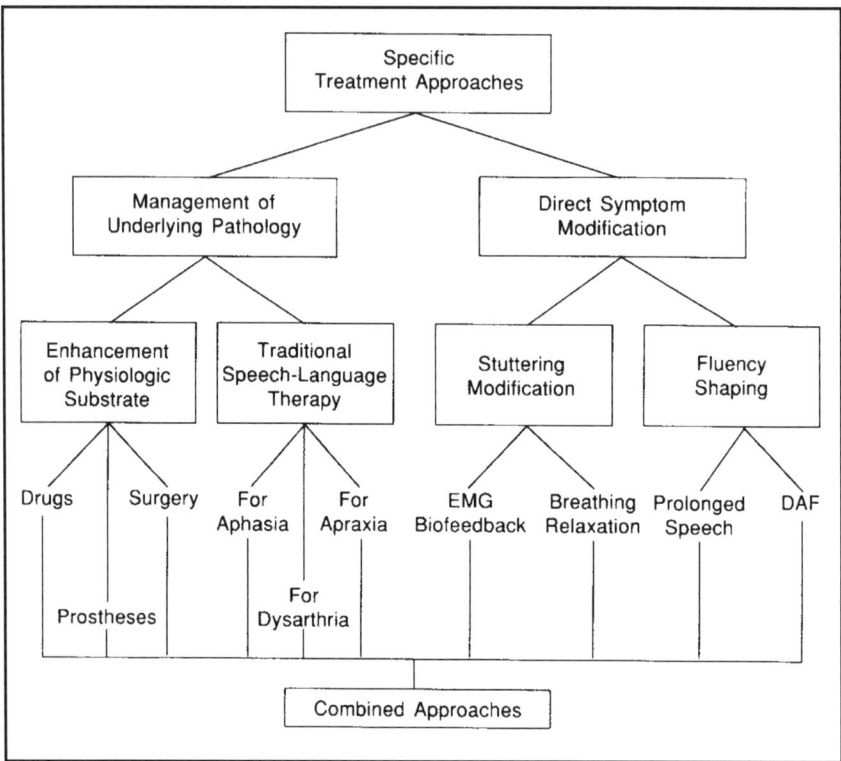

Figure 7.1. A framework for the treatment of acquired neurogenic dysfluency. The lowest labeled nodes represent treatments reported to have been successful in selected cases.

used in conjunction with the neurodiagnostic data will determine the presence of classical aphasias, dysarthrias, or apraxia of speech. Faced with dysfluency in the presence of these primary communicative deficits, addressing the primary deficit first may be the preferred procedure. If, however, dysfluency exists in isolation or is the most salient presenting problem, the clinician may elect to target direct modification of dysfluent symptoms. In such instances, an additional decision must be made as to whether to draw upon fluency-shaping or stuttering modification techniques, or both. In cases in which there is little evidence of struggle behavior, avoidance, or speech anxiety, fluency shaping may be indicated. Because these procedures are heavily operant in nature, they may also be preferable for patients with restricted cognitive capacity. In contrast, stuttering modification is intellectually demanding, rooted as it is in psychotherapeutic tradition. As discussed previously, anxiety, struggle, and secondary behaviors have been reported in some patients with aquired neurogenic dysfluency. If cognitive capacity is adequate, stuttering modification therapies may be more appropriate for such patients. Market et al. (1990) report the use of Van Riperian techniques (i.e., stuttering modification) by 17% of respondents and attitude/relaxation techniques by 27%. Finally, assistive devices, such as pacing boards and tactile stimulators, may prove beneficial to some patients and appear to be the treatment of choice for palilalia. As Helm-Estabrooks (1986) has stated, "Successful management of neurogenic stuttering requires differential treatment as well as differential diagnosis" (p. 211).

Yet, we should not paint too rosy a picture. Many authors report cases of neurogenic dysfluency in which specific treatments either did not generalize (Marshall & Neuberger, 1987) or were generally ineffective (Helm-Estabrooks, 1986; Rosenbek et al., 1978). There are at present no proven prognostic indicators. As our knowledge of acquired neurogenic dysfluency increases through controlled clinical experimentation, it seems likely that differential diagnostic profiling (incorporating data from neurology, psychology, and speech–language pathology) may come to guide the selection of a therapeutic plan. In the meantime, it is encouraging to note that there is no shortage of field-tested approaches for remediation of acquired neurogenic dysfluency, and all of them have contributed successfully to the management of selected cases.

References

Albert, M. L., Goodglass, H., Helm, N. A., Rubens, A. B., & Alexander, M. P. (1981). *Clinical aspects of dysphasia*. New York: Springer-Verlag.

Andrews, G., Quinn, P. T., & Sorby, W. A. (1972). Stuttering: An investigation into cerebral dominance for speech. *Journal of Neurology, Neurosurgery, and Psychiatry, 35*, 414–418.

Andy, O. J., & Bhatnagar, S. C. (1992). Stuttering acquired from subcortical pathologies and its alleviation from thalamic perturbation. *Brain and Language, 42*, 385–401.

Arend, R., Handzel, L., & Weiss, D. (1962). Dysphatic stuttering. *Folia Phoniatrica, 14,* 55–66.

Attanasio, J. S. (1987). A case of late-onset acquired stuttering in adult life. *Journal of Fluency Disorders, 12,* 287–290.

Baratz, R., & Mesulam, M. M. (1981). Adult-onset stuttering treated with anticonvulsants. *Archives of Neurology, 38,* 132.

Baumgartner, J., & Duffy, J. R. (1997). Psychogenic stuttering in adults with and without neurologic disease. *Journal of Medical Speech—Language Pathology, 5,* 75–95.

Bhatnagar, S. C., & Andy, O. J. (1989). Alleviation of acquired stuttering with human centermedian thalamic stimulation. *Journal of Neurology, Neurosurgery, and Psychiatry, 5,* 1182–1184.

Canter, G. J. (1971). Observations on neurogenic stuttering: A contribution to differential diagnosis. *British Journal of Disorders of Communication, 6,* 139–143.

Caplan, L. (1972). An investigation of some aspects of stuttering-like speech in adult dysphasic subjects. *Journal of South African Speech and Hearing Association, 19,* 52–66.

Critchley, M. (1927). On palilalia. *Journal of Neurological Psychopathology, 8,* 23–31.

Culatta, R., & Goldberg, S. A. (1995). *Stuttering therapy: An integrated approach to theory and practice.* Needham Heights, MA: Allyn & Bacon.

Culatta, R., & Leeper, L. (1988). Dysfluency isn't always stuttering. *Journal of Speech and Hearing Disorders, 53,* 486–488.

Dalton, P., & Hardcastle, W. J. (1989). *Disorders of fluency and their effects on communication* (2nd ed.). London: Cole and Whurr Limited.

Darley, F. L., Aronson, A. E., & Brown, J. R. (1975). *Motor speech disorders.* Philadelphia: Saunders.

Deal, J. L. (1982). Sudden onset of stuttering: A case report. *Journal of Speech and Hearing Disorders, 47,* 301–304.

Deal, J. L., & Doro, J. M. (1987). Episodic hysterical stuttering. *Journal of Speech and Hearing Disorders, 52,* 299–300.

Dempsey, G. L., & Granich, M. (1978). Hypno-behavioral therapy in the case of a traumatic stutterer: A case report. *International Journal of Clinical and Experimental Hypnosis, 16*, 125–133.

DeNil, L. F. (1999). Stuttering: A neurophysiological perspective. In N. B. Ratner & E. C. Healey (Eds.), *Stuttering research and practice: Bridging the gap* (pp. 85–102). Mahwah, NJ: Erlbaum.

DeNil, L. F., Kroll, R. M., Kapur, S., & Houle, S. (2000). A positron emission tomography study of silent and oral single word reading in stuttering and nonstuttering adults. *Journal of Speech, Language, and Hearing Research, 43*, 1038–1053.

Donnan, G. A. (1979). Stuttering as a manifestation of stroke. *Medical Journal of Australia, 1*, 44–45.

Downie, A. W., Low, J. M., & Lindsay, D. D. (1981). Speech disorders in parkinsonism: Use of delayed auditory feedback in selected cases. *Journal of Neurology, Neurosurgery, and Psychiatry, 44*, 852–853.

Duffy, J. D. (1994). Neurogenic stuttering and lateralized motor deficits induced by tranylcypromine. *Behavioral Neurology, 7*, 171–174.

Elliot, R. L., & Thomas, B. J. (1985). A case report of alprazolam-induced stuttering. *Journal of Clinical Psychopharmacology, 5*, 159–160.

Fairbanks, G. (1954). A theory of the speech mechanism as a servo-system. *Journal of Speech and Hearing Disorders, 19*, 133–139.

Fleet, W. S., & Heilman, K. M. (1977). Acquired stuttering from a right hemisphere lesion in a right-hander. *Neurology, 35*, 1343–1346.

Fox, P. T., Ingham, R. J., Ingham, J. C., Hirsch, T. B., Downs, J. H., Martin, C., Jerabek, P., Glass, T., & Lancaster, J. L. (1996). A PET study of the neural systems of stuttering. *Nature, 382*, 158–162.

Freund, H. (1966). *Psychopathology and the problem of stuttering*. Springfield, IL: Thomas.

Guitar, B. (1998). *Stuttering: An integrated approach to its nature and treatment*. Baltimore: Williams & Wilkins.

Hanson, W., & Metter, J. (1980). DAF as instrumental treatment for dysarthria in progressive supranuclear palsy: A case report. *Journal of Speech and Hearing Disorders, 45*, 268–276.

Head, H. (1926). *Aphasia and kindred disorders of speech*. London: Cambridge University Press.

Helm, N. A. (1979). Management of palilalia with a pacing board. *Journal of Speech and Hearing Disorders, 44*, 350–353.

Helm, N. A., & Butler, R. B. (1977). Transcutaneous nerve stimulation in acquired speech disorders. *Lancet, 8049*, 1177–1178.

Helm, N. A., Butler, R. B., & Benson, D. F. (1978). Acquired stuttering. *Neurology, 28*, 1159–1165.

Helm, N. A., Butler, R. B., & Canter, G. J. (1980). Neurogenic acquired stuttering. *Journal of Fluency Disorders, 5*, 269–279.

Helm-Estabrooks, N. (1986). Diagnosis and management of neurogenic stuttering in adults. In K. O. St. Louis (Ed.), *The atypical stutterer: Principles and practices of rehabilitation* (pp. 193–217). Orlando, FL: Academic Press.

Helm-Estabrooks, N. (1992). *Aphasia diagnostic profiles*. Chicago: Applied Symbolix.

Helm-Estabrooks, N. (1999). Stuttering associated with acquired neurological disorders. In R. F. Curlee (Ed.), *Stuttering and related disorders of fluency* (2nd ed., pp. 255–268). New York: Thieme Medical.

Helm-Estabrooks, N., & Hotz, G. (1998). Sudden onset of "stuttering" in an adult: Neurogenic or psychogenic? *Seminars in Speech and Language, 19*, 23–29.

Heuer, R. J., Sataloff, R. T., Mandel, S., & Travers, N. (1996). Neurogenic stuttering: Further corroboration of site of lesion. *Ear, Nose, and Throat Journal, 75*, 161–168.

Horner, J., & Massey, E. W. (1983). Progressive dysfluency associated with right hemisphere disease. *Brain and Language, 18*, 71–85.

Ingham, R. J., Fox, P. T., Ingham, J. C., Zamarripa, F., Martin, C., Jerabek, P., & Cotton, J. (1996). Functional-lesion investigation of developmental stuttering with positron emission tomography. *Journal of Speech and Hearing Research, 39*, 1208–1227.

Johns, D. F., & Darley, F. L. (1970). Phonemic variability in apraxia of speech. *Journal of Speech and Hearing Research, 13*, 553–583.

Kent, R. D., & LaPointe, L. L. (1982). Acoustic properties of pathologic reiterative utterances: A case study of palilalia. *Journal of Speech and Hearing Research, 25*, 95–99.

Koller, W. C. (1983). Dysfluency (stuttering) in extrapyramidal disease. *Archives of Neurology, 40*, 175–177.

LaPointe, L. L., & Horner, J. (1981). Palilalia: A descriptive study of pathological reiterative utterances. *Journal of Speech and Hearing Disorders, 46*, 34–38.

Lebrun, Y., & Leleux, C. (1985). Acquired stuttering following right-brain damage in dextrals. *Journal of Fluency Disorders, 10*, 137–141.

Lebrun, Y., Leleux, C., Rousseau, J. J., & Devereux, F. (1983). Acquired stuttering. *Journal of Fluency Disorders, 8*, 323–330.

Lebrun, Y., Retif, J., & Kaiser, G. (1983). Acquired stuttering as a forerunner of motor-neuron disease. *Journal of Fluency Disorders, 8*, 161–167.

Luchsinger, R., & Arnold, G. E. (1965). *Voice–speech–language.* Belmont, CA: Wadsworth.

Market, K. E., Montague, J. C., Jr., Buffalo, M. D., & Drummond, S. S. (1990). Acquired stuttering: Descriptive data and treatment outcome. *Journal of Fluency Disorders, 15*, 21–33.

Marshall, R. C., & Neuburger, S. I. (1987). Effects of delayed auditory feedback on acquired stuttering following head injury. *Journal of Fluency Disorders, 12*, 355–365.

Marshall, R. C., & Starch, S. A. (1984). Behavioral treatment of acquired stuttering. *Australian Journal of Human Communication Disorders, 12*, 87–91.

Mazzuchi, A., Moretti, G., Carpeggiani, P., Parma, M., & Paini, P. (1981). Clinical observations on acquired stuttering. *British Journal of Disordered Communication, 16*, 19–30.

McClean, M. D., & McClean, A. J. (1988). Case report of stuttering acquired in association with phenytoin use for post-head injury seizures. *Journal of Fluency Disorders, 10*, 241–255.

Meghji, C. (1994). Acquired stuttering. *Journal of Family Practice, 39*, 325–326.

Nowack, W. J., & Stone, R. E. (1987). Acquired stuttering and bilateral cerebral disease. *Journal of Fluency Disorders, 12,* 141–146.

Nurnberg, H. G., & Greenwald, B. (1981). Stuttering: An unusual side effect of phenothiazines. *American Journal of Psychiatry, 138,* 386–387.

Perkins, W. H., Kent, R. D., & Curlee, R. F. (1991). A theory of neuropsycholinguistic function in stuttering. *Journal of Speech and Hearing Research, 34,* 734–752.

Pool, K. D., Devous, M. D., Freeman, F. J., Watson, B. C., & Finitzo, T. (1991). Regional cerebral blood flow in developmental stutterers. *Archives of Neurology, 48,* 509–512.

Quader, S. E. (1977). Dysarthria: An unusual side effect of tricyclic antidepressants. *British Medical Journal, 9,* 97.

Quinn, P. T., & Andrews, B. (1977). Neurological stuttering: A clinical entity? *Journal of Neurology, Neurosurgery and Psychiatry, 40,* 699–701.

Rentschler, G. J., Driver, L. E., & Callaway, E. A. (1984). The onset of stuttering following drug overdose. *Journal of Fluency Disorders, 9,* 265–284.

Ringo, C. C., & Dietrich, S. (1995). Neurogenic stuttering: An analysis and critique. *Journal of Medical Speech–Language Pathology, 3,* 111–122.

Rosenbek, J. (1980). Apraxia of speech: Relationship to stuttering. *Journal of Fluency Disorders, 5,* 233–253.

Rosenbek, J. C. (1984). Stuttering secondary to brain damage. In R. F. Curlee & W. H. Perkins (Eds.), *Nature and treatment of stuttering: New directions.* Austin, TX: PRO-ED.

Rosenbek, J. C. (1985). Treating apraxia of speech. In D. F. Johns (Ed.), *Clinical management of neurogenic communicative disorders* (pp. 267–312). Austin, TX: PRO-ED.

Rosenbek, J., & LaPointe, L. L. (1985). The dysarthrias: Description, diagnosis and treatment. In D. Johns (Ed.), *Clinical management of neurogenic communicative disorders* (pp. 97–152). Austin, TX: PRO-ED.

Rosenbek, J., McNeil, M. R., Lemme, M. L., Prescott, T. E., & Alfrey, A. C., (1975). Speech and language findings in a chronic hemodyalsis patient: A case report. *Journal of Speech and Hearing Disorders, 40,* 245–252.

Rosenbek, J., Messert, B., Collins, M., & Wertz, R. T. (1978). Stuttering following brain damage. *Brain and Language, 6,* 82–96.

Rosenfield, D. B. (1972). Stuttering and cerebral ischemia. *New England Journal of Medicine, 287,* 991.

Schiller, F. (1947). Aphasia studied in patients with missile wounds. *Journal of Neurology, Neurosurgery and Psychiatry, 10,* 183–197.

Schreiber, S., & Pick, C. G. (1997). Paroxetine for secondary stuttering: Further interaction of serotonin and dopamine. *Journal of Nervous and Mental Disease, 185,* 465–466.

Schuell, H., Jenkins, J. J., & Jimenez-Pabon, E. (1964). *Aphasia in adults: Diagnosis, prognosis, and treatment.* New York: Harper & Row.

Shapiro, D. A. (1999). *Stuttering intervention: A collaborative journey to fluency freedom.* Austin, TX: PRO-ED.

Trost, J. E. (1971, November). *Apraxic dysfluency in patients with Broca's aphasia.* Paper presented at the annual convention of the American Speech and Hearing Association, Chicago.

Van Riper, C. (1971). *The nature of stuttering.* Englewood Cliffs, NJ: Prentice Hall.

Wallen, V. (1961). Primary stuttering in an 18-year-old adult. *Journal of Speech and Hearing Disorders, 16,* 394–395.

Watson, B. C., & Freeman, F. J. (1997). Brain imaging contributions. In R. F. Curlee & G. M. Siegel (Eds.), *Nature and treatment of stuttering: New directions* (pp. 143–166). Needham Heights, MA: Allyn & Bacon.

Watson, B. C., Pool, K. D., Devous, M. D., Freeman, F. J., & Finitzo, T. (1992). Brain blood flow related to acoustic laryngeal reaction time in adult developmental stutterers. *Journal of Speech and Hearing Research, 35,* 555–561.

Watson, B. C., Freeman, F. J., Devous, M. D., Chapman, S. B., Finitzo, T., & Pool, K. D. (1994). Linguistic performance and regional cerebral blood flow in persons who stutter. *Journal of Speech and Hearing Research, 37,* 1221–1228.

Weiner, A. E. (1981). A case of adult onset of stuttering. *Journal of Fluency Disorders, 6,* 181–186.

Wertz, R. T., Rosenbek, J. C., & LaPointe, L. L. (1983). *Apraxia of speech.* Philadelphia: Saunders.

Wood, F., Stump, D., McKeehan, A., Sheldon, S., & Proctor, J. (1980). Patterns of regional cerebral blood flow during attempted reading aloud by stutterers both on and off Haloperidol medication: Evidence for inadequate left frontal activation during stuttering. *Brain and Language, 9,* 141–144.

Wu, J. C., Maguire, G., Riley, G., Fallon, J., LaCasse, L., Chin, S., Klein, E., Tang, C., Cadwell, S., & Lottenberg, S. (1995). A positron emission tomography deoxyglucose study of developmental stuttering. *NeuroReport, 6,* 501–505.

Yairi, E., Gintautas, J., & Avent, J. R. (1981). Dysfluent speech associated with brain damage. *Brain and Language, 14,* 49–56.

Chapter 8

Neurogenic Disorders of Prosody

Samuel Amebu Seddoh and Donald A. Robin

The authors discuss disorders of prosody in patients with focal cerebral lesions. After a review of the relevant literature, they detail the steps involved in diagnosis of prosodic disturbances. The discussion focuses on the importance of acoustic measures to complement perceptual judgments and on the need to examine both the production and the perception of prosody. A look at different treatment approaches and case descriptions follows the assessment section.

1. *What is gained by using acoustic measures in diagnosing and treating prosodic disturbances?*

2. *How can acoustic measures be used to examine prosodic changes over time?*

3. *What stimuli should be used to assess and treat functional deficits in prosody?*

✧ ✧ ✧

Statements about disturbances in language that affect prosody can be traced to Jackson (1874) and Pick (1919; cited in Monrad-Krohn, 1947a, 1947b) who noted that language is more than words; it contains melodies through which meaning may be conveyed. Perhaps Monrad-Krohn (1947a, 1947b, 1963) was the first researcher to give detailed descriptions of different types of impaired speech prosody related to nervous system lesions. Yet, given the historical significance of prosody in the literature, this aspect of language remains a neglected area of clinical concern. Few clinicians routinely assess prosody, and it is often treated as an afterthought.

It is important to stress that prosodic impairments may contribute to abnormal speech or language performance in patients with neurological disease. Myers (1984) and Robin, Jordan, and Rodnitzky (1986) have pointed out that patients and their families must be counseled as to the effect prosodic impairment has on communication successes and failures. In order to provide appropriate counseling, clinicians must have as detailed a picture as possible of a patient's prosodic profile.

This chapter examines prosodic disturbances related to neurological lesions. Although the authors acknowledge impairments of prosody that accompany the various dysarthrias, the chapter is aimed at "higher" level disturbances related to focal lesions of the cerebral hemispheres and the corpus callosum. Disorders of the production and perception of different aspects of prosody are described for various patient groups. Furthermore, the role of acoustic measures as clinical tools is examined. It is our opinion that the clinician must make use of all possible knowledge that can be gained about a patient's speech and language and that acoustic studies of prosody are now mandatory in clinical practice.

This chapter is divided into five sections. The first section is an overview of normal prosody. The second section involves a brief review of the history of the study of prosodic disorders from Monrad-Krohn's (1947a, 1947b, 1963) pioneering work to the present. In the third section, suggestions are made for the diagnosis of prosodic impairments. This is followed in the fourth section with suggestions for the treatment of prosodic disturbances. Finally, in the fifth section, case studies of patients with focal lesions of the nervous system and subsequent prosodic disabilities are presented.

Definition

Prosody has been called the "melody of speech" (Berry, 1969; Monrad-Krohn, 1947a, 1947b). It refers to the nonsegmental components of spoken language, such as pitch, loudness, and length. These perceptual features are related to variations in three acoustic properties of the speech waveform: fundamental frequency (F0), amplitude, and duration, respectively. Thus, prosody can be defined as changes in the speech waveform that relate to intonation, stress patterns, timing, or rhythm. Changes in these features give rise to variations in pitch patterns, such as intonation contours, stress patterns, and temporal or rhythmic patterns of speech.

Communicative Functions of Prosody

Prosody is part of the linguistic system, and it functions to convey linguistic distinctions. The difference between echo (intonation) questions and statements, for example, is conveyed mainly by changes in intonation (or F0). The use of prosody can also be observed in the assignment of stress to utterances (Cooper, Eady, & Mueller, 1985; Selkirk, 1984). In this case, a word might receive emphasis (or stress), as in *"Don* shot the puck to Kent" versus "Don shot the puck to *Kent.*" In the first sentence, *Don* is stressed and would be the appropriate answer to the question, "Who shot the puck to Kent?"; in the second sentence, *Kent* receives stress and would be used to answer the question, "Who did Don shoot the puck to?" Prosodic features, such as pause, also distinguish between different syntactic constructions, (Cooper & Sorensen, 1981; Lea, 1973). For example, the sentences, "If Jerry fought his brother, we'll be upset" and "If Jerry fought, his brother will be upset" have different meanings depending on the position of the pause.

Prosody may also serve to convey information about the emotional state or attitude of the speaker. Intonation is one component of prosody that is believed to contribute to the signaling of emotional states such as happiness, sadness, or anger (Couper-Kuhlen, 1986; Scherer, 1986; Tompkins & Mateer, 1985; Williams & Stevens, 1972).

Prosodic Disturbance Due to Cerebral Injury

Monrad-Krohn (1947a, 1947b, 1963) described three types of prosodic breakdown. In one case, he noted that a patient's pitch output may be flattened. He referred to this abnormality as *aprosody*, although this term gives the erroneous impression that there is a complete loss or absence of prosody (Ryalls & Behrens, 1988). According to Monrad-Krohn, patients with this disorder have a general reduction in their ability to vary pitch in speech. Monrad-Krohn also discussed a prosodic disorder that he termed *hyperprosody*. This disorder is characterized by abnormally increased variations in pitch. Monrad-Krohn's third prosodic disorder is called *dysprosody*. He illustrated this disorder by describing a subject with a "foreign accent syndrome" whose native Norwegian accent disappeared after a left hemisphere lesion. This subject reportedly sounded as if she had a German accent.

In the past few years, the study of prosodic disturbance related to neurological lesions has become more common. Recently, acoustic studies have appeared in the literature that further our knowledge of the neural control of prosody and assist in the ability of clinicians to diagnose and treat such problems. In the remainder of this section, some studies of prosody will be reviewed, and the effect of damage to the right hemisphere, the left hemisphere, and the corpus callosum on prosodic production and perception will be discussed.

Prosodic Disturbance Due to Right Hemispheric Lesions

Unilateral damage to the right hemisphere can result in impairment in the production of prosody, the comprehension of prosody, or both (e.g., Baum, 1998; Behrens, 1988, 1989; Bryan, 1989; Cancelliere & Kertesz, 1990; Emmorey, 1987; Gandour, Larsen, Dechongkit, Ponglorpisit, & Khunadorn, 1995; Heilman, Bowers, Speedie, & Coslett, 1984; Kent & Rosenbek, 1982; Pell, 1998; Perkins, Baran, & Gandour, 1996; Ross, 1981; Ross, Edmonston, Seibert, & Homan, 1988; Ross, Thompson, & Yenkosky, 1997; Shapiro & Danly, 1985; Tompkins, 1991; Tompkins & Flowers, 1985; Tompkins & Mateer, 1985; van Lancker & Sidtis, 1992; Weintraub, Mesulam, & Kramer, 1981). One commonly reported finding is the abnormal production of aspects of F0 associated with intonation (Baum & Pell, 1997; Behrens, 1989; Blonder, Pickering, Heath, Smith, & Butler, 1995; Kent & Rosenbek, 1982; Ross et al., 1988; Ross et al., 1997; Shapiro & Danly, 1985; Weintraub et al., 1981).

Kent and Rosenbek (1982) studied acoustic characteristics of prosodic patterns produced by patients with right hemisphere lesions. Using spectrographic records, they found that F0 and intensity were reduced across utterances in addition to limited variations in syllable durations. Shapiro and Danly (1985) also found that the typical F0 rise associated with yes–no questions was reduced in patients with right anterior lesions. Likewise, Weintraub et al. (1981) found that their subjects with right hemisphere damage were significantly impaired in the ability to produce intonation patterns over yes–no questions. Behrens (1989) also reported narrower than normal peak-to-valley F0 range in the preterminal portions of yes–no questions for a group of eight male patients with unilateral right hemisphere damage.

In contrast to the finding of flat F0, Shapiro and Danly (1985) reported that patients with posterior right hemisphere lesions exhibited exaggerated F0 values. Other investigators have, however, failed to find F0 differences between patients with anterior and patients with posterior right hemisphere lesions (Ryalls, Joanette, & Feldman, 1987). Differences between the results of these studies may be due to differences in the site and size of lesion, the type of treatment received, and the linguistic backgrounds of the patients. For example, the subjects studied by Ryalls and colleagues (1987) were native speakers of French, whereas those studied by Shapiro and Danly were native speakers of American English.

It has been suggested that the right and the left hemispheres are differentially specialized in processing the least and the most linguistically structured prosodic contrasts, respectively (van Lancker, 1980). Ross and colleagues (e.g., Gorelick & Ross, 1987; Ross, 1981; Ross & Mesulam, 1979; Ross et al., 1988; Ross et al., 1997) have also argued that intonation (F0) associated with utterances that convey emotional meaning is lateralized to the right hemisphere. In one intriguing study, Ross et al. (1988) examined intonation production in five subjects who underwent a right-sided Wada Test (WT; Wada & Rasmussen, 1960). The subjects were asked to repeat the sentence, "I am going to the other movies" using six different affects—neutral, sad, happy, surprised, bored, and angry—by modeling the examiner's voice (p. 132). The patients' productions—which were recorded prior to, during, and after the WT—were analyzed acoustically. Results showed that all five subjects exhibited significant reductions in various measures of F0 during the WT. This outcome was interpreted by Ross and colleagues as an indication of "loss of the ability" (p. 130) to produce affective prosody on the part of the subjects. The investigators, however, showed no comparative data to demonstrate that the ability of the subjects to produce nonaffective prosody was intact. Given that the right hemisphere is also involved in processing intonation in nonemotional context (e.g, Behrens, 1989; Blonder et al., 1995; Blumstein & Cooper, 1974; Bryan, 1989; Shapiro & Danly, 1985; Weintraub et al., 1981), the absence of such data makes it difficult to assess objectively the validity of the view that what the patients failed to produce was specifically affective prosody.

The findings of a growing number of studies are inconsistent with the view that intonation associated with emotional utterances is lateralized to the right hemisphere (e.g., Baum & Pell, 1997; Cancelliere & Kertesz, 1990; Pell, 1998; Pell & Baum, 1997a; Schlanger, Schlanger, & Gertsman, 1976; Seron, van der Kaa, van der Linden, Remits, & Feyereisen, 1982; van Lancker & Sidtis, 1992). Impairment has been reported in emotional (e.g., Baum, & Pell, 1997; Cancelliere & Kertesz, 1990; Ross et al., 1997; Shapiro & Danly, 1985; Tucker, Watson, & Heilman, 1977) as well as nonemotional (Behrens, 1989; Blonder et al., 1995; Bryan, 1989; Heilman et al., 1984; Shapiro & Danly, 1985; Weintraub et al., 1981) domains, not only for right hemisphere–damaged patients, but also for left hemisphere–damaged patients (Cancelliere & Kertesz, 1990; Cooper, Soares, Nicol, Michelow, & Goloskie, 1984; Danly, Cooper, & Shapiro, 1983; Danly & Shapiro, 1982; Heilman et al., 1984; Pell, 1998; Ross et al., 1997).

In addition to production, patients with focal right hemisphere lesions have demonstrated impairments in the ability to perceive or comprehend variations in intonation. Perhaps inspired by Ross's (1981) view (see also Ross & Mesulam, 1979) that "the functional-anatomic organization of affective language in the right hemisphere mirrors that of proposition language in the left hemisphere" (p. 561), most investigations of intonation perception in the right hemisphere–damaged population focused on the ability of these patients to recognize different emotions conveyed through intonation (e.g., Bowers, Coslett, Bauer, Speedie, & Heilman, 1987; Bradvik et al., 1990; Denes, Caldognetto, Semenza, Vagges, & Zettlin, 1984; Ehlers & Dalby, 1987; Heilman et al., 1984; Pell, 1998; Pell & Baum, 1997a, 1997b; Ross et al., 1988; Tompkins & Flowers, 1985; Tompkins & Mateer, 1985; van Lancker & Sidtis, 1992). In a number of these studies, it was found that patients with right hemisphere lesions were more impaired than patients with left hemisphere damage in the identification of intonation that conveyed happy, sad, angry, or indifferent meanings (Bowers et al., 1987; Ehlers & Dalby, 1987; Heilman et al., 1984; Heilman, Scholes, & Watson, 1975; Tompkins & Flowers, 1985; Tucker et al., 1977). In some studies, no evidence was found for intonation impairment in emotional speech for right or left hemisphere–damaged patients (Bradvik et al., 1990; Lebrun, Lessinnes, De Vresse, & Leleux, 1985; Pell & Baum, 1997a). Results of other studies suggest that approximately the same degree of intonation impairment in emotional utterances may occur following damage to either the right or left hemisphere (Cancelliere & Kertesz, 1990; Pell, 1998; Ross et al., 1997; Schlanger et al., 1976; Seron et al., 1982; van Lancker & Sidtis, 1992).

A few investigators also reported impaired perception of intonation in nonemotional stimuli for right hemisphere–damaged patients (e.g., Heilman et al., 1984; Pell, 1998; Pell & Baum, 1997a; Perkins et al., 1996). Heilman and colleagues found that the studied right and left hemisphere–damaged patients were comparably impaired on the identification of intonation in nonemotional contexts. Pell and Baum (1997a) also reported that whereas the right and left hemisphere–damaged patients in their study performed as well as normal subjects on the identification of emotions conveyed through intonation, they performed poorly on the identification of aspects of intonation in nonemotional utterances.

The reasons for the discrepancies in the results of intonation investigations in patients with right hemisphere damage are unclear. Baum's (1998) view is that prosodic processing "by individuals with brain damage reflects a complex interaction of perceptual deficits and higher level linguistic and/or cognitive deficits" (p. 39). It should be noted, however, that studies devoted to understanding the basis of intonation processing (Seddoh, 1997a, 2000) are limited. Thus it is unclear whether the discrepancies in results are attributable to differential underlying deficits in perception, language, or cognition for different subjects. Differences in time post onset, as well as site and size of lesion, may account for the discrepancies. Also, because normal intonation is itself poorly understood, it is possible that inferences made about brain-damaged subjects' performances have been misguided by inappropriate theoretical assumptions.

Van Lancker and Sidtis (1992) have shown that patients with right hemisphere lesions rely mainly on temporal information in processing intonation (but see Pell & Baum, 1997b). This suggests that these patients may be using temporal information to compensate for their deficit in processing the spectral components of the acoustic signal (Robin, Tranel, & Damasio, 1990).

One critical point is that the course of recovery from prosodic impairment in right hemisphere–damaged patients has not been addressed to any great degree. Colsher, Cooper, and Graff-Radford (1987) found that patients tested in the acute period following the insult had reduced F0 contours, but patients tested at 6 months post onset of the insult appeared hypermelodic or normal. Further study of this issue is clearly warranted, as it is apparent that differences in the results of the studies on speech prosody following brain injury may be related to the time post onset that a particular patient is studied (Kertesz, 1979). In addition, the effects of treatment on recovery from prosodic impairment have not been examined extensively. Another critical problem is that in the literature to date, in most studies the neuroanatomical localizations of the lesions have been poorly described. It is hoped that future studies will be based on more reliable methods, such as structural and functional brain imaging techniques for analyzing lesion location.

Disturbance of Prosody Due to Left Hemispheric Lesions

There have been fewer studies of speech prosody in patients with left hemisphere lesions than in patients with right hemisphere lesions. Unfortunately, the results of these studies are equivocal. Results of some studies have indicated that intonation production ability may be relatively spared for aphasic patients (e.g., Baum & Pell, 1997; Seddoh, 2000). Others have reported abnormalities that suggest either underlying phonetic–motoric (e.g., Cooper et al., 1984; Ryalls, 1982; Seddoh, 2000) or linguistic processing deficit (Danly & Shapiro, 1982; Danly et al., 1983).

Similar to the finding reported by Shapiro and Danly (1985) for patients with posterior right hemisphere lesions, Danly and Shapiro (1982) found that patients with Broca's aphasia had exaggerated F0 contours. The same finding was reported by Ryalls (1984) whose subjects, like those of the Danly and Shapiro (1982) study, were native speakers of English who also had Broca's aphasia. By contrast, Ryalls (1982) found that F0 ranges were significantly restricted and durations were abnormal for eight French-speaking patients with Broca's aphasia. Cooper et al. (1984) similarly found that their English-speaking subjects with Broca's aphasia exhibited "relatively flat F0 peak contours" (p. 19).

The finding of diminished F0 ranges in patients with Broca's aphasia (Ryalls, 1982) is consistent with clinical descriptions of the speech of these patients as "monotonous" (Goodglass, 1973; Goodglass & Kaplan, 1983). The contradictory findings of exaggerated F0 (Danly &

Shapiro, 1982; Ryalls, 1984) and restricted F0 (Ryalls, 1982) in the same category of (Broca's) aphasic patients may be due to differences in methodology and/or intersubject F0 variability (see Cooper & Klouda, 1987). Danly and Shapiro (1982) examined F0 variation by measuring peak-to-valley fluctuations within specific words in the stimuli, whereas Ryalls (1982) measured overall F0 range across entire sentences. Possibly, these measurement differences affect the results.

Patients with Wernicke's aphasia have also been reported to exhibit greater than normal F0 production. Cooper, Danly, and Hamby (1979) found "unusually large" (p. 269) initial F0 peaks and peak-to-valley variations in F0 for their Wernicke's aphasic subjects. Similarly, Cooper et al. (1984) found "abnormally high F0 values" (p. 19) in stressed syllables produced by the Wernicke's aphasic patients who participated in their study. Taken together with the abnormalities reported for patients with Broca's aphasia, it appears that phonetic or motoric deficit may underlie prosodic impairment in aphasia (Ryalls, 1982; Seddoh, 2000). Ross and colleagues (Ross, 1992; Ross et al., 1997) suggested that F0 abnormalities exhibited by aphasic patients in utterances that are emotional may be due to articulatory difficulties. This possibility may apply to the production of intonation in nonemotional contexts as well.

One striking prosodic characteristic of normal speech is a gradual downward trend in the F0 contour from the beginning to the end of declarative sentences. This phenomenon, referred to as *declination* (Cohen & t'Hart, 1965), was first reported by Pike (1945) for speakers of American English. Since then it has been noted for speakers of several other languages (for review, see Cohen, Collier, & t'Hart, 1982; Vaissiere, 1983), thus causing speculation that it might be a universal feature of verbal communication (Couper-Kuhlen, 1986; Cruttenden, 1986; Ohala, 1978; but see also Lieberman, Katz, Jongman, Zimmerman, & Miller, 1985 for a different view). In one of the earliest studies of intonation production in English-speaking patients with aphasia, Danly, de Villiers, and Cooper (1979) examined declination as well as utterance-final F0 fall in two-word utterances produced by subjects with Broca's aphasia. In addition to the F0 measures, the durations of initial and final words were evaluated. Results showed that the patients were severely impaired in durational control but exhibited both aspects of F0 in their utterances, thus suggesting that the production of F0 and duration may be differentially controlled (Seddoh, 1999).

Danly and Shapiro (1982) also found that although their subjects with Broca's aphasia were impaired in durational control, they exhibited declination in short, but not in long sentences. Based on this finding, these researchers concluded that "Broca's aphasics patients have a narrower-than-normal scope for linguistic planning" (p. 189). It should be noted, however, that Danly and Shapiro's long stimuli were confounded by syntactic complexity. As is often the case, the longer the sentence, the greater the syntactic complexity. Patients with Broca's aphasia are known to have syntactic processing problems. It may be that the primary problem for the subjects studied by Danly and Shapiro was syntactic, and this problem might have affected their F0 production in general. A growing number of studies on neurologically normal subjects indicate that F0 associated with intonation is influenced by linguistic structure, particularly syntax (Eady & Cooper, 1986; Nagel, Shapiro, & Nawy, 1994; O'Shaugnessy, 1979; Seddoh, 1997a; Shapiro & Nagel, 1995).

Evidence for underlying linguistic involvement in intonation processing problems exhibited by patients with aphasia is indicated by studies on both Wernicke's and Broca's aphasic patients. Danly, Cooper, and Shapiro (1983) found that performances of their Wernicke's aphasic subjects on the production of aspects of F0 tended to be normal when they corresponded to utterance length, but they were abnormal when they corresponded to the processing of syntactic information. Similarly, Danly and Shapiro (1982) reported poor performance on F0 resetting (new F0 contour initiation following a major syntactic boundary) for their Broca's aphasic subjects.

The ability of aphasic patients to decode affective meaning on the basis of intonation also has been investigated. Similar to the results of studies on right hemisphere–damaged patients, impairment has been reported in this aspect of intonation for aphasic patients (Cancelliere & Kertesz, 1990; Pell, 1998; Ross et al., 1997; Schlanger et al., 1976; Seron et al., 1982; van Lancker & Sidtis, 1992). This finding suggests that intonation deficit in aphasia may not be limited to nonemotional contexts as was previously assumed. Other investigators, however, failed to find any evidence for intonation impairment in emotional contexts for left or right hemisphere–damaged patients (Bradvik et al., 1990; Lebrun et al., 1985; Pell & Baum, 1997a). Still other reports indicate less impairment for patients with left hemisphere damage compared to patients with right hemisphere damage (Bowers et al., 1987; Ehlers & Dalby, 1987; Heilman et al., 1984).

A number of studies have also examined F0 production in patients with aphasia who are native speakers of tone languages, such as Chinese and Thai (for review, see Gandour, 1987, 1988). Languages that are tonal differ from intonation languages—such as English, French, German, and Spanish—in one major respect: the use of F0. Although the acoustic correlate of both tone and intonation is F0, in tone languages, F0 (tone) functions primarily at the lexical or syllable level and it often contrasts one word or syllable with another. (For similar information on the use of F0 in pitch accent languages, such as Norweigian, see Moen, 1991.) In intonation languages, on the other hand, F0 (intonation) functions primarily at the sentence or phrase level to convey verbal information. Unlike the findings reported on F0 production for patients who are native speakers of English (which is an intonation language), investigations of F0 in patients with aphasia who are native speakers of tone languages indicate that in general, F0 associated with tone is largely spared in this population (e.g., Gandour, Petty, & Dardarananda, 1988; Gandour et al., 1992; but see also Eng, Obler, Harris, & Abramson, 1996; Packard, 1986; Yui & Fok, 1995 for contradictory data).

Gandour and his colleagues (e.g., Gandour, 1987; Gandour et al., 1988; Gandour et al., 1992) suggested that differences between the relatively normal F0 reported and abnormal F0 for patients who speak tone languages may be explained in terms of timing. According to these researchers, the "critical variable" (Gandour et al., 1988, p. 238) in F0 production in speech is the temporal domain over which the F0 spans. That is, F0 production depends on the ability to control timing over the length of the utterance with which the F0 is associated. Gandour and his colleagues considered that the relative resistance of tone to disruption in aphasia may be due to the fact that unlike intonation, which is produced over sentence- or phrase-sized linguistic units, tone is typically a syllable- or word-level linguistic phenomenon and consequently spans over shorter temporal domains. They argued that the successful production of intonation depends on the ability to control timing over sentence- or phrase-sized units, whereas the successful production of tone depends on the ability to control timing over word- or syllable-sized units. Consequently, they claimed that "deviant timing at the sentence level necessarily disrupts F0 contours associated with intonation. However, in a tone language, deviant timing at the sentence level does not necessarily disrupt F0 contours associated with tone" (Gandour et. al., 1988, p. 238).

Gandour and his colleagues' view implies that there is a dependent relationship between F0 production and speech timing at the sentence level in intonation languages. Seddoh (1997a, 1997b) argued against this view, claiming that it is difficult to reconcile it with data on speech timing and intonation production in neurologically normal (Cooper & Sorensen, 1981; Seddoh, 1977a) or brain-damaged patients (Danly et al., 1979; Danly & Shapiro, 1982; Klouda, Robin, Graff-Radford, & Cooper, 1988; Niemi, 1998; Seddoh, 1999). Although intonation may be considered to be "a succession of fundamental frequency curves in time" (Couper-Kuhlen, 1986, p. 63), there is a lack of evidence for the general notion that a dependent relationship exists between intonation and speech timing. Danly et al. (1979) and Danly and Shapiro (1982) found that their subjects with Broca's aphasia exhibited severe impairment in durational control, yet the same subjects exhibited terminal F0 fall and declination in syntactically simple and short utterances. Klouda et al. (1988), who studied the effect of callosal damage on intonation production, also reported that their subject exhibited difficulty in the production of intonation in declarative and interrogative sentences even though timing ability was intact. In an acoustic study of intonation (F0) and duration in two groups of English-speaking subjects with fluent and nonfluent aphasia, Seddoh (2000) also found that, although the performance of both groups of subjects on various components of the F0 contours was largely comparable to normal performance, measures of various aspects of duration revealed severe impairment particularly for the patients with nonfluent aphasia. Findings like these do not support the view that "deviant timing at the sentence level necessary disrupts F0 contours associated with intonation" (Gandour et al., 1988, p. 238).

Results of perceptual studies of patients who speak a tone language (e.g., Gandour & Dardaranda, 1983; Gandour et al., 1988) suggest that there may be some degree of dissociation between the perception and the production of tone. In this population, the perception of tone has been found to be more severely impaired than the production of tone (but see also Packard, 1986).

Stress is another prosodic element that has been studied in brain-damaged patients (Baum, 1998; Baum, Daniloff, Daniloff, & Lewis, 1982; Behrens, 1988; Bryan, 1989; Emmorey, 1987; Grela & Gandour, 1999; Weintraub et al., 1981). In general, patients with left hemisphere damage have been found to be more impaired in stress production of perception compared to patients with right hemisphere damage (e.g., Baum, 1998; Baum et al., 1982; Emmorey, 1987; Ouellette & Baum, 1993; although the opposite finding has also been reported in Bryan, 1989). Baum et al. (1982) found that patients with Broca's aphasia performed worse than normal subjects in comprehending phonemic stress contrasts. A similar finding has been reported for both fluent and nonfluent aphasic patients by Emmorey (1987) and Baum (1998).

Acoustic studies (e.g., Emmorey, 1987; Ouellette & Baum, 1993) suggest that unlike the case for right hemisphere–damaged patients, stress disturbances in patients with left hemisphere damage may be related to a primary difficulty with the manipulation of durational cues. For example, Ouellette and Baum (1993) found that although left hemisphere–damaged patients performed comparably with their right hemisphere–damaged counterparts and normal subjects on the use of F0 and amplitude to encode stress, their performance on the use of durational cues for the same purpose differed significantly from the performance of the right hemisphere–damaged and normal subjects. Impairment of patients with left hemisphere damage on the manipulation of durational cues in stress production is consistent with reports that suggest that the left and right hemispheres may be differentially specialized in processing durational and spectral information, respectively (Robin et al., 1990; van Lancker & Sidtis, 1992).

Studies of stress converge with the data on intonation to highlight the possibility that the underlying deficit in prosodic impairment in general may be either linguistic (Baum, 1998) or nonlinguistic (Grela & Gandour, 1999). Reports of impairment in the ability to identify phonemic stress contrasts by patients with left hemisphere damage (Baum, 1998; Emmorey, 1987) suggest that underlying deficit for these patients may be linguistic in nature. Recently, however, Grela and Gandour (1999) reported results that suggest a different interpretation. These investigators found that although perceptual judgments of stress produced by a male subject with fluent aphasia indicated relatively normal performance on the application of Rhythm Rule (a phonological phenomenon in which adjacent stresses in word sequences are adjusted to avoid "stress clash"), acoustic measures revealed some abnormalities. By comparison, another subject with nonfluent aphasia failed to produce stress appropriately not only in contexts requiring the application of the Rhythm Rule, but also in those that did not require it. These outcomes led Grela and Gandour to suggest that rather than being indicative of phonological impairment, the errors for both patients might originate from phonetic-motoric deficit.

Kent and Rosenbek (1982), arguing that prosodic disturbance is a primary symptom of apraxia of speech, reported acoustic data for patients with left hemisphere lesions and apraxia. They found that apraxic speakers had a dissociated spectrographic pattern in which syllable durations were uniform and the F0 pattern assumed a similar shape within syllables. The syllables tended to be separated by lengthy but consistent intervals.

In general, studies that investigated duration in the left hemisphere–damaged population indicate that patients with damage anterior to the Rolandic fissures are more impaired than their counterparts with a lesion posterior to the Rolandic fissures (e.g., Balan & Gandour, 1999; Baum & Boyczuk, 1999; Cooper et al., 1984; Danly & Shapiro, 1982; Gandour & Dardarananda, 1984; Gandour et al., 1992; McNeil, Liss, Tseng, & Kent, 1900; Seddoh et al., 1996). One issue that has been left almost unexplored is whether there is any relationship between speech timing and other elements of prosody such as intonation and tone (Seddoh, 1999). Such studies might contribute to a better understanding of the nature of the disorders of the production and/or perception of individual prosodic elements.

Disturbance of Prosody Due to Lesions of the Corpus Callosum

There is very little evidence to support a role of the corpus callosum in speech prosody. However, given the belief that the right hemisphere is dominant for the processing of intonation (Blumstein & Cooper, 1974), and because intonation is part of the linguistic system, there is a strong possibility that intonation processed in the right hemisphere might be transferred to the left hemisphere to be integrated with the overall message. It has been suggested that this transfer of prosodic information might occur across the corpus callosum (Ross, Harney, deLacoste-Utamsing, & Purdy, 1981; Speedie, Coslett, & Heilman, 1984). Watson and Heilman (1983) reported that a patient with callosal disconnection was unable to repeat intonation associated with emotional utterances.

In a case that will be described in greater detail in the case reports section of this chapter, Klouda et al. (1988) studied prosody in a patient who had a pericallosal aneurysm that resulted in callosal disconnection. The patient was impaired in her ability to produce appropriate intonation in both affective and nonaffective contexts. Acoustically, the most prominent changes were in the F0 contours while durational measures remained intact. Her F0 production ability improved, however, over the period of a year. This patient's initial inability to produce appropriate F0 in her utterances suggested that the transfer of F0 contours from the right to the left hemisphere might have been disrupted.

Summary of Cortical Contributions to Prosody

This brief review of the literature on neurogenic disorders of prosody points out the importance of the ability to comprehend and produce prosodic variations in speech. Disorders of prosody have been documented in patients with right and left hemispheric lesions and in patients with lesions in the corpus callosum. The study of higher prosodic disturbances is still in its infancy, and numerous questions remain unanswered. For example, it is unclear if the prosodic disturbances described previously represent a higher-level cognitive linguistic deficit in which patients are unable to meaningfully label the prosodic contour of an utterance, or if there exist some perceptual deficits that may account for the impairment. Differential diagnosis might be possible in that the relative contribution of the right hemisphere to prosody may be related predominantly to the processing of F0 information (e.g., van Lancker & Sidtis, 1992). Left hemispheric contributions to prosody may also be predominantly related to durational aspects of prosody.

Robin et al. (1990) reported that patients with right hemisphere lesions were impaired in their ability to perceive frequency information but were normal in their ability to perceive durational information in nonlinguistic stimuli. In direct contrast, patients with left hemisphere lesions were able to perceive frequency changes but were abnormal in their performance on all tasks of temporal perception. As van Lancker and Sidtis (1992) have shown, it appears that this separation of processing capacities exists for prosodic stimuli as well. Finally, Kent and Rosenbek (1982) found different spectrographic patterns depending on the site of the lesion in the nervous system, a finding that suggests differential diagnosis on the basis of abnormal acoustic parameters may be warranted.

What seems critical to the clinical endeavor is that carefully controlled evaluations of prosodic disturbances are performed. In order to do this successfully, clinicians need to consider using acoustic measures to define the specific parameters of prosody and develop stimuli that assess a range of emotive and nonemotive conditions. Acoustic, coupled with perceptual, data may provide information needed for differential diagnosis and for the development of therapeutic programs for individual patients.

Assessment of Prosodic Production

The production of prosody can be measured perceptually, acoustically, and physiologically. This section will focus on perceptual and acoustic measures for the reason that clinicians may find it easier to obtain the instrumentation for perceptual and acoustic measures than for physiological measures. In addition to assessing prosody in speech production, clinicians should examine the patient's ability to perceive differences in prosody in the speech of others. This is an area of prosody that frequently has been overlooked.

Perceptual measures are those that rely on the listener's ear to determine prosodic accuracy and acceptability. It can be argued that if an impairment is not perceptually relevant, it does not constitute a disorder and should not be treated. However, it has been demonstrated that the human ear may be a poor judge of acoustic reality (Breckenridge, 1977; Lieberman, 1965). That is, predictable prosodic changes in language are so ubiquitous that we hear them even when they are absent from the acoustic signal, or we may not be able to judge which acoustic parameter is changing even when we accurately identify a prosodic change.

The specific acoustic parameter that is disordered—the duration, F0, or intensity—cannot be determined without acoustic measures. Furthermore, although a patient may "sound" normal to the clinician during the treatment or diagnostic session, the clinician is operating within a restricted context. Often the patient or family members complain that under more natural conditions, the patient seems to have "lost" the ability to convey humor or emotion through the voice. They may state that the patient's speech is "different" in that the tone of voice is no longer meaningful. The critical point is that both perceptual and acoustic measures of speech prosody should be used; they complement one another, and their combination adds an important dimension to the diagnostic endeavor.

Table 8.1 lists examples of stimuli that may be used to examine the production of prosody in neurologically impaired patients. The battery is designed to assess different uses of prosody. The distinction between question and statement can be assessed using the sentences in Section I. Also, the patient can be asked to read or repeat a sentence in a happy (Section IIa) or angry (Section IIb) mood.

A patient's ability to use prosody to convey emphatic stress placed on the initial or final words of a sentence may also be assessed using stimuli of the type shown in Table 8.1 (Section III). The patient is asked to read a sentence after being primed by a question. A set of three priming questions was composed for each of the sentences in Table 8.1 (Section III). For example, for the sentence "Don shot the puck to Kent," we ask the patient, "Who shot the puck to Kent?" (to focus stress on the first word of the sentence); "Who did Don shoot the puck to?" (to focus stress on the final word of the sentence); and "What happened?" (to elicit a neutral version of the sentence).

Another prosodic production test can be designed to assess a patient's ability to use syntactic juncture to convey meaning (Klouda, 1986). Examples of these stimuli are also listed in Table 8.1 (Section IV). Subjects are requested to read the sentences as they are written. They are told to read the sentences to themselves and to read them aloud only when they are sure of the responses. In summary, the use of these tests allows for examination of prosody across different functional domains in patients with neurological dysfunction.

The data obtained from patients on these production tests are analyzed using two different measurement techniques: perceptual and acoustic. In order to assess the perceptual accuracy of the speech of the patient, an audio recording is made in which the patient's utterances are randomly interspersed with utterances from normal speakers who have performed the same task. A group of normal listeners judge the accuracy of each item, and the sentences are digitized on a computer that randomly plays back the utterances. If such equipment is not available, clinicians can simply play back the tape of the patient's sentence production, leaving out identifying information such as the priming question. Listeners are asked to listen to the tape and judge whether a sentence is a question or a statement, the mood of the speaker, where the stress in a sentence falls, and the meanings of the

Table 8.1
Examples of Stimuli Used for Assessment of Prosody

I. Statement and question forms

Statement	Question
1. His dog came here.	His dog came here?
2. Jane came back home.	Jane came back home?
3. Tom stole a doll.	Tom stole a doll?
4. She sells cookies.	She sells cookies?

II. Emotive stimuli

(a) Happy

1. The bird flew away.
2. Tomorrow I'm leaving for Chicago.
3. My daughter will graduate this fall.
4. The weather is lovely today.

(b) Angry

1. I hate that man.
2. She made me mad.
3. That's ridiculous.
4. Get off my shoulder.

III. Emphatic stress

1. *Don* shot the *puck* to *Kent*.
2. The *salesman* sold the *couch* to my *father*.
3. *Mary* typed the *paper* for *Kate*.
4. *Chuck* ate *supper* with *George*.

IV. Syntactic juncture (pause location) sentence pairs

1. If Jerry fought his brother, we'll be upset.
   If Jerry fought, his brother will be upset.
2. If the teacher forgot, Jim would remind him.
   If the teacher forgot Jim, we'd remind him.
3. When John left Cindy, we'd be upset.
   When John left, Cindy would be upset.
4. When Dan marries Amy, we'll attend the reception.
   When Dan marries, Amy will attend the reception.

sentences with syntactic juncture. It has been our experience that forced choice is one of the best ways to obtain listener responses. Samples from our response forms for the perceptual analysis of the production tasks are shown in Figure 8.1. It is important to obtain judgments from a number of different listeners. Clinicians may wish to use naive listeners or family members as judges of the patient's prosody. This may allow the clinician to gain an index of the disability that the prosodic problem creates.

Acoustic measures are also made from the data obtained from the patients. Acoustic measures allow for an examination of F0, durational, and relative intensity components of speech prosody. In our research protocols, we have been concerned with the measurement of F0 and durational elements of prosody. Clinically, however, we have begun to examine relative intensity changes related to prosodic variation. These acoustic measures necessitate the use of a sound spectrograph, computer software such as Cspeech (Milenkovic, 1994), or other commercially available equipment such as the Visi-Pitch (Kay Elemetrics, Inc.). A microcomputer to assist in data analysis is quite valuable, and clinicians should purchase instrumentation with this in

---

I. **Emotive Stimuli**

Please circle the word you consider to describe best the mood of the speaker in the sentence. Make sure to select one of the descriptive labels. If you are unsure, select your best guess and circle "Best Guess" along with your answer.

Happy   Angry   Best Guess

% Correct:_____ Total % Correct:_____

II. **Emphatic Stress**

Please circle the word that is emphasized. If there is no emphasis, circle "No Emphasis." If you are unsure, select your best guess and circle "Best Guess" along with your answer.

Initial Emphatic Word   Final Emphatic Word   No Emphasis   Best Guess

% Correct: Initial Stress:_____

% Correct: Final Stress:_____

% Correct: Unstressed:_____

Figure 8.1. Listener Response Form examples.

mind. In our view, these instrumental measures are critical to the clinical endeavor and provide a detailed sampling of the patient's speech.

Table 8.2 lists the acoustic features we examine most often in the speech of our patients. By using Cspeech software, we obtain data such as F0 contour and durational information of a patients' speech. Frequency values of specific points on the contour are determined by placing a cursor on the point and then reading the F0 value of the point displayed on the computer screen. Individual words of each sentence are located by viewing the waveform and by simultaneously playing back the auditory signal in order to listen to the sample. The peak F0 values for each word, as well as other measures, are determined. The F0 contours can also be visually inspected for flattening and other abnormalities.

Eady, Cooper, Klouda, Mueller, and Lotts (1986) reported that F0 in normal speakers decrease an average of 53 Hz following the first stressed word in a sentence. These authors also found that when focus is placed on the final word of a sentence, the decrease in frequency

Table 8.2
Acoustic Measures

I. Fundamental frequency measures

1. Peak fundamental frequency of each word
2. Terminal F0 change
3. Terminal final frequency

II. Nonsegmental durational measures

1. Sentence duration
2. Word duration
3. Syllable duration
4. Pause duration

III. Segmental durational measures

1. Voice onset time
2. Vowel duration
3. Formant frequency duration
4. Stop-gap duration

between Word 1 and Word 2 is only 23 Hz, but there is an average increase of 12 Hz over the final word. Echo (intonation) questions show a rise in F0 on the last word of the utterance to an average of 80 Hz. Statements, in contrast, show a drop in F0 over the terminal portion of the sentence (Seddoh, 1997a, 1997b). Examples of F0 analyses of patient's speech are included in the case reports section of this chapter.

Both segmental and nonsegmental durational measurements of the utterances can also be made. At the prosodic (nonsegmental) level, total sentence, word, and pause durations can be examined. The final words of questions are usually longer in duration compared to statements (Eady & Cooper, 1986). Similarly, stressed words are longer than the unstressed counterparts of the same words (Eady et al., 1986). Clause boundary may be signaled in normal speech by the insertion of pause and by increasing the duration of the word preceding the pause (Cooper & Sorensen, 1981).

Segmental analysis involves a variety of within-word measurements (see, for example, Seddoh et al., 1996). We obtain measures of voice onset time (VOT), which reflects the time between the initial onset of acoustic energy for a consonant and the onset of vocal fold vibration. It is well known that voiced sounds have VOTs in the 0–3 ms range, whereas voiceless sounds have VOTs in the 40–70 ms range. These numbers vary depending on context. Also, one can measure vowel duration, format frequency duration, closure duration (the time between the offset of acoustic energy associated with a vowel and the onset of energy for a following consonant), fricative duration, spirantization, and nasalization. These measures allow us to examine the integrity of detailed aspects of the speech waveform.

Assessment of Prosodic Perception

The complete assessment of prosody includes the examination of perception in addition to the production of prosodic variations in speech. Stimuli used in these tests of perception are similar to those used in the production tasks. The patient's ability to perceive emotive and nonemotive speech is assessed. Currently, the neurologically impaired patients seen, both in our clinic and for our research protocols, are tested for their ability to perceive differences in stress placement in sentences. For this test, the patient listens to the utterances and reports which word in the sentence received primary stress. The patient's performance is compared to the performance of normal subjects who can identify the utterances with better than 95% accuracy.

Summary of Prosodic Evaluation

The results of these production and comprehension tests allow for systematic analysis of each patient's prosodic ability. A summary sheet of results is shown in Figure 8.2. This sheet allows the clinician quick reference to the overall prosodic pattern demonstrated by a given individual.

Treatment of Prosodic Disorders

Myers (1984) pointed out the lack of literature regarding treatment of prosodic disturbances related to right hemisphere lesions. In fact, there are no reports of treatments for primary prosodic disturbances for focal cerebral lesions in general. However, suggestions for treatment of prosodic disturbances of production in dysarthric and apraxic patients do exist in the literature (e.g., Rosenbek & LaPointe, 1985; Wertz, LaPointe, & Rosenbek, 1984) and can serve to guide prosodic treatment with the types of neurogenically based prosodic disorders discussed in this chapter. No known approaches to treatment of prosodic perception deficits exist. The following section focuses on counseling and treatment of disorders of prosodic comprehension and production.

I. F0 Measures

Stimulus Type

	% Correct	Variable	Increased	Decreased
Perception	_____			
Production	_____	_____	_____	_____

II. Durational Measures

_____ _____ _____

Figure 8.2. Prosody summary sheet.

Counseling

Counseling of patients and their families about the effect of prosodic disturbances on communication success and failure is one goal of treatment. Myers (1984) and Robin et al. (1986) have suggested that patients and their family members can benefit from counseling. Such counseling might focus on making the communication partners aware that the patient is impaired in the ability to use prosodic cues and, therefore, cannot be expected to reliably produce those cues in his or her own speech or perceive them in the speech of others.

Many family members feel that their relative no longer has a sense of humor, or that they are no longer able to tell what the relative wants based on his or her "tone of voice." The need for patience and understanding when communicating with the patient is stressed to family members, as is the need for specifying messages clearly and unambiguously. In short, in their communicative interactions with the patient, the nature of the patient's speech and language deficit must be taken into consideration. (For additional cues that may aid family members in successfully communicating with neurologically impaired patients, see Vogel, Miller, & Garcia, Chapter 4, this volume.)

Treating Disorders of Prosodic Perception

Problems associated with the perception of prosody must be addressed before or concurrently with attempts to remediate production deficits. The clinician should begin treatment by using different aspects of prosody to facilitate discrimination of the various cues. Visual cues, such as pictures of faces portraying different emotions, can be used and then gradually faded. It is important to introduce the patient to perceptual protocols involving utterances spoken by a variety of different individuals in different ways.

The use of a device such as the Visi-Pitch (Kay Elemetrics, Inc.) can provide knowledge of results for the patient and the clinician, as well. For example, rather than rely on the auditory feedback alone, the F0 contour of the utterance can be displayed on the Visi-Pitch. Of course, eventually, the visual cue should be faded as the patient responds to the auditory feedback alone.

Contrasting two different prosodic cues also can be useful for remediation of prosodic comprehension. For example, the clinician can pair different types of stimuli (question versus statement or stress location differences) with visual cues to assess the patient's understanding of these differences, and then gradually fade the visual cues.

As research in the area of prosodic comprehension proceeds, it may be found that assessment of pitch and duration perception is essential for estimating the level of impairment (low-level perception versus high-level comprehension) and for planning treatment. If a patient has difficulty discriminating differences in absolute pitch, the clinician may opt to treat this problem prior to treating specific prosodic abnormalities. Moreover, if the problem in understanding prosody is confined to one acoustic dimension, then the clinician can focus treatment on that feature.

Treatment of Prosodic Production Deficits

Treatment of prosodic production disturbances may involve the use of two contrastive intonation types. Visual and auditory stimuli can be paired. A graphic representation of F0 contour associated with a particular sentence type can be presented. A device that displays frequency, intensity, and timing information (such as the Visi-pitch) may be useful in facilitating prosodic change. For example, treatment may proceed in the following way: First, the clinician models the prosodic contour using a graphic (visual) as well as an auditory cue. Next, the clinician and patient repeat the intonation type together. When an accepted level of accuracy is achieved, the patient is instructed to alter stress or prosodic patterns using self-monitoring skills.

In the absence of a feedback device, the constrastive stress procedures outlined by Rosenbek and LaPointe (1985) may be useful in treating prosodic disturbances. These authors noted that the stimuli should be selected to meet the needs of individual patients. The complexity, length, and phonetic composition of the utterance must be considered. Initially the patient imitates the clinician. Treatment then moves to the question-and-answer format described previously in this chapter. Rosenbek and LaPointe suggested that once stress patterning is accurate in the contrastive stress drills, clinicians should move to a "preplanning activity," which is the first stage of carryover. Here, a conversation is instigated in which the questions and responses of the clinician elicit varying stress and other prosodic patterns. Finally, real dialogues are used in which the patient is asked to maintain stress patterns. Also, it is important also to provide homework composed of contrastive stress drills.

As part of the treatment process, clinicians must be able to monitor behavioral change objectively. Evaluation of prosody using acoustic measures may be useful in monitoring small changes over time. The evaluation may be conducted during the acute phase (1–3 weeks post onset), at 3 months post onset, and at 1 year post onset. Of course the number of reevaluations will depend on the needs of the individual patient. Thus, subtle changes in frequency or durational cues that are not yet apparent to the ear may be detected by acoustic measures.

Case Studies

In this section, three case studies are presented. These patients are presented in regard to their prosodic profiles.

 RIGHT HEMISPHERE LESION

Patient W.G. was a 68-year-old, right-handed male who sustained a stroke-related right temporoparietal lobe lesion. We evaluated W.G.'s ability to produce intonation 10 years post onset. He was tested with stimuli in Sections I and II listed in Table 8.1. His productions of 10 statements and 10 matched questions were recorded. Acoustic analyses of F0 and durational measures were performed on these recorded utterances.

Figure 8.3 shows the initial F0 peak (P1) for the two sentence types. Performance of the task by 5 neurologically normal subjects (age 64–76 years) was plotted for comparison. The graph shows that W.G. had exaggerated P1 in his productions. This exaggeration in P1 (and perhaps other aspects of the F0 contour as well) may be a compensatory strategy used by W.G., who might have been aware of his prosodic deficits.

It is interesting to note that unlike P1, which was measured on the earlier portions of the F0 contour (preterminal F0 contour), the values of the other measures on the terminal portion of W.G.'s F0 contours for questions were below normal levels. These measures are Terminal Final F0 (Figure 8.4) and Terminal F0 Change (Figure 8.5). According to Seddoh (1997a, 1997b) who developed these measures, Terminal Final F0 (TFF) is the highest and the lowest frequency limits of the end of the F0 contours for questions and statements, respectively. Terminal F0 Change (or F-delta) is the amount of the

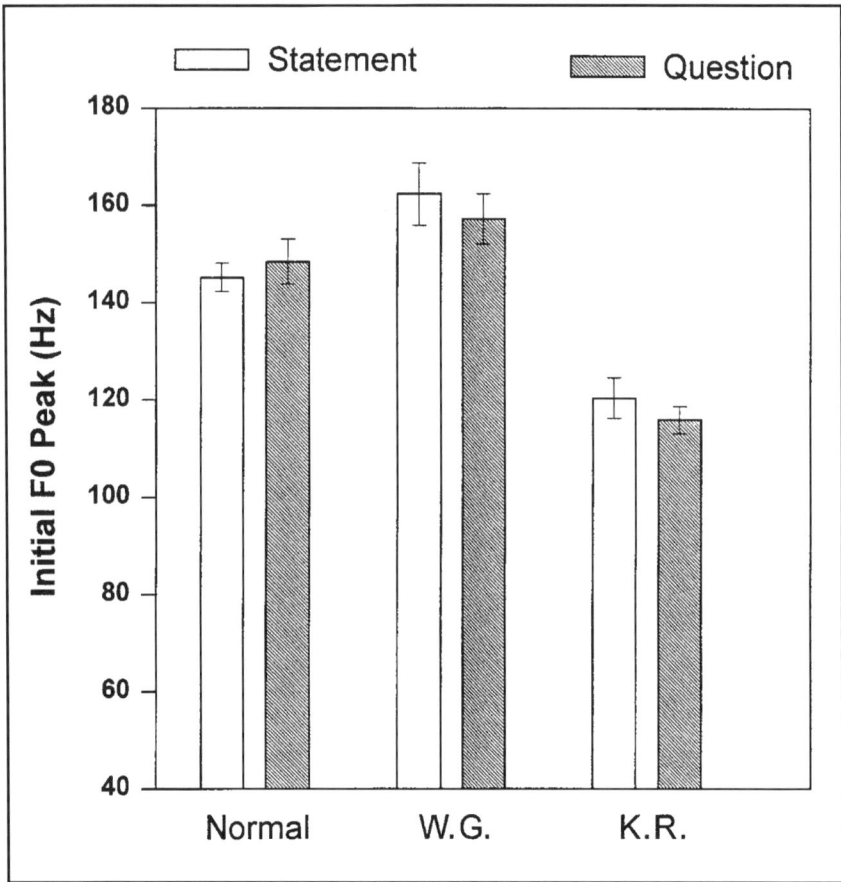

Figure 8.3. Initial F0 peak for statements versus question.

frequency fall or rise exhibited at the terminal portion of the F0 contour. It is measured as the difference between the frequency value of the point at which the F0 contour begins to rise or fall toward the end of the utterance, and the value of TFF. (For further discussion of these measures, see Seddoh, in press-a.)

Poor performance on the production of TFF for questions is a prosodic impairment frequently reported for brain-damaged patients. It appears that it is the production of the higher F0 values associated with the rising portion of the terminal F0 contours (for questions) that is a problem for these patients. This impairment seems to occur irrespective of the site of lesion (Seddoh,

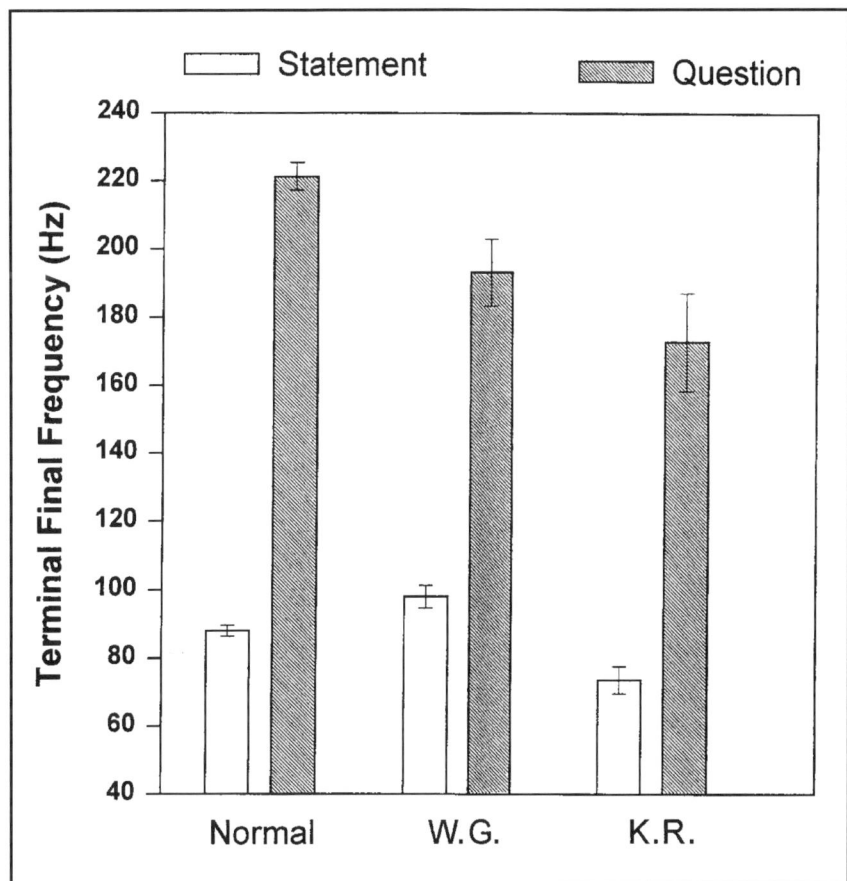

Figure 8.4. Terminal-final F0 for statement versus question.

1997a, 1997b). Thus, W.G.'s relatively poorer performance on TFF and F-delta for questions may be an effect of general brain damage.

Figure 8.4 shows the nonsegmental durations for the same utterances. The durational difference between questions and statements exhibited by W.G. was less than it was for the normal subjects. As noted earlier, studies with neurologically normal subjects indicate that questions tend to have longer durations than do statements. This tendency is also revealed for the performance of the normal subjects in Figure 8.6.

Treatment may begin with question-statement utterances because of the large difference in terminal F0 demonstrated in these type of utterances. Or,

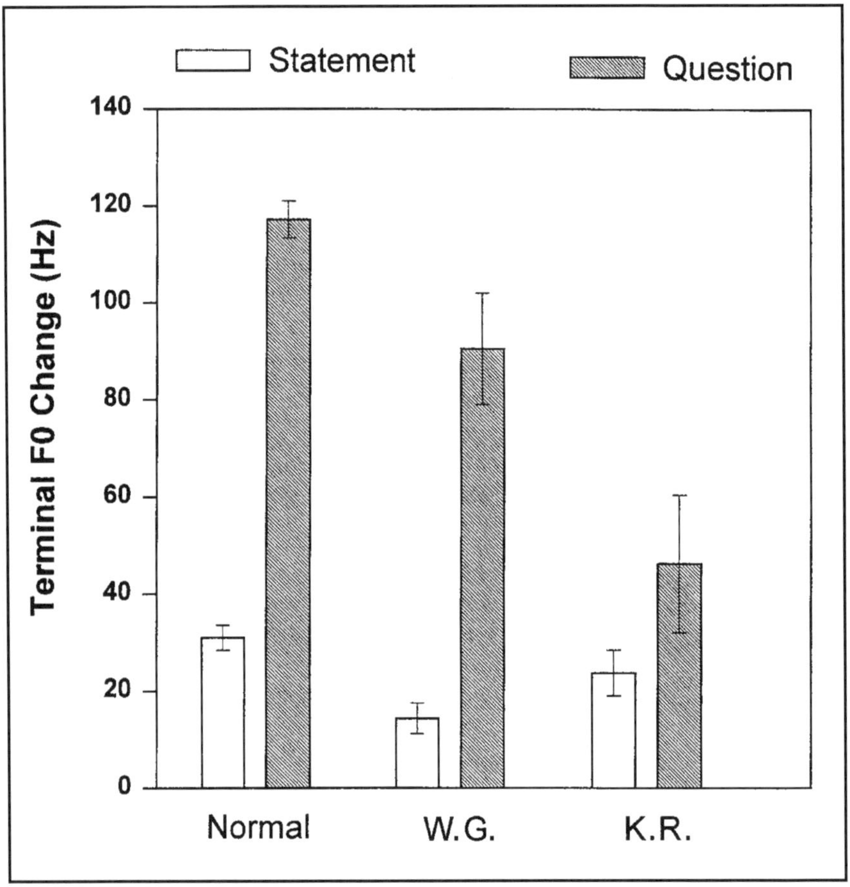

Figure 8.5. Amount of terminal F0 change for statement versus question.

treatment may begin with nonspeech stimuli, encouraging the patient to produce contrastive F0 patterns with prolonged vowels. A Visi-Pitch could be used to provide visual feedback of the F0 patterns.

 CALLOSAL DISCONNECTION

Robin, an author of this chapter, participated in the study of a patient (C.D.) with a callosal disconnection (Klouda et al., 1988). C.D. was a 39-year-old,

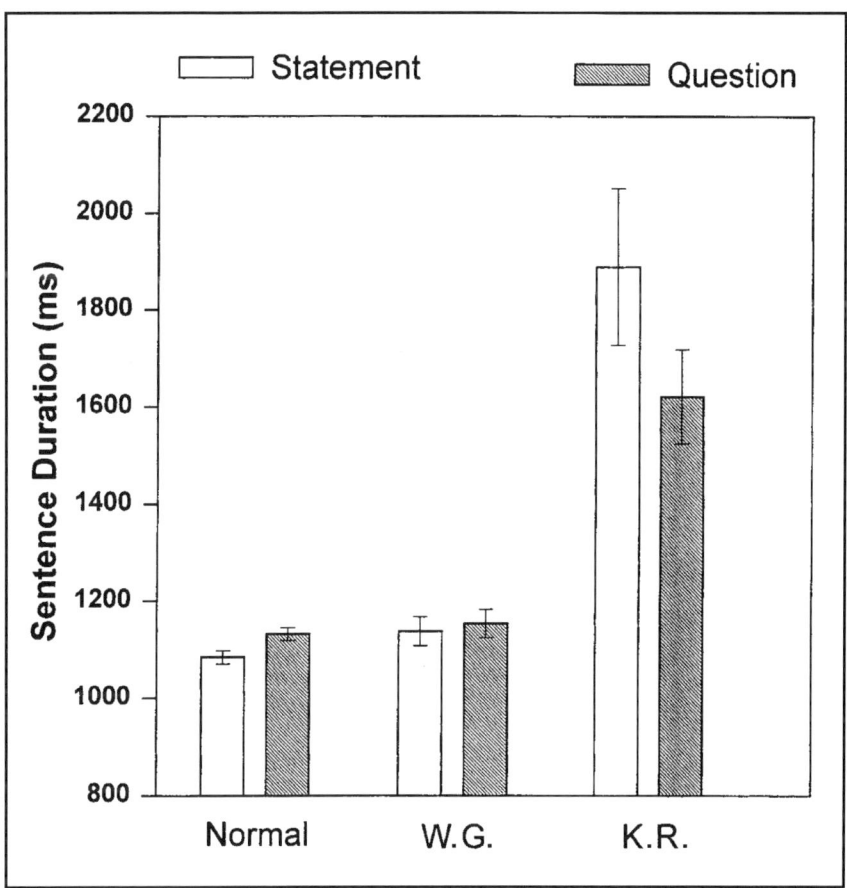

Figure 8.6. Sentence duration for statement versus question.

right-handed woman who had sustained a subarachnoid hemorrhage from a left pericallosal aneurysm. The aneurysm was clipped. The lesion involved the anterior four fifths of the corpus callosum but spared the splenium. Initially the patient was mute. By 4 weeks post onset, she showed no focal neurological signs but spoke with inappropriate prosody. Her prosody was tested at 4 weeks, at 4 months, and at 1 year post onset. Comprehension of prosody was intact at all test periods. Figure 8.7 shows that C.D.'s F0 contours for emotive stimuli were relatively flat. However, at Times 2 and 3 her use of F0 had improved dramatically. It should be noted that this recovery did not reach normal levels. Although normal listeners' perceptions of C.D.'s speech improved over time, at Time 3 listeners continued to make errors in their

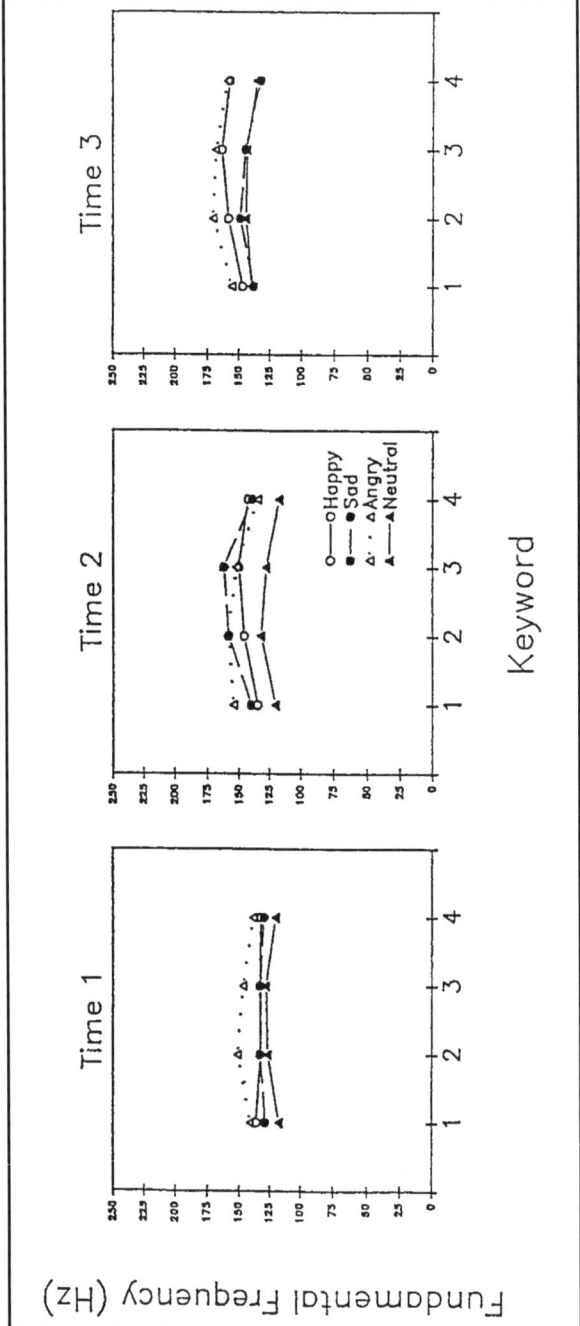

Figure 8.7. Average F0 peaks for emotionally intoned sentences at three different test times for C.D. *Note.* From "The Role of Callosal Connections in Speech Prosody," by G. V. Klouda, D. A. Robin, N. R. Graff-Radford, and W. E. Cooper, 1988, *Brain and Language, 35*(1), p. 160. Copyright 1988 by Academic Press. Reprinted with permission.

perception of C.D.'s speech. Nonsegmental durational measures were intact at all three test periods.

Figure 8.8 shows F0 contours for the question and statement stimuli used to assess prosody. Although C.D. made a distinction between them, the F0 was clearly attenuated at Time 1, although improvement was noted at Times 2 and 3. Further, normal listeners' perceptions of questions was less accurate (79%) at Time 1 than at Times 2 and 3. Durational cues for questions were intact.

Figure 8.9 shows C.D.'s F0 contours for the sentence focus tasks that were used to assess her prosody. At Time 1, the typical increase in F0 associated with initial and final stress was diminished. At Time 2, this improved somewhat but did not become normal. This distinction was more pronounced at Time 3 than at Time 2. The decrease in frequency following the initial stressed word was present, but was less than normal at Times 1 and 2 and nearly normal at Time 3. All durational cues were intact at all three test periods. Listeners were 100% accurate in judging stress in these stimuli, suggesting that durational cues were salient in producing sentence focus, and these cues might serve to compensate for the reduction in frequency level in these utterance types. Segmental durational elements were essentially intact.

This patient made such prominent changes in F0 control over time that if treatment had been initiated, one would have expected success with that feature of prosody. Whether treatment would have enhanced the normal recovery of this patient is not known. However, because at 1 year post onset, listeners continued to have some difficulty perceiving her prosodic patterns, treatment might have been warranted for C.D.

 LEFT HEMISPHERE LESION

K.R. was a 65-year-old man who had sustained a left hemisphere stroke that involved the basal ganglia. We examined him at 4 years, 8 months post stroke. K.R.'s production and comprehension of language in general was clearly impaired when we saw him. For example, his production was perceptually determined to be dysprosodic, and he seemed to have disturbance in the rhythmic organization of speech output.

Figure 8.3 shows K.R.'s P1 output for statements and questions. Compared to the performance of the normal subjects, K.R.'s P1 values for both utterance types were clearly diminished. The other two F0 measures conducted, that is, TFF (Figure 8.4) and Terminal F0 Change (Figure 8.5), also showed similar decreases in magnitude.

What is particularly striking about K.R.'s performance is that in all the measures, the F0 contours for questions were more adversely affected compared to the F0 contours for statements. This pattern of performance suggests that part of K.R.'s underlying problems may be motoric. Two pieces of

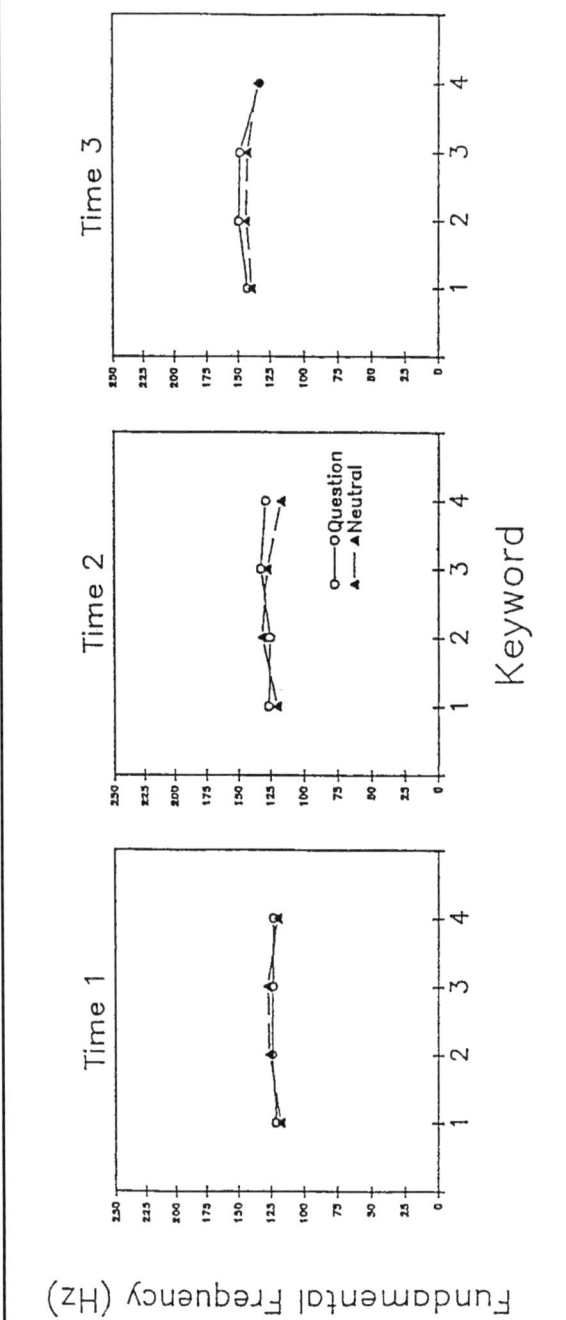

Figure 8.8. Average F0 peaks for statement and question intonation patterns at three different test times for C.D. Note. From "The Role of Callosal Connections in Speech Prosody," by G. V. Klouda, D. A. Robin, N. R. Graff-Radford, and W. E. Cooper, 1988, *Brain and Language*, 35(1), p. 161. Copyright 1988 by Academic Press. Reprinted with permission.

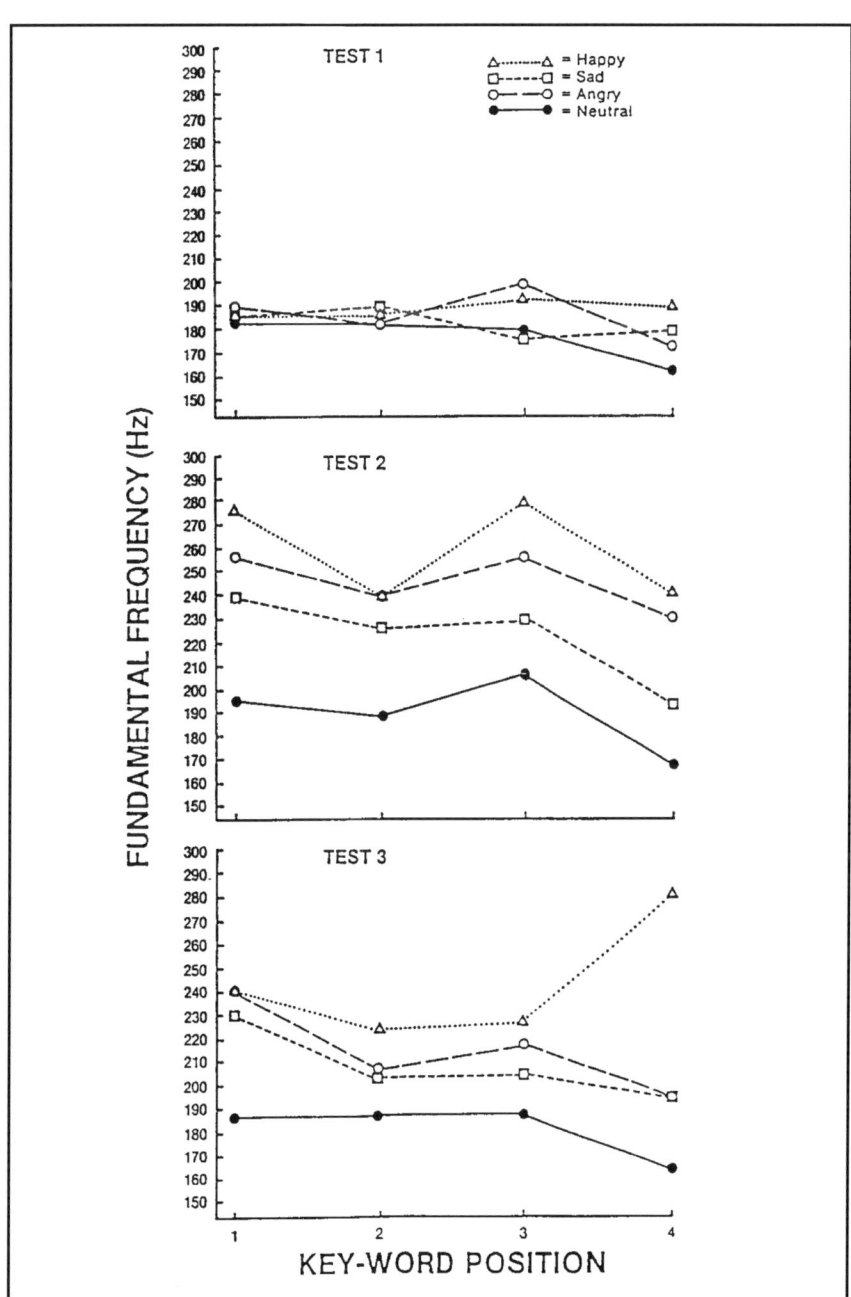

Figure 8.9. Average F0 peaks for sentences with different stress patterns at three different test times for CD. *Note.* From "The Role of Callosal Connections in Speech Prosody," by G. V. Klouda, D. A. Robin, N. R. Graff-Radford, and W. E. Cooper, 1988, *Brain and Language, 35*(1), p. 163. Copyright 1988 by Academic Press. Reprinted with permission.

evidence support this possibility. First, K.R. had a subcortical lesion in the basal ganglia, a structure known to be associated with motor control. Secondly, studies of neurologically normal subjects indicate that the production of rising intonation, such as that associated with echo (intonation) questions, is more effortful in comparison to the production of falling intonation, such as that associated with statements (Ohala & Ewan, 1973; Sundberg, 1979). Perhaps the most obvious evidence pointing to the possible involvement of an underlying motor control problem comes from the measurements of duration. Figure 8.6 revealed a clear impairment of prosody for K.R. His total sentence durations were much longer than normal. Perhaps more importantly, his durations for statements were abnormally longer than his durations for questions, a pattern of performance opposite to that exhibited by normal speakers. This pattern of performance also suggests that K.R. might have difficulty in programming the linguistic difference between questions and statements in terms of timing.

K.R.'s prosody impairment was most evident in durational abnormalities. Therefore, treatment should focus on those durational aspects of prosody. However, given that his comprehension of prosody was impaired, treatment might involve the perception of sentence stress along with the treatment of sentence stress production errors. To target his perceptual ability, various stress patterns could be presented and treatment could focus on identifying the portion of the stimulus that contains the greatest amount of stress. Exaggerated stress patterns could be used in conjuction with visual representation of the patterns. Eventually, the visual cues would be faded and the stress patterns normalized.

For treatment of prosody production, global timing features of prosody—such as word and pause length—can be targeted. Treatment might begin with nonspeech stimuli; the patient could be encouraged to produce vowels of different lengths while using instrumentation such as the Visi-Pitch to provide visual feedback. Then, treatment would progress to the use of word combinations and sentence length material. Eventually, other stimulus types could be added.

Summary

Patients with cortical and subcortical lesions often display disturbances in prosody. These prosodic impairments may involve comprehension or production, or both. Accurate assessment of prosodic disorders is essential to realizing a complete picture of a patient's communication profile and to the development of appropriate treatment strategies. One of the most common prosodic problems for patients with brain damage is the production of the higher components of rising F0 contours, such as those associated with echo questions. It appears that this difficulty occurs regardless of the site of lesion or type of communication disorder. On the other hand, the production of falling F0 contours, such as those associated with statements, may be relatively preserved for these patients. Comprehension of aspects of prosody, such as intonation and tone, have also been reported to be impaired in patients with aphasia. For aphasic speakers of tone languages, deficits in tone comprehension are reportedly more pronounced than deficits in tone production. Treatment of prosodic disorders should include couseling of patients and their significant others as well as therapies aimed at eliminating specifc errors.

Acknowledgments

The research reported in this chapter was supported in part by NINCDS Program Project NS19632 and by NIH (NIDCD) grant #DC90076 (NCVS). The authors acknowledge the support of Dr. Antonio Damasio and Dr. Daniel Tranel.

References

Balan, A., & Gandour, J. (1999). Effect of sentence length on the production of liguistic stress by left- and right-hemisphere-damaged patients. *Brain and Language, 67*, 73–94.

Baum, S. R. (1998). The role of fundamental frequency and duration in the perception of linguistic stress by individuals with brain damage. *Journal of Speech and Hearing Research, 41*, 31–40.

Baum, S. R., & Boyczuk, J. P. (1999). Speech timing subsequent to brain damage: Effects of utterance length and complexity. *Brain and Language, 67*, 30–45.

Baum, S. R., Daniloff, K. J., Daniloff, R., & Lewis, J. (1982). Sentence comprehension by Broca's aphasics: Effects of some suprasegmental variables. *Brain and Language, 17*, 261–271.

Baum, S. R., & Pell, M. D. (1997). Production of affective and linguistic prosody by brain-damaged patients. *Aphasiology, 11*(2), 177–198.

Behrens, S. J. (1988). The role of the right hemisphere in the production of linguistic stress. *Brain and Language, 33*, 104–127.

Behrens, S. J. (1989). Characterizing sentence intonation in a right hemisphere-damaged population. *Brain and Language, 37,* 181–200.

Berry, M. F. (1969). *Language disorders of children.* New York: Appleton Century-Crofts.

Blonder, L. X., Pickering, J. E., Heath, R. L., Smith, C. D., & Butler, S. M. (1995). Prosodic characteristics of speech pre- and post-right hemisphere stroke. *Brain and Language, 51,* 318–335.

Blumstein, S. E., & Cooper, W. E. (1974). Hemispheric processing of intonation contours. *Cortex, 10,* 146–158.

Bowers, D., Coslett, H. B., Bauer, R. M., Speedie, L. J., & Heilman, K. M. (1987). Comprehension of emotional prosody following unilateral hemispheric lesions: Processing defect versus distraction defect. *Neurophyschologia, 25*(2), 317–328.

Bradvik, B., Dravins, C., Holtas, S., Rosen, I., Ryding, E., & Ingvar, D. H. (1990). Do single right hemisphere infarcts or transient ischaemic attacks result in aprosody? *Acta Neurologica Scandinavica, 81,* 61–70.

Breckenridge, J. (1977). *Declination as a phonological process.* Murry Hill, NJ: Bell Laboratories Technological Memo.

Bryan, K. L. (1989). Language prosody and the right hemisphere. *Aphasiology, 3* (4), 285–299.

Cancelliere, A. E. B., & Kertesz, A. (1990). Lesion localization in acquired deficits of emotional expression and comprehension. *Brain and Cognition, 13,* 133–147.

Cohen, A., Collier, R., & t'Hart, J. (1982). Declination: Construct or intrinsic feature of speech pitch? *Phonetica, 19,* 254–273.

Cohen, A., & t'Hart, J. (1965). Perceptual analysis of intonation patterns. *Proceedings of the 5th International Congress on Acoustics,* A16.

Colsher, P. L., Cooper, W. E., & Graff-Radford, N. R. (1987). *Intonational characteristics of right-hemisphere-damaged patients' speech and its perception by normal listeners.* Unpublished manuscript.

Cooper, W. E., Danly, M., & Hamby, S. (1979). Fundamental frequency (F0) attributes in the speech of Wernicke's aphasics. In J. J. Wolf &

D. H. Klatt (Eds.), *Speech communication: Papers presented at the 97th meeting of the Acoustical Society of America* (pp. 265–270). New York: The Acoustical Society of America.

Cooper, W. E., Eady, S. J., & Mueller, P. R. (1985). Acoustical aspects of contrastive stress in question-answer contexts. *Journal of the Acoustical Society of America, 77,* 2142–2156.

Cooper, W. E., & Klouda, G. V. (1987). Intonation in aphasic and right hemisphere-damaged patients. In J. H. Ryalls (Ed.), *Phonetic approaches to speech production in aphasia and related disorders* (pp. 59–80). Austin, TX: PRO-ED.

Cooper, W. E., Soares, C., Nicol, J., Michelow, D., & Goloskie, S. (1984). Clausal intonation after unilateral brain damage. *Language and Speech, 27,* 17–24.

Cooper, W. E., & Sorensen, J. M. (1981). *Fundamental frequency in sentence production.* New York: Springer-Verlag.

Couper-Kuhlen, E. (1986). *An introduction to English prosody.* London: Edward Arnold.

Cruttenden, A. (1986). *Intonation.* Cambridge, MA: Cambridge University Press.

Danly, M., Cooper, W. E., & Shapiro, B. (1983). Fundamental frequency, language processing, and linguistic structure in Wernicke's aphasia. *Brain and Language, 19,* 1–24.

Danly, M., de Villiers, J. G., & Cooper, W. E. (1979). Control of speech prosody in Broca's aphasia. In J. J. Wolf & D. H. Klatt (Eds.), *Speech communication: Papers presented at the 97th meeting of the Acoustical Society of America* (pp. 259–263). New York: The Acoustical Society of America.

Danly, M., & Shapiro, B. (1982). Speech prosody in Broca's aphasia. *Brain and Language, 16,* 171–190.

Denes, G., Caldognetto, E. M., Semenza, C., Vagges, K., & Zettin, M. (1984). Discrimination and identification of emotions in human voice by brain damaged subjects. *Acta Neurologica Scandinavica, 69,* 154–162.

Eady, S. J., & Cooper, W. E. (1986). Speech intonation and focus location in matched statements and questions. *Journal of the Acoustical Society of America, 80,* 402–415.

Eady, S. J., Cooper, W. E., Klouda, G. V., Mueller, P. R., & Lotts, D. W. (1986). Acoustical characteristics of sentential focus: Narrow versus broad and single versus dual focus environments. *Language and Speech, 29,* 233–251.

Ehlers, L., & Dalby M. (1987). Appreciation of emotional expressions in the visual and auditory modality in normal and brain-damaged patients. *Acta Neurologica Scandinavica, 76,* 251–256.

Emmorey, K. D. (1987). The neurological substrates for prosodic aspects of speech. *Brain and Language, 30,* 305–320.

Eng, N., Obler, L. K., Harris K. S., & Abramson, A. S. (1996). Tone perception deficits in Chinese-speaking Broca's aphasics. *Aphasiology, 10*(6), 649–656.

Gandour, J. (1987). Tone production in aphasia. In J. H. Ryalls (Ed.), *Phonetic approaches to speech production in aphasia and related disorders* (pp. 45–57). Boston: College-Hill.

Gandour, J. (1998). Aphasia in tone language. In P. Coppens, Y. Lebrun, & A. Basso (Eds.), *Aphasia in atypical populations* (pp. 117–141). Mahwah, NJ: Erlbaum.

Gandour, J., & Dardarananda, R. (1983). Identification of tonal contrasts in Thai aphasic patients. *Brain and Language, 18,* 98–114.

Gandour, J., & Dardarananda, R. (1984). Voice onset time in aphasia: Thai II. Production. *Brain and Language, 23,* 177–205.

Gandour, J., Larsen, J., Dechongkit, S., Ponglorpisit, S., & Khunadorn, F. (1995). Speech prosody in affective contexts in Thai patients with right hemisphere lesions. *Brain and Language, 51,* 422–443.

Gandour, J., Petty, H. S., & Dardarananda, R. (1988). Perception and production of tone in aphasia. *Brain and Language, 35,* 201–240.

Gandour, J., Ponglorpisit, S., Khunadorn, F., Dechongkit, S., Boongird, P., Boonklam, R., & Potisuk, S. (1992). Lexical tones in Thai after unilateral brain damage. *Brain and Language, 43,* 275–307.

Goodglass, H. (1973). Studies on the grammar of aphasics. In H. D. Goodglass & S. E. Blumstein (Eds.), *Psycholinguistics and aphasia* (pp. 183–215). Baltimore: Johns Hopkins University Press.

Goodglass, H., & Kaplan, E. (1983). *The assessment of aphasia and related disorders* (2nd ed.). Philadelphia: Lea & Febiger.

Gorelick, P. B., & Ross, E. D. (1987). The aprosodias: Further functional-anatomic evidence for the organization of affective language in the right hemisphere. *Journal of Neurology, Neurosurgery, and Psychiatry, 50*, 553–560.

Grela, B., & Gandour, J. (1999). Stress shift in aphasia: A multiple case study. *Aphasiology, 13*(2), 151–166.

Heilman, K. M., Bowers, D., Speedie, L., & Coslett, H. B. (1984). Comprehension of affective and noneffective prosody. *Neurology, 34*, 917–921.

Heilman, K. M., Scholes, R., & Watson, R. T. (1975). Auditory affective agnosia: Disturbed comprehension of affective speech. *Journal of Neurology, Neurosurgery, and Psychiatry, 38*, 69–72.

Kent, R. D., & Rosenbek, J. C. (1982). Prosodic disturbance and neurologic lesion. *Brain and Language, 15*(2), 259–291.

Kertesz, A. (1979). *Aphasia and associated disorders: Taxonomy, localization, and recovery*. New York: Grune & Stratton.

Klouda, G. V. (1986). *Speech production in stutterers*. Unpublished doctoral dissertation, University of Iowa, Iowa City.

Klouda, G. V., Robin, D. A., Graff-Radford, N. R., & Cooper, W. E. (1988). The role of callosal connections in speech prosody. *Brain and Language, 35*, 154–171.

Lea, W. A. (1973). Segmental and suprasegmental influences on fundamental frequency contours. In L. M. Hyman (Ed.), *Consonant types and tone* (pp. 15–70). Los Angeles: University of Southern California Press.

Lebrun, Y., Lessinnes, A., De Vresse, L., & Leleux C. (1985). Dysprosody and the nondominant hemisphere. *Language Sciences, 7*(1), 41–52.

Lieberman, P. (1965). On the acoustic basis of the perception of intonation by linguists. *Word, 21,* 40–54.

Lieberman, P., Katz, W., Jongman, A., Zimmerman, R., & Miller, M. (1985). Measures of the sentence intonation of read and spontaneous speech in American English. *Journal of the Acoustical Society of America, 77,* 549–657.

McNeil, M. R., Liss, J., Tseng, C. H., & Kent, R. (1990). Effects of speech rate on the absolute and relative timing of apraxic and conduction aphasic sentence production. *Brain and Language, 38,* 135–158.

Milenkovic, P. H. (1994). *Cspeech.* Madison: University of Wisconsin.

Moen, I. (1991). Functional lateralization of pitch accents and intonation in Norwegian: Monrad-Krohn's study of an aphasic patient with altered "melody of speech." *Brain and Language, 41,* 538–554.

Monrad-Krohn, G. H. (1947a). Altered melody of language ("dysprosody") as an element of aphasia. *Acta Psychiatrica et Neurologica Scandinavica, 47*(Suppl.), 204–212.

Monrad-Krohn, G. H. (1947b). Dysprosody or altered "melody of language." *Brain, 70,* 405–415.

Monrad-Krohn, G. H. (1963). The third element of speech prosody and its disorders. In L. Halpern (Ed.), *Problems of dynamic neurology* (pp. 101–117). Jerusalem: Hebrew University Press.

Myers, P. S. (1984). Right hemisphere impairment. In A. Holland (Ed.), *Language disorders in adults* (pp. 177–208). Austin, TX: PRO-ED.

Nagel, H. N., Shapiro, L. P., & Nawy, R. (1994). Prosody and the processing of filler-gap sentences: Sentence processing III. *Journal of Psycholinguistic Research, 23,* 473–485.

Niemi, J. (1998). Modularity of prosody: Autonomy of phonological quantity and intonation in aphasia. *Brain and Language, 61,* 45–53.

Ohala, J. J. (1978). Production of tone. In V. A. Fromkin (Ed.), *Tone: A linguistic survey* (pp. 5–39). New York: Academic Press.

Ohala, J. J., & Ewan, W. G. (1973). Speed of pitch change. *Journal of the Acoustical Society of America, 53,* 345 (Abstract).

O'Shaughnessy, D. (1979). Linguistic features in fundamental frequency patterns. *Journal of Phonetics, 7,* 119–145.

Ouellette, G., & Baum, S. R. (1993). Acoustic analysis of prosodic cues in left- and right-hemisphere-damaged patients. *Aphasiology, 8,* 257–283.

Packard, J. L. (1986). Tone production deficits in nonfluent aphasic Chinese speech. *Brain and Language, 29,* 212–223.

Pell, M. D. (1998). Recognition of prosody following unilateral brain lesion: Influence of functional and structural attributes of prosodic contours. *Neurophsychologia, 36*(8), 701–715.

Pell, M. D., & Baum, S. R. (1997a). The ability to perceive and comprehend intonation in linguistic and affective context by brain-damaged adults. *Brain and Language, 57,* 80–99.

Pell, M. D. & Baum, S. R. (1997b). Unilateral brain damage, prosodic comprehension deficits and the acoustic cues to prosody. *Brain and Language, 57,* 195–214.

Perkins, J. M., Baran, J. A., & Gandour, J. (1996). Hemispheric specialization in processing intonation contours. *Aphasiology, 10,* 343–362.

Pike, K. L., (1945). *The intonation of American English.* Ann Arbor: University of Michigan Press.

Robin, D. A., Jordan, L. S., & Rodnitzky, R. L. (1986, February). *Prosodic impairment in Parkinson's disease.* Paper presented at the Third Biennial Clinical Dysarthria Conference, Tucson, AZ.

Robin, D. A., Tranel, D., & Damasio, H. (1990). Auditory perception of temporal events in patients with left and right cerebral damage. *Brain and Language, 39,* 539–555.

Rosenbek, J. C., & LaPointe, L. L. (1985). The dysarthrias: Description, diagnosis, and treatment. In D. F. Johns (Ed.), *Clinical management of neurogenic communicative disorders* (pp. 97–152). Austin, TX: PRO-ED.

Ross, E. D. (1981). The aprosodias: Functional-anatomic organization of the affective components of language in the right hemisphere. *Archives of Neurology, 38,* 561–569.

Ross, E. D. (1992). Lateralization of affective prosody in brain. *Neurology, 42*(Suppl. 3), 411 (Abstract).

Ross, E. D., Edmonston, J. A., Seibert, G. B., & Homan, R. W. (1988). Acoustic analysis of affective prosody during right-sided Wada test: A within-subjects verification of the right hemisphere's role in language. *Brain and Language, 33,* 128–145.

Ross, E. D., Harney, J. H., deLacoste-Utamsing, C., & Purdy, P. D. (1981). How the brain integrates affective and prepositional language into a unified behavioral function. *Archives of Neurology, 38,* 745–748.

Ross, E. D., & Mesulam, M. M. (1979). Dominant language functions of the right hemisphere? *Archives of Neurology, 36,* 144–148.

Ross, E. D., Thompson, R. D., & Yenkosky, J. (1997). Lateralization of affective prosody in brain and the callosal integration of hemispheric language functions. *Brain and Language, 56,* 27–54.

Ryalls, J. H. (1982). Intonation in Broca's aphasia. *Neuropsychologia, 20,* 355–360.

Ryalls, J. H. (1984). Some acoustic aspects of fundamental frequency of CVC utterances in aphasia. *Phonetica, 41,* 103–111.

Ryalls, J. H., & Behrens, S. J. (1988). An overview of changes in fundamental frequency associated with cortical insult. *Aphasiology, 2,* 107–115.

Ryalls, J. H., Joanette, Y., & Feldman, L. (1987). An acoustic comparison of normal and right hemisphere damaged speech prosody. *Cortex, 23,* 685–694.

Scherer, K. R. (1986). Vocal affect expression: A review and model for future research. *Psychological Bulletin, 99,* 143–165.

Schlanger, B. B., Schlanger, P., & Gertsman, L. J. (1976). The perception of emotionally toned sentences by right hemisphere damaged and aphasic subjects. *Brain and Language, 3,* 396–403.

Seddoh, S. A. (1997a). Basis of intonation production: An acoustic investigation of two hypotheses. *Proceedings of the International Conference on Cognitive Science '97 (ICCS'97).* Seoul, South Korea: The Korean Society for Cognitive Science.

Seddoh, S. A. (1997b). *Intonation in aphasia: An acoustic and perceptual investigation.* Unpublished doctoral dissertation, University of Iowa, Iowa City.

Seddoh, S. A. (1999). Intonation and speech timing: Association of dissociation? *Journal of the Acoustical Society of America, 106* (4), 2246 (Abstract).

Seddoh, S. A. (2000). Basis of intonation disturbance in aphasia: Production. *Aphasiology, 14,* 1105–1126.

Seddoh, S. A. K., Robin, D. A., Sim, H.-S., Hageman, C., Moon, J. B., & Folkins, J. W. (1996). Speech timing in apraxia of speech versus conduction aphasia. *Journal of Speech and Hearing Research, 39,* 590–603.

Selkirk, E. O. (1984). *Phonology and syntax: The relation between sound and structure.* Cambridge, MA: MIT Press.

Seron, X., van der Kaa, M. A., van der Linden, M., Remits, A., & Feyereisen, P. (1982). Decoding paralinguistic signals: Effect of semantic and prosodic cues on aphasic comprehension. *Journal of Communication Disorders, 15,* 223–231.

Shapiro, B., & Danly, M. (1985). The role of the right hemisphere in the control of speech prosody in propositional and affective contexts. *Brain and Language, 25,* 19–36.

Shapiro, L. P., & Nagel, H. N. (1995). Lexical properties, prosody and syntax: Implications for normal and disordered language. *Brain and Language, 50,* 240–257.

Speedie, L. J., Coslett, B., & Heilman, K. M. (1984). Repetition of affective prosody in mixed transcortical aphasia. *Archives of Neurology, 41,* 268–270.

Sundberg, J. (1979). Maximum speed of pitch changes in singers and untrained subjects. *Journal of Phonetics, 7,* 71–79.

Tompkins, C. A. (1991). Automatic and effortful processing of emotional intonation after right or left hemisphere brain damage. *Journal of Speech and Hearing Research, 34,* 820–830.

Tompkins, C. A., & Flowers, C. R. (1985). Perception of emotional intonation by brain-damaged adults: The influence of task processing levels. *Journal of Speech and Hearing Research, 28,* 527–538.

Tompkins, C. A., & Mateer, C. A. (1985). Right hemisphere appreciation of prosodic and linguistic indications of implicit attitude. *Brain and Language, 24,* 185–203.

Tucker, D. M., Watson, R. T., & Heilman, K. M. (1977). Discrimination and evocation of affectively intoned speech in patients with right parietal disease. *Neurology, 27,* 947–950.

Vaissiere, J. (1983). Language-independent prosodic features. In A. Cutler & D. R. Ladd (Eds.), *Prosody: Models and measurements* (pp. 53–66). New York: Springer-Verlag.

van Lancker, D. (1980). Cerebral lateralization of pitch cues in the linguistic signal. *Papers in Linguistics, 13*(2), 201–277.

van Lancker, D., & Sidtis, J. J. (1992). The identification of affective-prosodic stimuli by left- and right-hemisphere-damaged subjects: All errors are not created equal. *Journal of Speech and Hearing Research, 35,* 963–970.

Wada, J., & Rasmussen, T. (1960). Intracartoid injection of sodium amytal for the lateralization of cerebral speech dominance. *Journal of Neurosurgery, 17,* 226–282.

Watson, R. T. , & Heilman, K. M. (1983). Callosal apraxia. *Brain, 106,* 391–403.

Weintraub, S., Mesulam, M.-M., & Kramer, L. (1981). Disturbances in prosody: A right-hemisphere contribution to language. *Archives of Neurology, 38,* 742–744.

Wertz, R. T., LaPointe, L. L., & Rosenbek, J. C. (1984). *Apraxia of speech in adults: The disorder and its management.* Orlando, FL: Grune & Stratton.

Williams, C. E., & Stevens, K. N. (1972). Emotions and speech: Some acoustical correlates. *Journal of the Acoustical Society of America, 52,* 1238–1250.

Yui, E. M. L., & Fok, A. Y.-Y. (1995). Lexical tone disruption in Cantonese aphasic speakers. *Clinical Linguistics and Phonetics, 9*(1), 79–92.

Chapter 9

Neurological Aspects of Spasmodic Dysphonia

Michael P. Cannito

In this chapter, Cannito critically reviews the numerous potential sites of neurologic lesion that have been proposed as underlying the signs and symptoms of spasmodic dysphonia. Some are found to be more credible than others. When viewed in conjunction with other behavioral and neurophysiological research, a model of variable supranuclear pathology emerges as the most viable interpretation of this mysterious voice disorder. Clinical implications for both assessment and management, supported with an actual case study of spasmodic dysphonia, are presented.

1. *Given our present state of knowledge, why are lower brainstem and peripheral nerve explanations of spasmodic dysphonia unjustifiable?*

2. *What aspects of spasmodic dysphonia symptoms are best explained by an appeal to limbic system function?*

3. *How might a supranuclear dysarthria model of spasmodic dysphonia influence treatment decisions in a manner that is differentiated from traditional hyperfunctional voice therapy? From psychotherapy?*

꙳   ꙳   ꙳

Spasmodic (spastic) dysphonia (SD) is an enigmatic disturbance of vocal motor control characterized by intermittent voice stoppage in a context of strained-strangled (laryngealized) and/or breathy (aspirate) phonatory perturbations (Cannito & Johnson, 1981).

These disruptions are typically speech specific, imparting a bizarre, labored, and dysfluent quality. Aronson (1978) catalogs a diverse assortment of perceptual-acoustic symptoms, characterizing SD voice productions as "staccato or stuttering-like, intermittent, jerky, grunting, squeezed, groaning and effortful" (p. 533). In contrast, the majority of SD patients exhibit a more normal voice quality for nonspeech vocal gestures such as singing, paralanguage, yawning, and laughing, and when phonating in the higher ranges of their fundamental pitch (Aronson, 1985; Freeman, Cannito, & Finitzo-Hieber, 1985a). Furthermore, the supralaryngeal articulatory aspects of speech production appear to be relatively unimpaired. It is both its apparent focality and function specificity that make SD one of the most puzzling and controversial disorders of human communication.

Because SD is an uncommon disorder, its precise incidence and prevalence remain unknown; however, it appears to affect women more frequently than men. Onset has been reported as early as the teens and 20s, but the average age of SD onset falls nearer to 50 years (Aronson, 1985). Slow insidious onset is commonly reported, although some SD patients have experienced an abrupt initial deterioration of the voice. The disorder is notoriously resistant to speech therapy and other behavioral interventions (Boone, 1977); however, many patients report that they have acquired beneficial compensatory strategies as a result of the therapies they have explored (Freeman, Cannito, & Finitzo-Hieber, 1985b). For a few years, it appeared that surgical treatment (recurrent laryngeal nerve resection) would solve the problem of SD; however, postoperative return of symptoms and other complications have been reported in a substantial subset of surgically treated SD patients (Aronson & DeSanto, 1983; Dedo & Izdebski, 1983).

Prior to 1973, voice clinicians tended to regard SD as a single clinical entity whose primary defining feature was intermittent voice stoppage (Aronson, Brown, Litin, & Pearson, 1968a) or periodic breaks in phonation (Fox, 1969), suggestive of involuntary muscular contraction at the level of the vocal folds. More recently, however, attempts have been made to specify the perceptual acoustic characteristics of SD in greater detail.

Aronson (1973) identified two forms of SD: the adductor and abductor types. He described the predominant characteristic of the *adductor type* (ADSD) as a strained-strangled hoarseness due to irregular hyperadduction of the vocal folds. The salient characteristic of the *abductor type* (ABSD) was described as intermittent breathy phonation or intermittent aphonia. To further objectify the acoustic characteristics of SD, a number of authors have conducted spectrographic case studies of these patient types (Cannito & Johnson, 1981; Merson & Ginsberg, 1979; Wolfe & Bacon, 1976; Zwitman, 1979). Review of these reports suggests a striking variability of vocal symptoms across patients (even within the same subcategory). Indeed, one is tempted to conclude that heterogeneity of vocal symptoms within SD is at least as great as that between SD and other voice pathologies from which it is differentiated. Such a conclusion, however, is probably unwarranted. Cannito and Johnson (1981) suggested that SD may be more parsimoniously considered a *continuum disorder* amenable to scaling along two continuous dimensions of harshness and breathiness, rather than to strict binary categorization. This hypothesis has been supported by subsequent research indicating that both variants of SD share many phonetic similarities as well as differences (Freeman et al., 1985a; Freeman, Cannito, Finitzo, & Schaefer, 1985). In addition, Aronson (1985) suggests that the continuum hypothesis "is not only plausible, but one that would help to explain their similarities pertaining to nature of onset, factors influencing severity, and multiple etiologies" (p. 190). At present, however, the heterogeneity versus homogeneity issue continues to be controversial (see Cannito et al., 1997; Watson, MacIntire, Roark, & Schaefer, 1995).

Other challenges to an explanatory model of SD include its dramatic intermittency and affect sensitivity, or waxing and waning of symptoms as a function of the emotional context. Because of the striking variability of SD symptoms—including (a) intermittency of dysphonia during connected speech, (b) vocal deterioration under psychological stress, and (c) marked improvement for nonspeech vocalizations—SD was long considered to be of psychogenic etiology (Aronson, 1978; Brodnitz, 1976; Murphy, 1964; Traube, 1871). It has often been suggested that SD patients are significantly depressed (Aronson et al., 1968a). Accumulating evidence, however, has linked SD with a variety of neuropathological symptoms (Aronson, Brown, Litin, & Pearson, 1968b; Feldman, Nixon, Finitzo-Hieber, & Freeman, 1984; McCall, 1974).

Acknowledging that, as with other motor speech disorders, a psychogenic "mimic" form of SD is at least possible (Darley, 1978; but see also Sapir, 1995), this chapter focuses upon explanations of a neurogenic etiology in SD. Although the literature suggests that the neurogenic etiology is the more prevalent one, researchers disagree as to the specific type and localization of neuropathology underlying the symptom complex of SD. Hypothetical lesion loci have included peripheral nerve, medulla, midbrain, basal ganglia, cerebral cortex, and the limbic system. The levels of CNS involvement in SD that have been posited by various authors are summarized in Figure 9.1. Each of these levels will be discussed in detail in the remainder of this chapter. For a review of neuroanatomical structure and function, the reader is referred to Chapter 3 in this volume.

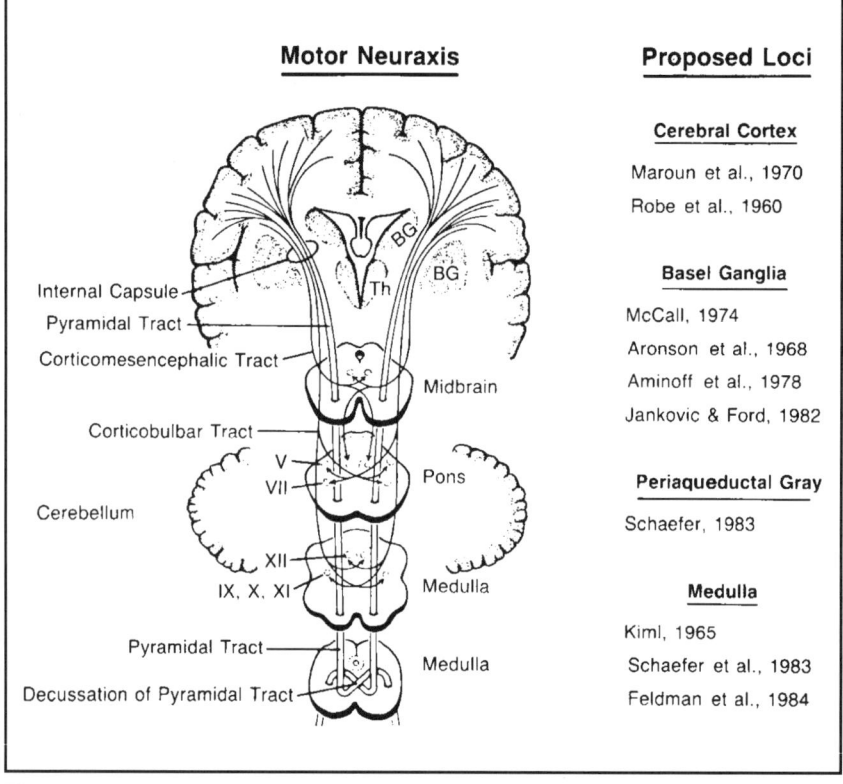

Figure 9.1. Possible sites of central nervous system lesions, proposed by various authors, to account for the pathology of spasmodic dysphonia. *Note.* Adapted from "Neuropathologies of Speech and Language: An Introduction to Patient Management," by T. Wertz, in *Clinical Management of Neurogenic Communicative Disorders* (pp. 1–96), edited by D. F. Johns, 1985, Austin, TX: PRO-ED. Copyright 1985 Little, Brown. Adapted with permission.

It is clear, however, that an adequate neuropathological model of SD must account for its apparent focality, function specificity, heterogeneity, intermittency, and affect sensitivity. In the review that follows, it will be argued that infranuclear explanations implicating lower motor neurons or peripheral nerves are inadequate to account for vocal and other symptoms exhibited in SD. In contrast, supranuclear explanations, particularly those involving the pyramidal/extrapyramidal voluntary motor system, do indeed provide a coherent basis for a model of this enigmatic disorder. Finally, implications of such a model for clinical management, as well as an SD patient treated within a neuromotor framework, are discussed.

Proposed Lesion Loci

Peripheral Nerve

In an effort to explain the positive response of SD patients to surgical sectioning of the recurrent laryngeal nerve, Dedo, Townsend, and Izdebski (1978) compared recurrent laryngeal nerves of SD patients with control recurrent laryngeal nerves taken at autopsy and at laryngectomy. Based on light microscopy and histological staining techniques, atypical fiber bundles were reported in the SD sample, but no active demyelinization or other abnormalities were found. Boccino and Tucker (1978) subsequently reported evidence of demyelinization in the recurrent laryngeal nerves of SD patients. These findings, however, were refuted by Ravits, Aronson, DeSanto, and Dyck (1979), who used more sensitive histometric and "teased fiber" morphology techniques in conjunction with electron microscopy. Results yielded "no significant difference between the disease and control groups in morphology, median fiber diameter, density or size distribution of fibers, or morphology of teased fibers" (p. 1380).

Explanations implicating peripheral neuropathy are inadequate on symptomatic grounds as well. It is well known that peripheral neuropathy can result in the slowing of conduction of neural impulses (in the case of demyelinization) or their complete disruption (Rowland, 1982). Disruption of the final common pathway to the intrinsic laryngeal musculature results in consistent adductor or abductor fixation of the vocal fold(s), rather than in an intermittent abnormality that is restricted to speech (Luchsinger & Arnold, 1965). It is generally felt, at present, that the neurologic locus of dysfunction underlying SD must be at least at the level of the brainstem within the central nervous system (Shipp, Izdebski, Reed, & Morrissey, 1985).

Medulla

Evidence of abnormal reflex behavior mediated by brainstem (cranial) sensorimotor nuclei has been reported in SD for middle ear (stapedial) reflexes (Hall, 1981; Hall & Jerger, 1976; McCall, 1974), as well as parasympathetic efferent vagal stimulation of the stomach and the heart (Feldman et al., 1984). In addition, abnormal auditory brainstem responses (ABR) have been reported in SD patients (Finitzo-Hieber, Freeman, Gerling, Dodson, & Schaefer, 1981; Hall, 1981; Schaefer, Finitzo-Hieber, Gerling, & Freeman, 1983; Sharbrough, Stockard, & Aronson, 1978). These abnormalities potentially implicate cochlear, trigeminal, facial, and vagal dorsal motor nuclei of the pons and medulla, and the polysynaptic brainstem auditory pathway to the level of inferior colliculus in the midbrain.

These factors, combined with frequent somatic complaints by SD patients implicating a varity of cranially innervated structures, led Schaefer et al. (1983) to posit that SD may be a generalized brainstem syndrome involving multiple cranial nerve nuclei. Suggested mechanisms included either a "shared" lesion affecting adjacent structures or a "skip" lesion affecting more distal structures.

It is clear, however, that a lesion involving a significant portion of the cranial sensorimotor neuron pool would result in widespread, crippling consequences. A variety of such brainstem syndromes are well documented in the neurologic literature (Clark, 1975). A lateral medullary syndrome, for example, can be characterized by a loss of pain and thermal sense of the ipsilateral half of the face and contralateral half of the body, vertigo, nausea, disequilibrium, persistent hiccup, and vocal hoarseness (Carpenter, 1978). For the majority of SD patients, these symptoms are simply not present. Because SD does not resemble the effects of a gross structural medullary lesion, a disease process implicated at this level must be both subtle and diffuse. For example, dysfunction of a number of specific neurotransmitter systems may be inferred (Schaefer, 1983). With respect to vocalization, however, medullary lesions are, in general, maximally disruptive of species-specific vocalization in monkeys (Kirzinger & Jurgens, 1985); therefore, even a subtle and diffuse lesion at this level would seem inadequate to account for the selective disruption of speech that is apparently exhibited by patients with SD.

A second attempt at a brainstem localization hypothesis has been offered by Izdebski and Shipp (1985), who suggest dysfunction in an unspecified "comparator" mechanism localized to the brainstem. This comparator receives afferent somatosensory input from subglottal mechanoreceptors that are sensitive to air pressure and flow. The comparator then uses this information for regulation of efferent adductor laryngeal control. These authors hypothesize that in SD there is an enhancement of the threshold level for subglottal pressure necessary to trigger an adductory reflex response. Thus, when the critical subglottal pressure value is exceeded during speech, the result is an immediate hyperadduction of the vocal folds. The positive response of many SD patients to recurrent laryngeal nerve resection, which reduces overpressure by fixation of one vocal fold, has been offered as evidence in support of this position.

There are, however, a number of problems associated with this hypothesis. It has been demonstrated in animals that the mechanoreceptors in question do indeed exist and that they project, along with other laryngeal somatosensory receptors, to secondary neurons housed primarily in the caudal portion of nucleus solitarius and secondarily in the main sensory and spinal nuclei of the trigeminal nerve (Dubner, Sessle, & Storey, 1978). It is plausible that a disease process could affect these structures locally, resulting in an afferent hypersensitivity of the type proposed. Axelrod (1974), for example, has demonstrated hypersensitivity in postsynaptic pineal neurons, either by presynaptic denervation or a long-term pharmacologic (reserpine) blockade, altering at a molecular level "the 'avidity' with which the receptor binds the neurotransmitters" (p. 9). It seems unlikely, however, that a destructive process would be selective for only those cell bodies associated with subglottal pressure and flow detection. A destructive lesion should logically implicate other functions mediated by the brainstem nuclei in question. Nucleus solitarius mediates taste, visceral pain, and general laryngopharyngeal proprioception; the trigeminal nuclei mediate general somasthesia for the head and neck (Dubner et al., 1978). Abnormalities of these functions (i.e., taste, vocal tract somasthesia, and visceral pain) have not been reported typically in the SD literature (see Schaefer et al., 1983). Cannito (1986) found no difference in oral stereognosis, oral 2-point discriminations, or facial tactile number recognition between 18 SD females and matched normal controls.

On the aerodynamic side, the afferent hypersensitivity hypothesis would predict an increased frequency of vocal perturbations in SD specific to phonetic environments in which subglottal pressure is particularly increased. Two obvious instances of this include the early portions of sustained vowels and the vocalic nuclei of strongly stressed syllables. No published studies have reported such distributions. Further, some SD patients exhibit quite the opposite effect. Thus, the afferent hypersensitivity hypothesis is dissatisfying on both anatomic and aerodynamic grounds.

A third theory implicating the brainstem focuses on the medullary reticular formation. The reticular formation is a phylogenetically primitive structure that traverses the length of the brainstem and forms its inner core. In addition to its role in the reticular activating system, which subserves arousal, the reticular formation functions as an interneuronal pool analogous to the intermediate gray area of the spinal cord (House, Pansky, & Siegal, 1979). Maximal overlap of afferent fibers from different sources occurs in the medullary reticular formation and subserves associative sensory functions. For example, parvicellular reticular nucleus receives fibers from secondary cranial nerve nuclei, including the cochlear, trigeminal, solitary, and vestibular. At this level, reticular interneurons participate in control of autonomic cardiovascular and respiratory responses (House et al., 1979). Because of its important role as a lower center for cranial sensorimotor convergence, some authors have logically inferred that a lesion in the medullary reticular formation could explain the diversity of symptoms associated with SD. As early as 1965, Kiml speculated on the possible role of brainstem reticular formation in SD due to its enormous cytoarchitectural possibilities for interaction. Among more recent neural models considered for SD, Schaefer (1983) also hypothesizes a lesion of reticular formation neurons of the brainstem predicated on the role of reticular formation in mediating respiration and interneuronal convergence.

Despite its logical appeal, a gross lesion in medullary reticular formation is probably unsupportable as an underlying etiology of SD. Experimentally induced lesions of the lateral medullary reticular formation surrounding nucleus ambiguous (as well as lesions in nucleus ambiguous itself) have been shown to abolish all elicited species-specific vocalizations in squirrel monkeys (Jurgens & Pratt, 1979a, 1979b). These primitive mammalian vocalizations are more comparable to human vocal gestures, such as laughing and crying, than to speech (Jurgens & Ploog, 1981). Therefore, a lateral reticular lesion would most likely predict either a total loss of phonatory function or a loss of non-speech vocal function. In addition, clinical neuropathology of lateral brainstem reticular formation frequently results in loss of consciousness, accompanied by respiratory and cardiovascular disturbances that often become fatal (House et al., 1979). Thus, although the medullary reticular formation remains of interest to an understanding of SD, abnormalities at this level may reflect abnormal neuronal processing interactions that occur under the modulating influence of impaired supranuclear structures.

Midbrain

Another locus that potentially has some explanatory power in relation to SD is the reticular formation of the midbrain tegmentum. This region houses a number of critical nuclear masses that might be implicated in the symptom complex of SD. These include (a) auditory nuclei and pathways of the lower midbrain thought to be major contributors to Wave 5 of the auditory brainstem response (Stillman, 1980); (b) the periaqueductal gray, a midline reticular nucleus that is a coordinating center for mammalian species-specific vocalization (Jurgens & Ploog, 1981; Jurgens & Pratt, 1979b; Kelley, Beaton, & Magoun, 1946); (c) midbrain reticular substance, wherein experimental lesions in primates have been associated with postural tremors, spasmodic torticollis, and intermittent losses of postural muscle tone (Bril, Sharpe, & Ashby, 1979; Foltz, Knopp, & Ward, 1959; Pechadre, Larochelle, & Poirier, 1976); (d) the substantia nigra, associated with movement control and motor deterioration in Parkinson's disease (Carpenter, 1978); and (e) mesencephalic nucleus of the trigeminal nerve, thought to be associated with jaw proprioception (House et al., 1979). Although the reputed functions of all these structures may appear related to SD symptoms, lesions in even a subset of them would produce more striking clinical abnormalities than are typical of the SD patient. For example, a midbrain lesion should result in severe abnormalities of more rostral components of the auditory brainstem response, whereas a periaqueductal lesion would abolish all species-specific vocalizations (Jurgens & Pratt, 1979a, 1979b;

von Cramon, 1981). The auditory brainstem response of the SD patient is not markedly abnormal, but rather exhibits merely a prolongation of Wave 5 latency at higher repetition rates of acoustic stimulation; Vocal perturbations are intermittent and specific to purposeful speech. Although it is possible that a very subtle and diffuse lesion in these areas may not have such gross consequences as have been portrayed, even a minimal lesion at the midbrain level would seem unable to explain the functional specificity and focality that is characteristically attributed to SD.

Because of the synaptic possibilities it offers for diverse interneuronal processing interactions among multiple midbrain and other rostro-caudal structures, midbrain reticular formation seems to be a reasonable candidate for localization of dysfunction, if not a structural lesion, in SD. Actual lesions of midbrain reticular formation frequently produce coma and are associated with large-amplitude slow waves in the cortical EEG (House et al., 1979). Thus, it again appears that if there are abnormalities at this level, they are probably restricted to deviant interneuronal processing, again perhaps under the modulating influence of impaired higher-level structures. One such structure, the globus pallidus of the basal ganglia, projects a major outflow (via the ansa lenticularis) to the pedunculopontine nucleus of the midbrain reticular formation. This is the only directly descending output of the basal ganglia, and it may mediate basal gangliar modulation of motor function (House et al., 1979). Along similar lines, Jankovic (1983) has reported two cases of blepharospasm in humans secondary to focal midbrain lesions, resulting in denervation hypersensitivity of the facial nucleus. Although spasmodic blinking is obviously not a speech-specific disorder, the parallel with a midbrain interpretation of SD is intriguing. Clinical cases of aphonia and dysphonia secondary to midbrain lesions have also been reported (Botez & Barbeau, 1971; Vogel & von Cramon, 1982). In any case, a midbrain locus would indicate a supranuclear disorder with respect to laryngo-pharyngeal motor neurons subserving vocal function.

Basal Ganglia and Related Structures

Although the term *extrapyramidal* is unfortunately ambiguous, in routine clinical parlance it has come to be associated with the basal ganglia (caudate, putamen, and globus pallidus) and other intimately related subcortical motor centers of the diencephalon and midbrain, including the subthalamic nucleus and substantia nigra. Disorders of the extrapyramidal motor system result in a variety of dyskinesias wherein the smoothly modulated control of voluntary movement is impeded by fast or slow spontaneous alternations of muscular tone. For definitions of the extrapyramidal movement disorders and a discussion of their pathophysiology, the reader is referred to Chapter 2 in this volume. A variety of hyperkinesias affecting oral-facial-cervical structures have been described in the neurology literature (Jankovic, 1981; Marsden, 1976). These include blepharospasm, oral-mandibular dystonia, spasmodic torticollis, and essential tremor. Cooper (1976) has suggested a model for the dystonias that involves a variety of lesions disrupting complex motor feedback circuits that subserve communication among subcortical motor programming structures. These structures include the globus pallidus, red nucleus, midbrain reticular formation, brachium conjunctivum (cerebellar-cortical pathway), and dentate nucleus. What these lesions have in common is that they all affect the pathways of convergence upon the ventrolateral nucleus of the thalamus.

Interestingly, there is a high incidence of SD among such movement-disordered subgroups (Jankovic & Ford, 1982). When spontaneous onset of oral-facial-cervical dystonia occurs, the disorder is termed Meige's syndrome (also known as Breugel's syndrome). According to Jankovic and Ford (1982), "Spasmodic dysphonia, usually described separately, is now considered a focal dystonia occasionally associated with other features of Meige's syndrome . . . [which] may begin as blepharospasm, oromandibular dystonia, tongue protrusion, or spasmodic dysphonia and over a period of months or years may progress to a more generalized dystonia" (p. 410). In a study of 12 SD patients referred for routine neurologic examination, Dedo et al. (1978) reported that 50% exhibited dyskinetic movement disorders, including postural tremor, blepharospasm, idiopathic torsion dystonia, and buccolingual dyskinesia. Similarly, Rosenfield (1988) reported that of 41 patients referred for SD, 59% exhibited essential tremors external to the larynx or Meige's syndrome or both. The view that SD represents a focal dystonia resulting from extrapyramidal motor pathology has been aired by many (Aronson et al., 1968b; Critchley, 1939; Freeman et al., 1985a; Marsden & Sheehy, 1982; McCall, 1974). In addition, SD has been noted as an early symptom of adult onset torsion dystonia (Jankovic & Ford, 1982) and a late symptom in Gilles de la Tourette syndrome (Lang &

Marsden, 1983). SD has also been likened to dystonic writer's cramp, with the implication that as a dystonia it must be a basal ganglia disorder (Blitzer, Lovelace, Brin, Fahn, & Fink, 1985). It must also be acknowledged, however, that the CNS pathophysiology underlying dystonic writer's cramp and similar function-specific dystonias remains essentially unknown.

In a series of studies of extrapyramidal motor involvement in SD, McCall (1974) used a combination of fluoroscopic, acoustic-phonetic, and electromyographic measures. Fluoroscopic assessments indicated that SD "can occur as a manifestation of apparent isolated, phonatory-related laryngospasms or may appear in association with a more general problem that affects the behavior of the larynx, hypopharynx, tongue and soft palate" (p. 127). Descriptive electromyography (EMG) was performed on eight SD patients with non-tremor-related dysphonia. Recordings were obtained from bipolar hooked wire electrodes inserted in the cricothyroid, sternothyroid, and thyrohyoid muscles. Results indicated that intermittent voice stoppage in the acoustic records was associated with sharp, burst-like increases in electromyographic activity in the cricothyroid muscle and occasionally the sternothyroid and thyrohyoid muscles. McCall interpreted these findings as suggestive of laryngeal dystonia "consistent with the hypothesis of involvement of the extrapyramidal motor system" (p. 136). Abnormal fluctuations in laryngeal EMG activity in the interarytenoid, thyroarytenoid, and cricothyroid have also been described in one SD patient by Shipp et al. (1985).

Findings of these early qualitative studies have not been consistently replicated when contemporary quantitative EMG techniques have been employed (Schaefer et al., 1992; van Pelt, Ludlow, & Smith, 1994; Watson et al., 1991). Schaefer et al. (1992) reported significantly abnormal increases in normalized peak amplitudes of thyroarytenoid muscle activation during speech (but not during quiet breathing or sustained phonation) for a group of individuals with SD. In contrast, van Pelt et al. (1994) found no such differences between SD and normal vocal folds. Findings have been inconsistent across subjects within studies and equivocal across studies. Overall, no clear pattern of abnormality in SD during speech had been observed. A recent study by Nash and Ludlow (1996) may explain some of this variability. This study used quantitative EMG to compare words produced by

11 speakers with ADSD to normal controls, but differentiated between words in which voice breaks did and did not occur. Abnormal muscle activation was found to be restricted to the thyroarytenoid muscles in these cases and only occurred during words in which voice breaks were perceptually and acoustically identified. In previous studies using quantitative EMG, the procedure of averaging across break and nonbreak words may have statistically washed out differences in EMG activation during speech in SD. Abnormal fluctuations in laryngeal muscle tone during speech, but not during nonspeech activity (such as valsalva or resting respiration), seem more consistent with an extrapyramidal dystonia explanation than with general spasticity or flaccidity of the vocal folds. Alternatively, heterogeneity of vocal symptoms of SD (see Sapienza, Murry, & Brown, 1998), within or between studies, as well as small sample sizes may also account for the equivocal results.

Considerable similarity of symptoms has been noted in SD and essential tremor (Aronson et al., 1968b). Aronson and Hartman (1981) demonstrated that SD patients, with rhythmic voice arrests during vowel prolongations, share many commonalities with essential voice tremor patients, including virtually identical voice tremor frequencies of 5 to 6 Hz, high incidence of extralaryngeal tremor, and a high percentage of other associated neurological soft signs. The resemblance is so striking that they suggest that this subgroup be differentiated diagnostically as "spastic dysphonia of essential tremor" (p. 57).

Although the precise underlying mechanisms of essential tremor remain unknown, converging physiologic evidence suggests a more central rather than peripheral site of origin (Jankovic & Fahn, 1980). A high incidence of postural tremor reminiscent of benign essential tremor has been noted throughout the spectrum of dystonic disorders (Marsden, 1976). Thus, laryngeal tremors have been viewed as consistent with a diagnosis of focal dystonia in many patients with SD. A focal dystonia model of SD is appealing in that it establishes the notion that disruption at various locations within an integrated system of feedback loops can have similar consequences for the output of the system. A focal dystonia model does not explain, however, the speech specificity of SD or some of the associated sensory findings or the fact that a subset of SD patients does not appear to have associated dystonias, vocal tremors, or extralaryngeal tremors.

Cerebral Cortex and Its Projections

The classical pyramidal motor system has its cell bodies in the fifth and sixth layers of the perirolandic (frontoparietal) sensorimotor cortex, and descending axons project via the internal capsule and cerebral penduncles to brainstem and spinal lower motor neuron pools. Lesions in this system result in supranuclear palsy, spastic paralysis, and associated spastic dysarthria when the crainial musculature subserving speech is involved (Darley, Aronson, & Brown, 1975). It is quite possible to obtain a truly "spastic" dysphonia as an early symptom of a gradual onset dysarthria (Aronson, 1978) or as a chronic residual of dysarthria that has otherwise resolved.

A significant number of neurologic signs suggestive of pyramidal motor dysfunction have been reported in SD. Aronson et al. (1968a) reported hyperreflexia, dysdiadochokinesis of tongue and extremities, increased jaw and sucking reflexes, and asymmetry of face and palate as symptoms in their SD group. However, pyramidal soft signs were less common than extrapyramidal soft signs and were more typical of older patients. A similarly high incidence of pyramidal soft signs, in excess of five per patient, were reported by Robe, Brumlik, and Moore (1960), in contrast to a comparatively low incidence of other potentially localizing signs (i.e., cerebellar or brainstem symptoms).

In an effort to explore the possibility of cortical involvement in SD, a number of researchers have used electroencephalographic (EEG) techniques. The results of these studies are equivocal. In the early study of Robe et al. (1960), 9 of the 10 EEGs obtained were interpreted to be abnormal. The types of deviations noted were quite heterogeneous; however, 50% of the patients exhibited "burst-like" discharges in the absence of clinical history of seizures. Electrical deviations tended to arise from the posterior temporoparietal electrode placement, but results were not particularly informative with respect to lateralization. These results are problematic due to the fact that the EEG technique employed is obsolete (pre-International 10–20 standardization) and, therefore, not directly comparable to more contemporary research. (This does not imply, a priori, that in the hands of an experienced clinician the technique was necessarily invalid.) More recent reports of EEG activity in SD patients have been less impressive. Kiml (1965) reported EEG abnormalities of various types in 4 of 10 SD patients. Aronson et al. (1968a) reported EEG abnormalities in 5 of

22 SD patients. Four of these exhibited mild nonspecific dysrhythmia, and one was clearly abnormal (i.e., bilateral, independent spike foci during sleep). Dedo et al. (1978) reported normal EEG recordings in all 12 SD patients studied. Taken in combination, these later studies suggest approximately 20% incidence of EEG abnormalities in SD. The absence of control group data obfuscates interpretation of the findings.

In an important but neglected study, Maroun, Jacob, and Gowing (1970) reported dysphonic symptoms reminiscent of SD in patients undergoing surgery for neoplasms involving left frontoparietal and supplemental motor cortices. Based largely on the work of Penfield and Roberts (1976), these authors posited that a disruption of corticothalamic feedback loops involved in motor programming might provide the mechanism underlying vocal perturbation in SD. They write, "The dysphonia in these patients was clearly not due to edema or other local lesions in the larynx or pharynx, nor was there evidence of pseudobulbar palsy or dysfunction of lower cranial nerves. Therefore, the disturbance in phonation was considered to be 'cerebral' dysphonia" (p. 673). Subjective impressions of the patients' tape-recorded speech suggested a "strained hoarseness" at times associated with "explosive speech" and "facial flushing" during vocal efforts.

Other cortical areas related to vocalization in subhuman primates include the prefrontal motor cortex, the anterior temporal cortex, and the anterior cingulate gyrus. Franzen and Myers (1973) observed a dramatic reduction in socially directed vocalizations in free-ranging macaques secondary to bilateral ablations of either the prefrontal or anterior temporal cortices that spared subcortical structures (e.g., amygdala and uncinate fassiculus). Anterior cingulate lesions did not have this effect. Combined bilateral lesions of the frontal and anterior temporal regions almost completely abolished naturalistic vocal responses. Because of the massive interconnections of the frontotemporal regions via the uncinate fassiculus, these authors speculate on a functional system subserving vocalization for social interaction. A striking disassociation is seen in the work of Sutton, Larson, and Lindeman (1974), who demonstrated that anterior cingulate lesions abolish voluntary initiation of a conditioned vocalization in response to a "go signal," whereas lesions in the homologues of the human anterior and posterior speech areas had little effect. These findings have been replicated and extended by Kirzinger and Jurgens (1985).

Pathological involvement of vocalization cortex may be implicated in some patients with SD. It is potentially interesting that the anterior cingulate gyrus is intimately related, developmentally and anatomically, to the supplemental motor cortex that was discussed in relation to SD by Maroun et al. (1970). Supplemental motor cortex has been hypothesized by some authors to mediate the connection between the limbic "drive to speak" and the motor speech programmer in Broca's area (Freedman, Alexander, & Naeser, 1984; Rubens & Kertesz, 1983). It is also known, however, that large acute structural lesions in the left supplemental motor area typically result in transcortical motor aphasia, whereas left frontal premotor cortex lesions result in Broca's aphasia (Benson, 1979) rather than SD. Yet, it is among the "higher cortical" disorders (e.g., alexia without agraphia) that one expects the degree of functional specificity for vocal language behavior that seems characteristic of SD, due to the increased spatial separation of functional centers on the convoluted surface of the hemispheres. If a cortical locus of dysfunction did exist in some individuals with SD, then it would be reasonable to hypothesize some coexisting impairment in language function. Preliminary evidence of subtle, higher-level language deficit that appears to interact with laryngeal reaction time has been reported for a small subgroup of individuals with SD by Watson et al. (1991). Interestingly, these speakers also exhibited abnormal cortical electrophysiological findings.

Evidence for a cortical motor component in SD can also be gleaned by analogy from electrical stimulation experiments performed in monkeys. Hast and Milojevic (1967) stimulated the laryngeal motor cortex of the inferolateral frontal operculum and recorded laryngeal muscle responses via strain gauge on a graphic-level recorder. Characteristic of their era, they delivered exaggerated voltage levels to the stimulating electrodes, effecting grossly aberrant movement patterns within the larynx. These consisted of sustained, synchronous oscillatory adduction-abduction of the vocal fold ending in complete adduction and a transient respiratory arrest. A subsequent study using microelectrode stimulation at low-current levels (Hast, Fischer, Wetzel, & Thompson, 1974) yielded no such aberrant oscillatory movements but did elicit differentiated contractions of the thyroarytenoid and cricothyroid muscles from discrete electrode placements in the laryngeal motor cortex. Curiously, however, cardiac slowing was also simultaneously obtained from those electrode placements effective in contracting the cricothyroid. These experiments suggest that in primates, both visceral motor responses and laryngeal tremor phenomena can be linked to a single cortical locus of abnormal electrical discharge. One is reminded that abnormal cardiac slowing and abnormal cricothyroid EMG activity have been demonstrated in patients with SD (Feldman et al., 1984; McCall, 1974). A cortical locus of motor dysfunction might account for some apparent visceral and extrapyramidal findings reported among SD patients. Upper motor neuron pathology may also account for the pyramidal symptoms (e.g., hypertonus, hyperreflexia) sometimes reported in association with SD, due to disinhibition of lower motor neuron pools deprived of regulatory supranuclear input.

Limbic System

Current concepts in neurophysiology stress the significance of multiple parallel sensorimotor pathways subserving related but unique processing activities within a given functional modality (Kelso & Tuller, 1981). Such afferent systems have been described with respect to audition, vision, and somesthesia (Diamond, 1979; Merzenich & Kaas, 1980). Multiple parallel systems have also been elucidated for extremity movement (Kuypers, 1982).

A growing body of converging evidence demonstrates the existence of multiple parallel pathways, apart from the classical pyramidal motor system, for mammalian species-specific vocalization (Jurgens, 1976; Jurgens & Ploog, 1970; Jurgens & Pratt, 1979a, 1979b; Kelley et al., 1946; Sutton et al., 1974). According to Jurgens and Ploog (1981), in primates the cortex of the anterior cingulate gyrus is considered the highest level of the system because it is required for learned vocalization. Reticular formation surrounding nucleus ambiguous is regarded as the lowest level of the system, because stimulation at this level yields phonation, wheras direct stimulation of the motor neurons yields only vocal fold movement. Intermediate levels of this system include subcortical limbic structures (i.e., dorsomedial and lateral hypothalamus, basal amygdaloid nucleus, and midline thalamus) that are necessary structures for involuntary vocal emotional reaction, as well as the periaqueductal gray of the caudal midbrain. This latter structure serves as a synaptic processing station that integrates diverse internal and external stimuli that result in the generation of a vocal call.

Clinical reports of dysphonia associated with midbrain lesions in humans reinforce the distinction of volitional motor versus limbic vocalizations. Botez and Barbeau (1971) report three patients with lesions of the periaqueductal gray region of the mesencephalic-pontine tegmentum resulting in total mutism and reduced faciovocal activity. A series of eight patients with dysphonia secondary to midbrain trauma has also been reported (Vogel & von Cramon, 1982; von Cramon, 1981). These patients were initially mute and unable to perform voluntary adduction of the vocal folds, whereas they did phonate reflexively during coughing and choking. Subsequently these patients recovered relatively normal affective vocalizations, but remained completely speechless, or anarthric. Later in recovery, these patients presented a profile of pseudobulbar dysarthria with speech-specific vocal characteristics that the authors considered to be reminiscent of SD. Symptoms included frequent laryngealization, monopitch, and hard glottal attacks. These defects were attributed to "a transitory lesion of the periaqueductal gray" causing "temporary inhibition within the brainstem vocalization system" (von Cramon, 1981, p. 804).

Alluding to this limbic vocalization literature, Schaefer (1983) has posited a "direct model" for spasmodic dysphonia involving "a lesion along any of these pathways or in the region of the periaqueductal gray or reticular formation" (p. 1199). Such an interpretation is contraindicated by the fact that lesions of the periaqueductal gray and its descending pathway abolish all species-specific vocalizations in primates (Jurgens & Ploog, 1970; Jurgens & Pratt, 1979a), whereas pyramidal system lesions are specifically disruptive to human speech. Regarding this phenomenon, Jurgens and Ploog (1981) write, "Speech must be learned, whereas monkey vocalizations are essentially innate—that is, genetically programmed motor patterns. If this explanation is correct, then genetically preprogrammed vocal patterns in man, such as laughing and crying, should be preserved, even after bilateral lesions in cortical face area" (p. 137).

In summary, the parallel limbic vocalization pathway offers an explanation for the normal or nearly normal nonspeech vocalizations exhibited in SD, rather than the converse. This concept has been invoked in the recent neurologic literature to explain the positive affect-sensitivity and preservation of nonspeech vocalizations seen in other speech disorders, including pseudobulbar palsy (Jurgens & Ploog, 1981; Meyers, 1976), traumatic midbrain dysphonia (Vogel & von

Cramon, 1982), and stuttering (Rosenfield, 1982, 1984) in addition to SD. This interpretation lends support to the view that speech-specific vocal perturbation in SD results from impairment of the volitional motor system rather than limbic or lower brainstem centers for vocal motor control.

Comparison of SD with the Dysarthrias

It is plausible that disruption of neural structures subserving laryngeal motor control at various levels in the central nervous system could result in perceptually similar dysphonic symptoms. Dedo et al. (1978) have suggested that SD symptoms could result from various pathologies of the peripheral or central nervous system that were sufficient to cause "selective disturbances in conduction and control of neural impulses to the larynx" (p. 879). In addition, the possibility of multiple sporadic brainstem lesions, analogous to multiple sclerosis, has been suggested as a potential explanation of SD (Schaefer, 1983). According to these views, SD may be considered a selective dysarthria representing "several etiologically different disorders having similar voice signs" (Aronson, 1985, p. 168).

It has long been acknowledged that SD shares many vocal symptoms with dysarthrias that have more specific lesion localizations (Aronson et al., 1968b). According to Aronson et al. (1968a), the distinguishing feature differentiating SD from dysarthria in general is the lack of clinically significant involvement of the supraglottal articulators. Despite this now clinically accepted dogma, articulatory abnormalities have been reported in SD. Aronson et al. (1968a) state that "rate and fluency of articulation were profoundly influenced by the occurrence of spasm" (p. 210). Other abnormalities that the authors perceived included phoneme repetition and prolongation. Spectrographic verification of prolonged phoneme duration in SD has been reported (Cannito & Johnson, 1981; Merson & Ginsberg, 1979). Spectrographic evidence of variable consonantal errors in SD, including substitutions, omissions, and distortions, has also been presented by Freeman et al. (1985a). All of these authors have attributed the articulation difficulties to a loss of coordination among laryngeal and supralaryngeal structures associated with the dysphonic episodes. It should be acknowledged that this explanation represents a logical inference and not a quantitatively supported result. In contrast to this view, Cannito (1989) has demonstrated an abnormal degree of vocal tract unsteadiness in SD subjects who were sustaining vowels with an artificial voice source.

The failure of earlier Mayo Clinic studies (Aronson et al., 1968b) to provide a clear-cut indication of the relationship of SD symptoms to those exhibited by patients with dysarthrias is felt to stem from the dichotomous method of comparison that was employed. The occurrence of a particular symptom in SD and in other neurogenic voice disorders was simply indicated using a plus or minus scoring system. This type of approach obscures potentially valuable information regarding a symptom's relative prevalence and severity within any given disorder.

In order to clarify the relationship between SD and the dysarthrias, a reanalysis of the Mayo Clinic dysarthria data (Darley et al., 1975) was undertaken by this author, using the published mean perceptual ratings of subgroups of dysarthrics as the dependent measures. To accomplish this, 10 vocal symptoms characteristic of SD were selected from among the 38 dysarthric symptoms originally studied. These are listed in order of importance vertically in Table 9.1 (dysarthric subgroups are listed horizontally). Selection of SD vocal symptoms was based upon a careful literature review coupled with clinical experience. A crosscheck of this selection against the vocal symptoms of SD described by Aronson et al. (1968a) revealed good agreement with the symptoms reported in that study (see particularly the summary on p. 209). The first five symptoms may be characterized as cardinal, or differentiating, symptoms of SD. The last five may be viewed as frequently associated symptoms. For each of these symptoms, the mean perceptual ratings of the dyarthric groups (reported in the original study) were ranked and tabulated.

Inspection of Table 9.1 reveals that all dysarthrias except cerebellar ataxia and bulbar palsy occurred among the highest ranked for various SD-related symptoms. Some groups, however, appear to exhibit relatively more frequent distribution of the higher ranks than others. To quantify these relationships, the extension of the median test (a nonparametric equivalent of one-way ANOVA for independent samples; Siegel, 1956) was computed. If the rankings were randomly distributed among dysarthric subgroups, the frequency of occurrence of the higher rankings would not differ significantly across the subgroups. A chi-square statistic was derived from the frequency of occurrence of the

Table 9.1
Rank Ordering of the Mean Severity Ratings of Dysarthric Groups Across 10 Vocal Symptoms of Spasmodic Dysphonia

Spasmodic Dysphonia Symptoms	Pseudo-Bulbar Palsy	Dystonia	Huntington's Chorea	Amyotrophic Lateral Sclerosis	Parkinson's Disease	Cerebellar Ataxia	Bulbar Palsy
Cardinal Symptoms							
Vocal stoppages	6	7	5	2.5	2.5	2.5	2.5
Strain-strangle	7	6	4	5	1.5	3	1.5
Voice tremor	6	7	5	3	1.5	4	1.5
Transient breathiness	7	5	6	2	4	2	2
Monopitch	6	3	4	5	7	1	2
Associated Symptoms							
Reduced rate	6	4	2	7	3	5	1
Forced respiration	3.5	3.5	7	3.5	3.5	3.5	3.5
Harsh voice	7	5	4	6	2	3	1
Low pitch level	7	3	2	6	5	1	4
Reduced loudness	5	6	1	4	7	2	3

Note. Adapted from a reanalysis of the Mayo Clinic dysarthria data in *Motor Speech Disorders* (Appendix C), by F. Darley, A. Aronson, and J. Brown, 1975, Philadelphia: Saunders. Copyright 1975 by W. B. Saunders. Adapted with permission.

observed rankings in excess of the overall median among dysarthric groups. Cardinal and associated symptoms were tested alone and in combination. Resultant chi-square statistics were significant in all cases, $p < .005$. Paired comparisons were computed using Mann-Whitney U test (nonparametric equivalent of Fisher's t test) for both the combined SD symptoms and for cardinal symptoms only. For combined symptoms, the results indicated that pseudobulbar palsy and dystonia were significantly different from cerebellar ataxia and bulbar palsy, $p < .05$. Amyotrophic lateral sclerosis was significantly different from cerebellar ataxia. Figure 9.2 illustrates the total number of SD symptoms falling above the combined dysarthric median for each group.

Inspection of Figure 9.2 reveals a high degree of association between the vocal symptoms of SD and pseudobulbar palsy and dystonia, reflect-

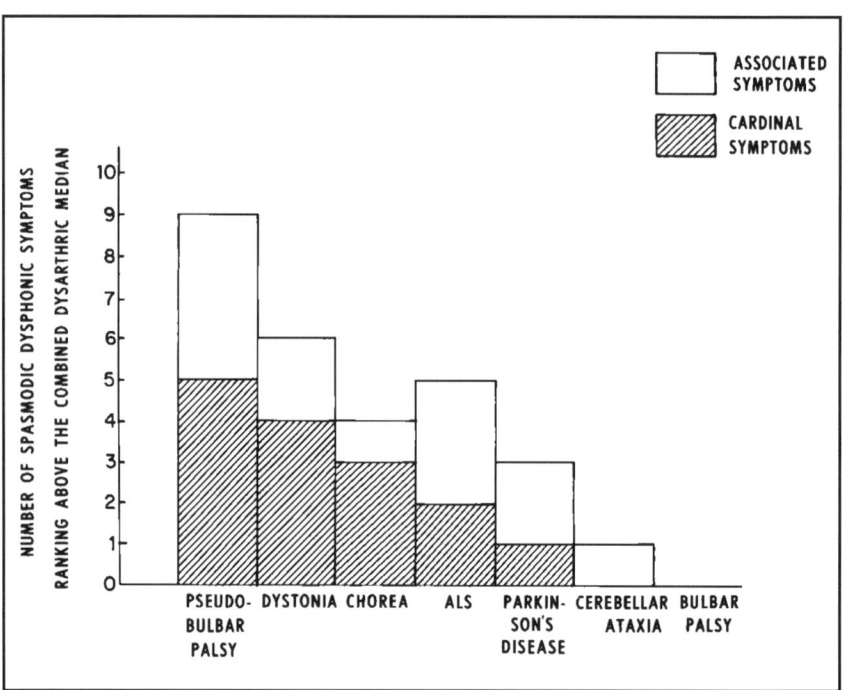

Figure 9.2. Comparison of the dysarthrias on the basis of vocal symptoms of spasmodic dysphonia. *Note.* Adapted from an analysis of the Mayo Clinic dysarthria data in *Motor Speech Disorders* (Appendix C) by F. Darley, A. Aronson, and J. Brown, 1975, Philadelphia: Saunders. Copyright 1975 by W. B. Saunders. Adapted with permission.

ing upper motor neuron and basal gangliar (pallidal) pathology, respectively. A moderate degree of association with the symptoms of SD is exhibited by chorea, also a basal gangliar (striatal) pathology. Relatively low association with SD was exhibited by amyotrophic lateral sclerosis, a variable disorder with both upper and lower motor neuron components, and parkinsonism, a midbrain (nigral) disorder. Virtually no association with SD was exhibited by cerebellar ataxia or bulbar palsy. The conclusion that emerges from this analysis is that the higher one ascends within the central nervous system, with respect to anatomical lesion locus, the more similar are the vocal symptoms to SD. This outcome argues not for multifocal pathogenesis of SD, but for a variable supranuclear lesion locus involving the pyramidal/extrapyramidal motor cortex and underlying basal ganglia structures deep within the cerebral hemispheres.

Extralaryngeal Motor Functions in SD

A variable supranuclear lesion model of SD, involving extrapyramidal motor cortex and basal ganglia or their interconnections, would appear to account for many of the speech and nonspeech motor symptoms associated with SD. Although numerous investigations have reported a high incidence of abnormal pyramidal and extrapyramidal motor signs and symptoms in SD patients, such findings are usually based on the subjective evaluation of one examiner, typically a neurologist. The major studies of this type are summarized in Table 9.2. In an attempt to more objectively quantify such clinical observations, Cannito (1986) compared upper extremity and vocal tract motor performance in 18 female subjects with SD with that of a group of 18 closely matched normal controls. Subjects were equated for sex, age, and handedness. Care was taken to rule out subjects with significant neurological or psychiatric histories (other than SD). Performance on 19 motor variables was measured using a computer-automated-assessment battery approach. See Table 9.3. It was hypothesized that the subjects with SD would perform more poorly than the controls on complex voluntary serial motor activities and sustained positional steadiness (as predicted by a higher-level, motor-processing model of SD), but would

Table 9.2
Summary of the Primary Studies Yielding a High Incidence
of Pyramidal-Extrapyramidal Neuromotor Signs
in Spasmodic Dysphonia

Study	N	Incidence (%)
Critchley (1939)	3	100
Robe, Brumlik, and Moore (1960)	10	100
Aronson, Brown, Litin, and Pearson (1968a)	27	74
Aminoff, Dedo, and Izdebski (1978)	12	50
Rosenfield (1988)	41	59
Total	93	68[a]

[a]Total percentage is weighted for variations in number of spasmodic dysphonia subjects across samples.

not differ from the controls for simple isolated ballistic movements. All measures were found to be sufficiently reliable, with test-retest reliability coefficients (estimated from the intertrial correlations using the Spearman-Brown procedure) ranging from .85 to .98.

Multivariate analyses using Hotelling's T^2 statistic indicated a significant between-groups effect in the anticipated direction for those measures for which differences had been predicted ($T^2 = 36.51$; $df = 2, 27$; $p = .045$), but no difference for those measures for which similar performance had been predicted ($T^2 = 12.34$; $df = 8, 27$; $p = .441$). A stepwise discriminate function analysis revealed that a linear combination of four of the nonspeech motor measures was able to differentiate the subject groups with 86% accuracy ($F = 7.22$; $df = 8, 27$; $p < .001$). The measures included in the discriminate equation were finger-lift reaction time (dominant hand), finger-tapping speed (dominant hand), Purdue pegboard test (nondominant hand), and visual pursuit ramp tracking (mandibular). The resultant classification matrix is presented in Table 9.4.

It is important to note that the SD group was characterized by a differential performance pattern with relatively poor performance on speed of finger tapping and peg placement, but relatively good performance on finger reaction time and slow ramp tracking. Although the results were striking, the a priori predictions were not entirely supported. Repeated-measures ANOVA ($p < .05$) indicated that significant

Table 9.3
Extralaryngeal Motor Variables and Hypotheses in Spasmodic Dysphonia

Variable Number	Experimental Task	Impaired Function	
		Predicted	Observed
	Simple Versus Complex Movement		
1	Finger reaction time (dominant hand)	No	No
2	Finger reaction time (nondominant hand)	No	No
3	Finger-tapping speed (dominant hand)	Yes	Yes
4	Finger-tapping speed (nondominant hand)	Yes	Yes
	Complex Movement Sequences		
5	Pegboard speed (dominant hand)	Yes	Yes
6	Pegboard speed (nondominant hand)	Yes	Yes
7	Whispered trisyllable speed	Yes	Yes
	Slow Visual Pursuit Tracking		
8	Slow ramp tracking (dominant hand)	Yes	No
9	Slow ramp tracking (nondominant hand)	Yes	No
10	Slow ramp tracking (jaw)	Yes	No
	Maintenance of Sustained Position		
11	Upper extremity steadiness (dominant hand)	Yes	No
12	Upper extremity steadiness (nondominant hand)	Yes	No
13	Second formant frequency steadiness	Yes	Yes
	Ballistic Visual Pursuit Tracking		
14	Step track initiation time (dominant hand)	No	No
15	Step track initiation time (nondominant hand)	No	No
16	Step track initiation time (jaw)	No	No
17	Step track movement time (dominant hand)	No	No
18	Step track movement time (nondominant hand)	No	No
19	Step track movement time (jaw)	No	No

Note. From *Extralaryngeal Functions in Spasmodic Dysphonia: Vocal Tract and Manual Control*, by M. P. Cannito, 1986, unpublished doctoral dissertation, University of Texas at Dallas. Copyright 1986 by M. Cannito. Reprinted with permission.

Table 9.4
Classification of Subjects as Spasmodic Dysphonic or Control on the Basis of the Stepwise Discriminant Function for Four Motor Variables

Actual Group	N of Cases	N Predicted	
		Group I (Control)	Group II (Spasmodic Dysphonic)
Group I: Control	18	16 (89%)	2 (11%)*
Group II: Spasmodic dysphonic	18 $X^2 = 18.84$	3 (17%)**	15 (83%) $p < .001$

Note. A total of 86% of cases were correctly classified.
*Probability of misclassification is .111.
**Probability of misclassification is .167.

differences were limited to rapid sequential movements of the upper extremities and vocal tract and vocal tract steadiness (Cannito, 1989; Cannito & Kondraske, 1990). Slow ramp visual pursuit tracking and sustained upper extremity steadiness remained unimpaired, as did the isolated ballistic movement tasks. In addition, the findings could not be accounted for on the basis of impaired affect (e.g., psychomotor retardation) inasmuch as the differentiating motor variables were uncorrelated with standardized psychometric tests of anxiety and depression (Spielberger, Gorusch, Lushene, Vagg, & Jacobs, 1983; Zung, 1967) that had also been administered. Although the findings are compatible with earlier observations of extralaryngeal motor abnormalities in SD, a selective impairment in speech motor behaviors and rapid sequential manual skills seems to imply a defect of very high levels of motor information processing within the CNS (Cannito & Kondraske, 1990).

With respect to extralaryngeal motor functions in SD, it is of considerable interest that quantitative measures of laryngeal motor performance have yielded analogous results. Reich and Till (1983) found that the phonatory reaction times of subjects with SD were abnormally prolonged for productions of a two-syllable word but not for an isolated vowel. Ludlow and Connor (1987) also demonstrated significant delays for phonation onset in their SD subjects; however, laryngeal movement initiation time was normal. It was complex coordination for voicing rather than vocal fold movement per se that was impaired. These authors also suggest a supranuclear abnormality to explain the pattern of findings that was observed. Taken together, studies of laryngeal and extralaryngeal motor performance suggest that many subjects with SD exhibit difficulty with coordination of rapid voluntary movements when task demands become sufficiently complex.

Neural Imaging in Spasmodic Dysphonia

Preliminary support for the variable pyramidal/extrapyrimidal lesion explanation of SD has also been provided by a series of neural imaging studies completed during the last several years by Freeman, Finitzo, and their associates (including the author) at the University of Texas at Dallas and Southwestern Medical Center. Among various techniques employed were nuclear magnetic resonance imaging (MRI) and brain electrical activity mapping (BEAM). This research is summarized in Finitzo and Freeman (1989).

MRI is a signal-processing technology that records perturbations induced in an electromagnetic field around the head and reconstructs images of brain slices analogous to those obtained from computerized tomography (CT) scans. Preliminary findings in subjects with SD have been reported by Schaefer et al. (1985). Both abductor and adductor patients were represented in their SD sample. Subsequently Cannito (1986) described a 25-patient series resulting in 16 normal and 9 (36%) abnormal MRI scans. Sites of lesion in the abnormal studies included one right thalamocortical gliosis (post-thalamotomy onset of SD), one enlarged pineal body (probably tumor), one cerebellar malformation (Arnold Chiari malformation, type 1), and deep supratentorial white matter lesions in six patients. The deep white matter lesions were typically multiple and of small volume. Examples of MRI scans of one such patient are presented in Figure 9.3. A breakdown of the distribution of these lesions by subject is provided in Table 9.5. A total of 30 deep white matter lesions were identified. Working closely with the neuroradiologist, the author has plotted the distribution of the 30

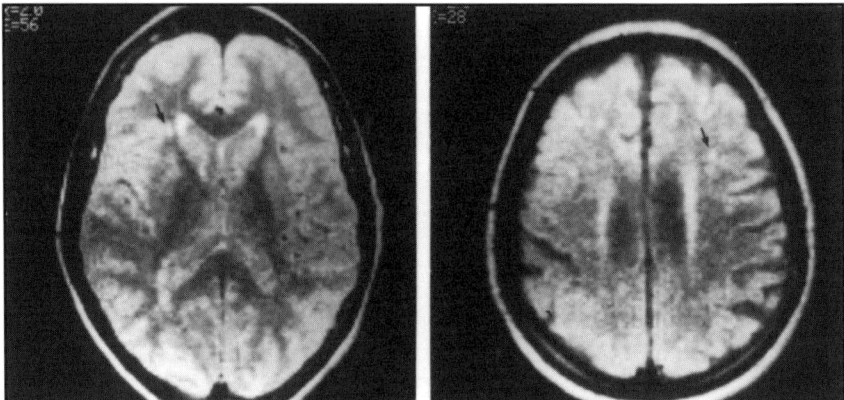

Figure 9.3. MRI of horizontal brain sections of an SD subject illustrating deep frontal white matter lesions. Left, callosal projection (forceps minor) level; right, coronal radiata level. *Note.* From *Extralaryngeal Functions in Spasmodic Dysphonia: Vocal Tract and Manual Control*, by M. P. Cannito, 1986, unpublished doctoral dissertation, University of Texas at Dallas. Copyright 1986 by M. P. Cannito. Reprinted with permission.

deep white matter lesions on conventional CT templates (patterned after those of Naeser & Hayward, 1978). The composite brain slices showing the distribution of these lesions are depicted in Figure 9.4. Primary involvement was noted in the frontal white matter, with secondary involvements in the basal ganglia/internal capsule and parietal-occipital juncture areas. It may be significant that the greatest lesion density underlies the frontal lobes. This finding corresponds well to the localization hypothesized on the basis of a comparison of SD with the dysarthrias.

Lesions in the white matter adjacent to the left frontal horn may disrupt the motor outflow from the cortical face area (Ross, 1980) and have been implicated in articulation problems associated with aphasia (Freedman et al., 1984). Lesions in the posterior corpus callosum cause disruption of bilateral sensorimotor integration or dyspraxia (Volpe, Sidtis, Holzman, Wilson, & Gazzaniga, 1982). It is possible that either or both of these mechanisms might result in loss of volitional laryngeal control. Despite careful scrutiny of lower regions, with the exception of a single cerebellar malformation, no brainstem lesions were observed. Radiological interpretation of probable etiologies included demyelinating, traumatic, vascular, neoplastic, and developmental causes.

Table 9.5
Distribution of Small Supratentorial White Matter Lesions Identified by MRI in Six Cases of Spasmodic Dysphonia

Case No.	Total No. of Lesions	Left Side	Right Side
1	6	Corona radiata (2)	Corona radiata (1)
		External capsule (1)	Posterior limb interna capsule (1)
		Occipito-parietal trigone (1)	
2	2	Corona radiata (1)[a]	
		Inferior basal ganglia (1)[b]	
3	10	Corona radiata (2)	Corona radiata (4)
		Frontal horn (1)	Frontal horn (1)
			Occipito-parietal trigone (2)
4	3	Frontal horn (1)	Frontal horn (2)
5	8	Corona radiata (1)	Corona radiata (1)
		Frontal horn (1)[b]	Frontal horn (2)
		Occipito-parietal trigone (2)	Occipito-parietal trigone (1)
6	1	Parietal white matter (1)[b]	

Note. From *Extralaryngeal Functions in Spasmodic Dysphonia: Vocal Tract and Manual Control*, by M. P. Cannito, 1986, unpublished doctoral dissertation, University of Texas at Dallas. Copyright 1986 by M. Cannito. Reprinted with permission.
[a]Adjacent to caudate body.
[b]Comparatively larger lesions.

These results suggest that some patients with SD exhibit gross lesions in supranuclear subcortical structures.

Cannito, Finitzo, Freeman, and Pool (1985) examined patterns of electrical brain activity thought to represent cerebral processing functions in 10 normal-hearing adductor SD patients using the recent BEAM technique. The equivocal nature of earlier EEG studies of SD may have reflected shortcomings of the traditional subjective method of visual inspection of the EEG recording. In contrast, the fully automated and probabilistic measurement strategy offered by the BEAM technique is intended to minimize subjective bias and provides precise

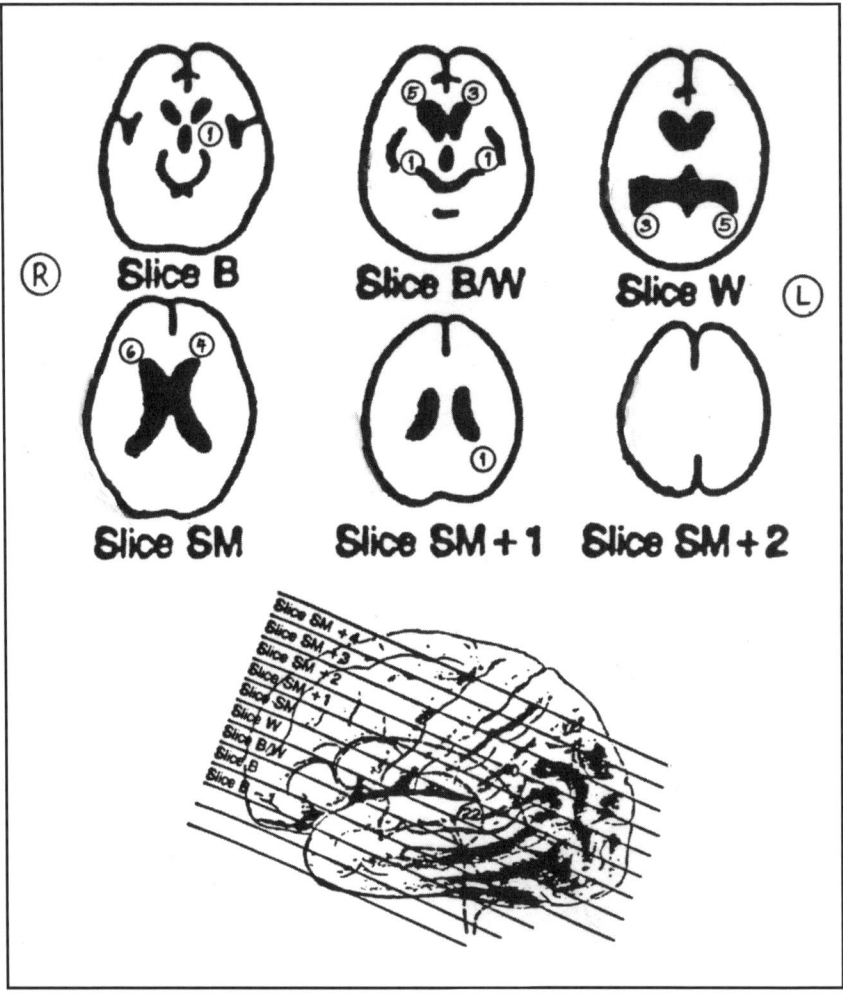

Figure 9.4. Neuroanatomic distribution of deep supratentorial white matter lesions identified in six cases of spasmodic dysphonia by MRI. *Note.* From *Extralaryngeal Functions in Spasmodic Dysphonia: Vocal Tract and Manual Control*, by M. P. Cannito, 1986, unpublished doctoral dissertation, University of Texas at Dallas. Copyright 1986 by M. P. Cannito. Reprinted with permission.

quantification of clinical electrocortical abnormality. It should be recognized, however, that topographic brain mapping is highly experimental and that its clinical validity has yet to be established (American Academy of Neurology, 1989).

The SD subjects were compared to control subject data from the BEAM standardization sample (Duffy, Bartels, & Burchfield, 1981), which included subjects from the third, fourth, fifth, and sixth decades of life. The experimental subjects ranged in age from 33 to 65 years, with a mean age of 48.2 ($SD = 8.97$). The sample included two males and eight females. Reported time post onset of SD ranged from 2 to 21 years. Results indicated abnormalities in excess of ±3 standard deviations from normal in the classic EEG spectral bands in 50% of the patients, auditory cortical-evoked potential abnormalities in 90%, and visual cortical-evoked potential abnormalities in 60% of the patients. Sixty percent of the combined evoked potential abnormalities were bilaterally distributed, 30% left-lateralized, and 10% right-lateralized. Typical localizations were left temporofrontal, medial frontal, and right parieto-occipital, pictured in Figure 9.5.

In addition to individual data, group effects were demonstrated for three electrodes during the 108–144 ms epoch following onset of the auditory tone stimulus. Electrode locations were left anterior temporal (T3), right anterior temporal (T4), and medial frontal (FZ). The raw amplitude data in microvolts from the SD subjects were compared with that of the normal controls, blocked by age in decades. The respective means and standard deviations are presented in Table 9.6. A between-subjects ANOVA was computed for each electrode by five subject groups. Resultant F-ratios were significant at the .001 level of probability. Paired means comparisons (Newman-Keuls) revealed significant differences between the SD subjects and all control groups for all three electrodes. Within the SD sample, abnormal activity from both the temporal lobe electrodes was highly correlated ($r = .71$), whereas the frontal activity was uncorrelated with that of either temporal lobe. Significant interhemispheric asymmetry of the evoked potential abnormality, with greater left-sided difference, was demonstrated using a t test for correlated samples with patient's z scores from the temporal lobe electrodes ($p = .016$).

These findings provide evidence of abnormal higher brain activity in the subjects with SD. Localization of these differences tended to occur over the left and right central and medial frontal electrode placements. It is intriguing to speculate on a relationship between these scalp distributions and underlying brain topography. For example, medial frontal cortex is now regarded as a "starter mechanism" of vocalization for speech (Freedman et al., 1984). Left central cortex is, of course, the

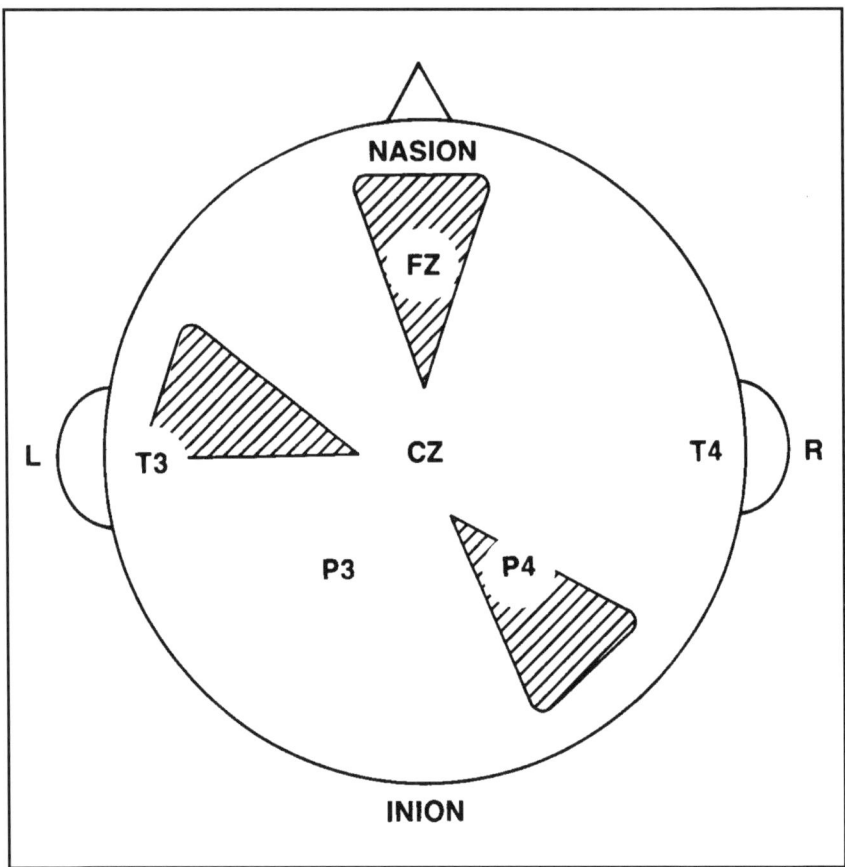

Figure 9.5. Composite diagram of the approximate scalp distributions of areas of overlapping electrocortical dysfunction in 10 cases of SD. *Note.* From *Extralaryngeal Functions in Spasmodic Dysphonia: Vocal Tract and Manual Control*, by M. P. Cannito, 1986, unpublished doctoral dissertation, University of Texas at Dallas. Copyright 1986 by M. P. Cannito. Reprinted with permission.

classical speech and language area. Recently, analogous functions for the processing of intonation have been hypothesized for the right central area (Ross, 1981). Despite all this, our present knowledge of the actual neural generators of so-called cortical EEG and evoked potential activity, as well as the localizing significance of such automated patient-tonormal comparisons (American Academy of Neurology, 1989), is limited, and we must acknowledge that attempts at such brain-behavior correlations in SD remain in the realm of speculation.

Table 9.6
Group Means, Standard Deviations, and Newman-Keuls Comparisons for Cortical Auditory Evoked Response at 108–144 ms

Group	x̄ (μV)	Standard Deviation	Degrees of Freedom	Significance
Electrode T3 by Groups (F = 8.03, p < .001)				
Spasmodic dysphonics	− 1.793	0.793		
30–39 yrs	+ 0.012	0.726	18	**
40–49 yrs	+ 0.353	0.421	12	**
50–59 yrs	+ 0.049	1.145	22	**
60–69 yrs	− 0.181	0.787	19	**
Electrode FZ by Groups (F = 13.25, p < .001)				
Spasmodic dysphonics	− 3.384	1.800		
30–39 yrs	+ 1.307	1.707	18	**
40–49 yrs	+ 2.160	1.888	20	**
50–59 yrs	+ 0.509	2.276	22	**
60–69 yrs	− 0.472	1.358	15	**
Electrode T4 by Groups (F = 5.59, p < .001)				
Spasmodic dysphonics	− 1.840	0.717		
30–39 yrs	− 0.166	0.905	22	**
40–49 yrs	+ 0.228	0.917	22	**
50–59 yrs	− 0.248	1.175	22	**
60–69 yrs	− 0.879	0.981	22	*

Note. From *Extralaryngeal Functions in Spasmodic Dysphonia: Vocal Tract and Manual Control*, by M. P. Cannito, 1986, unpublished doctoral dissertation, University of Texas at Dallas. Copyright 1986 by M. Cannito. Reprinted with permission.
*Spasmodic dysphonics differed from normals with probability less than .05.
**Spasmodic dysphonics differed from normals with probability less than .01.

Since the original studies, abnormal MRI and BEAM findings in SD have been extended to larger sample sizes (Finitzo & Freeman, 1989) and corroborated with regional cerebral blood flow (SPECT) imaging (Devous et al., 1990). Ruling out subjects with prior known neurological disorders, 12 of 51 patients with SD who were studied exhibited MRI abnormalites, with deep supratentorial, small volume white matter lesions being the most common. Quantitative topographic mapping of electrocortical activity using BEAM was ultimately accomplished in 43 of the subjects with SD. Using rigorous quantitative criteria, 24 of these subjects were deemed abnormal and most exhibited multiple abnormalites in the topographic regions noted in Figure 9.5. Resting regional cerebral blood flow abnormalities were observed in 37 of 49 subjects with SD, with the most common loci in the frontal and temporal lobes bilaterally. The results of these imaging studies, although intriguing, remain controversial (see Aronson & Lagerlund, 1991; Finitzo, Freeman, Devous, & Watson, 1991) and, as yet, have not been replicated. Additional neural imaging research in SD is now needed (a) to explore electro-cortical activation using contemporary dipole localization methodologies, in addition to topographic mapping, for both post-sensory and premotor processes, and (b) to examine functional imaging during speech activation tasks in comparison to resting state using positron emission tomography or functional MRI.

Recent Developments

Since the publication of the original version of this chapter in 1991, there has been a truly remarkable surge of research activity on SD. Much of this work has been driven by the widespread application of botulinum toxin (BOTOX) treatment to management of laryngeal dyskinesias. This topic will be adressed in the upcoming section on treatment. Unfortunately, this flurry of BOTOX treatment research seems to have deflected interest in neural mechanisms underlying the peripheral movement disorder, and comparatively few new studies have been published that elucidate basic pathologic processes. Some notable exceptions, however, have addressed the topics of localization of neurological dysfunction and extra-laryngeal involvement in SD.

Two critically important studies have recently been published by Ludlow and collegues (Deleyiannis, Gillespie, Bielamowicz, Yamashita, & Ludlow, 1999; Ludlow, Schulz, Yamashita, & Deleyiannis, 1995), wherein the technique of unilateral superior laryngeal nerve stimulation was used to evaluate differential levels of neurological dysfunction in SD. In normal subjects, the technique has been shown to elicit a relatively shorter latency response in the ipsilateral TA muscle as well as a longer latency bilateral TA response. This component of the evaluation examines the integrity of the afferent fibers in the peripheral nerve, the lower motor neuron pool, and the efferent limb of the peripheral reflex response. Pairing the initial stimulation (described as the "unconditioned stimulus") with subsequent stimulations at varying interstimulus intervals (described as the "conditioned stimulus") yields a normal reduction in amplitude and frequency of these responses. This component of the evaluation examines conditioned inhibition of the reflex response and is believed to evoke supranuclear control processes within the CNS. Two studies examining eight patients with ADSD and 10 patients with ABSD (in comparison to normal controls) indicated no significant differences from normal for the unconditioned stimuli. This was interpreted to indicate intactness of peripheral and brainstem reflex pathways in SD. For the conditioned stimuli, however, both types of SD patients differed significantly from normal inasmuch as there was decreased response inhibition in both patient groups. This was interpreted to suggest that higher-level modulation of the reflex pathways by CNS inhibitory mechanisms was abnormal. Moreover, there were qualitative differences within and between the SD patient groups, with a few abnormal responses elicited to the unconditioned stimuli.

Other recent studies have yielded additional support for the presence of extralaryngeal vocal tract involvement in individuals with SD. Velar postural abnormalities have been documented (Doody & Rosenfield, 1990; Lundy, Casiano, Lu, & Xue, 1996) using videonasoendoscopy. Abnormally increased variability of EMG activity occurring only during speech has been documented in the levator palatini muscle, but in the posterior genioglossus muscle only during sustained vowel production (Schaefer et al., 1992) for a group of 11 speakers with SD. In addition, abnormal vocal tract configuration was documented by Crary, Kotzur, Gauger, Gorham, and Burton (1996) using dynamic magnetic resonance imaging during prolongation of /i/ and /a/. Five women with ADSD exhibited abnormally high laryngeal position, abnormally increased pharyngeal constriction, and abnormal degrees of vocal tract instability over time. Following BOTOX treatment, these values improved but did not attain normal levels. A recent study of vowel formant frequencies during connected speech also revealed significant differences between 16 speakers with ADSD and matched normal controls, before and after BOTOX treatment, further supporting the notion of abnormal vocal tract configuration in this population (Buder, Cannito, Taylor, Woodson, & Murry, 1999). Kinematic data have been presented demonstrating abnormal movements during mandibular tracking in one speaker with ABSD (Boutsen, Bakker, & Cannito, 1998), whereas abnormal lip articulation profiles that were not contingent upon laryngeal spasms have been demonstrated for two of three selected cases of adductor and abductor SD (Tingley & Dromey, 2000). The collective findings of these recent studies are congruent with and supportive of the model of SD originally proposed in 1991, which is described in the next section of this chapter.

Summary

Although many neural explanations of SD have been proposed, it is apparent that some are less satisfactory than others on either logical or empirical grounds. Peripheral neuropathy is today generally rejected as an explanation for SD (Izdebski & Shipp, 1985). Bulbar-level explanations fail to account for the intermittent and speech-specific nature of the SD symptom complex, nor are SD symptoms similar to those exhibited by patients with documented bulbar disease. Although multiple cranially innervated structures frequently exhibit spasmodic abnormalities in SD, "cranial nerve spasmodic disorders cited are generally considered to be of supranuclear (basal ganglia) origin" (Hartman & Vishwanat, 1984, p. 403). The intactness of nonspeech, affective vocalization in SD appears to rule out limbic structures or the periaqueductal gray as primary lesion loci. Yet because the signs and symptoms that have been noted in association with SD are not exclusively basal gangliar, it is probably appropriate to hypothesize a more general type of supranuclear involvement. Specifically, abnormalities observed in structures innervated by the cranial motor neuron pool probably reflect deviant neuronal interactions conditioned by the descending, modulating influence of impaired structures projecting from higher levels within the CNS.

A variable supranuclear lesion locus appears appealing at this point in our understanding of SD. Premotor association cortex, pyramidal motor cortex, and the descending motor tracts lie in close proximity to the basal ganglia and share a common vascular supply. In addition, these structures interact as part of a single functional system during voluntary movement (Evarts, 1980; Kornhuber, 1984). A lesion variably affecting these structures might account for both spastic and dyskinetic vocal and nonvocal signs. These structures and their interactions are pictured schematically in Figure 9.6. Behavioral evidence from the dysarthrias, extralaryngeal motor findings in SD, and brain-imaging studies of SD are consistent with this view. Such an explanation is able

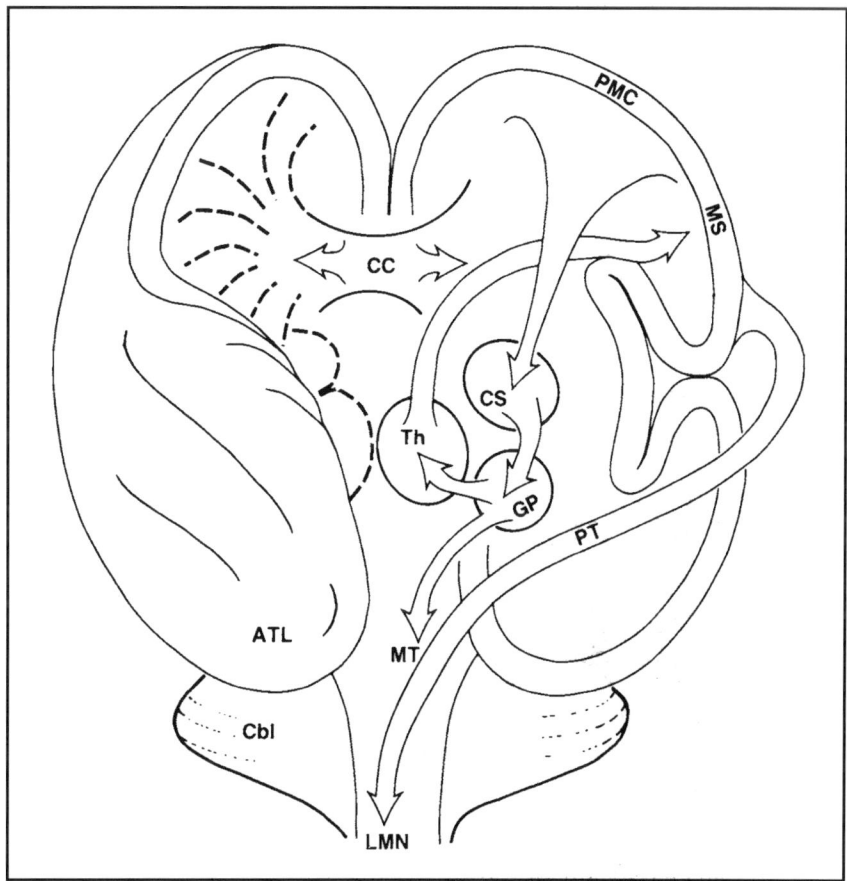

Figure 9.6. Semischematic diagram of proposed cerebral motor circuits that may be implicated in the spasmodic dysphonias: *pmc*, premotor association cortex; *ms*, motor strip; *cc*, corpus callosum; *cs*, corpus striatum; *gp*, globus pallidus; *th*, thalamus; *mt*, midbrain tegmentum; *lmn*, lower motor neuron; *atl*, anterior temporal lobe (landmark only); *cbl*, cerebellum (landmark only).

to accommodate the apparent focality, function specificity, heterogeneity, intermittency, and affect sensitivity of symptoms associated with this unusual voice disorder.

Implications for Management

It has been argued in this chapter that SD represents a supranuclear motor disturbance that predominantly affects the pathways for phonation for speech but may variably involve pathways for other cranial and somatic motor functions. Such a view places SD squarely within the realm of neuromotor speech disorders, which also encompasses the dysarthrias and apraxia of speech. Specifically, SD should be regarded as a family of focal, supranuclear dysarthrias. Whether SD represents a disorder of motor preprogramming or of execution and regulation of vocal motor commands remains unknown. Nevertheless, a supranuclear dysphonia of this type should probably be approached therapeutically somewhat differently from a voice disorder arising from either functional or peripheral vocal fold lesion etiologies. As Rosenbek and LaPointe (1985) have written, "Only if a dysarthric patient's nervous system returns to normal will speech return too. The return to normal—either because of natural or physiologic recovery or because of medical treatment—is a rare circumstance indeed. Therefore, the aim of all dysarthria treatment is compensated intelligibility. With professional guidance and by dint of individual effort, many dysarthric patients can learn to talk better. They can do so for two reasons: (1) physiologic support for a patient's speech can be enhanced; or (2) they can learn to make better use of whatever residual support is left to them" (p. 104).

These observations are germane to SD because the SD patient must recognize that the neural machinery is broken; the premorbid voice will never be achieved again; and rather than a return to normal voice, the goal of therapy should be to achieve the best compensatory voice possible. Thorough counseling in this regard is a critical prerequisite to progress in therapy. Many patients with SD will resist the compensatory voice, stagnant in mourning for their premorbid one. Maximization of the physiologic substrate can be achieved in specific cases by surgical fixation of one vocal fold, or by weakening the vocal fold(s) by botulinum toxin injection, or sometimes by pharmacologic treatment (Rosenfield, 1988). Although not a panacea, botulinum toxin injection of the intrinsic laryngeal musculature is now generally regarded as the treatment of choice for adductor SD and considered beneficial for many cases of abductor or mixed SD (Cannito & Woodson, 2000). Compensated intelligibility can be achieved using a variety of dysarthria therapy techniques, including reduced rate, exaggerated stress and articulation, phrasing, and airflow maintenance (see Darley et al., 1975; Yorkston, Beukelman, & Bell, 1988). Murry and Woodson (1995) demonstrated that a combined modality approach, incorporating botulinum toxin injection and behavioral voice therapy, significantly prolonged the period between injections for a group of speakers with adductor SD.

Counseling is also important for helping patients deal with the negative impact of SD on their professional and personal lives. Using the *Self-Rating of Depression Scale* (Zung, 1967) and the *State-Trait Anxiety Scale* (Spielberger et al., 1983), Cannito (1991) has demonstrated that over half of 18 spasmodic dysphonic females studied were clinically depressed or anxious. This is not to say that emotional problems cause SD in these patients any more than postmorbid depression would be regarded as causing aphasia in a stroke patient. However, depression and anxiety may well exacerbate an affect-sensitive neuromotor problem (see Chapter 2) and impede progress in therapy. These easy-to-administer paper-and-pencil scales served well as a preliminary screening (in conjunction with patient interview) for potential professional counseling referral. Since the original publication of this chapter, research has demonstrated that although emotional measures improved following botulinum toxin injection in adductor SD, they do not (on average) achieve a normal level (Cannito, Murry, & Woodson, 1994; Liu et al., 1998; Murry, Cannito, & Woodson, 1994). The psychosocial impact of dysarthria and the importance of counseling for dysarthric individuals and their families are discussed at length in Chapter 5 of this volume.

The guiding principles of therapy for apraxia of speech as described by Rosenbek (1985) include "(1) efforts to improve the speech programmer by specific concentration on programmer function, and (2) efforts to reorganize speech function by systematically incorporating intact or relatively intact systems into the function of the speech programmer" (p. 270). These observations may be germane to SD in that retraining of phonatory programming may be possible by repetitive contrastive drill (see Chapter 8). The well-established preservation of nonspeech vocalizations provides a broad repertoire of "relatively intact systems" that may be brought, through therapy, under volitional control. The facilatory effects of speech produced in a context of vegetative vocalization (i.e., yawning or laughing) in SD have been demonstrated acoustically by Freeman et al. (1985a). It seems reasonable to believe that approaching SD therapy within the broader context of treatment for other neuromotor speech disorders may provide some useful general strategies that may be adapted to the unique needs of the patient with SD. It should also be clear that the management of SD patients is a multidisciplinary endeavor involving otolaryngology, neurology, and in many cases psychotherapy, in addition to speech pathology.

Neuromotor-Oriented Treatment

SD has proven to be dramatically resistant to traditional voice therapy, leading some to question the wisdom of the speech pathologist even treating such individuals beyond, perhaps, a short trial course of laryngeal tension-reducing exercises. Implicit in this thinking has been the tenacious assumption that patients with SD are crazy and could speak just fine if they really wanted to! Approaching SD management within a motor speech disorders framework radically alters all phases of the clinical process—from diagnosis to selection of treatment goals, to counseling, to ongoing monitoring of treatment efficacy. The following case study, originally reported by Cannito, Louera, and Rosenfield (1989), describes a patient with SD who was treated within a context of dysarthria management in which the focus was shifted away from traditional voice therapy techniques toward enhancement of the physiologic substrate and compensated intelligibility. It also points out the value of intelligibility testing in the assessment and ongoing management of more severe manifestations of SD (Bender, Cannito, Matessich, Murry, & Woodson, 2000).

 CASE STUDY

M.M. is a 72-year-old retired businesswoman. Her voice disorder was originally diagnosed as a mixed (adductor-abductor) SD with voice tremor by an examining laryngologist in 1976. Tremors of the tongue and head were also noted. She began traditional voice therapy soon after and was treated for about a year. The dysphonia persisted. She subsequently tried periods of psychotherapy and biofeedback relaxation therapy without noticeable benefit. She was reinstated in voice therapy at the University of Texas Speech and Hearing Center in the summer of 1987, when she reported experiencing difficulty establishing new relationships following her retirement due to her voice disorder. Relaxation of the laryngeal area and loudness reduction were employed in treatment, in addition to the traditional voice therapy techniques of easy onset of phonation, tone focus, and control of breath support.

M.M. was seen by the author for evaluation in September 1987. Vocal quality was characterized by the presence of strained-strangled phonation and intermittent breathiness. Presence of frequent hard glottal attacks, intermittent breaks in phonation, glottal stops, vocal fry, and audible voice tremor were noted. She was unable to sustain a vowel for more than approximately 4 seconds. There was a ratio discrepancy of approximately 12 seconds between sustained /s/ and /z/. The timing of laryngospasms between syllables gave the perceptual impression of frequent omissions of initial consonants. Conversational speech was unintelligible and dysfluent.

M.M.'s phonation quality improved across a variety of nonspeech tasks including humming, paralanguage (e.g., "un-huh"), laughing, coughing, yawning, and grunting. Whispering was facilitory, but not spasm free. Better voice quality was noted for vowels sustained at high pitch, but duration remained dramatically curtailed, even in falsetto register. On examination, oral structure and function were unremarkable, with the exception that velar spasms were noted to occur in synchrony with the laryngospasms. A case history revealed no prior neurological or psychiatric involvement (other than SD). She admitted "stammering" as a child, but said dysfluency resolved with speech therapy by age 12.

M.M. continued voice therapy, but the treatment approach was modified somewhat. Rather than focusing attention on traditional dimensions of voice quality, improved intelligibility was targeted as the treatment goal. A soft, breathy phonatory pattern, prolonged syllable duration, and light articulatory contacts were incorporated into the therapy techniques. After 22 sixty-minute biweekly sessions, her speech intelligibility was evaluated using Yorkston and Beukelman's *Assessment of Intelligibility of Dysarthric Speech* (AIDS; Yorkston & Beukelman, 1984). It was found that when not actively using her "speech controls," her connected utterances were only 17% intelligible; however, when controls were employed her intelligibility score increased to 77%. The patient reported that the compensated speech was difficult and demanded excessively high levels of concentration.

In February 1988, while continuing the intelligibility-oriented speech therapy, M.M. was referred to Dr. David Rosenfield at Baylor College of Medicine in Houston for a comprehensive neurological evaluation. Neurologic examination indicated severe intention tremor of the upper extremities and axial (head-neck) tremor as well as phonatory tremor. Fiberoptic examination of the larynx indicated constant movement of laryngeal musculature, with significant starts and stops and hyperfunctional laryngeal contraction on adduction with overrelaxation with which she attempted to compensate. MRI revealed supranuclear white matter lesions in the deep cerebral white matter (centrum semiovale and periventricular regions) of the cerebral hemispheres as well as small bilateral lesions in the pontine region of the brainstem. These were associated with biopsy-proved arteritis, but may or may not have been related to the laryngeal tremor disorder. Alcohol was reported to improve the condition, whereas stress worsened it. A diagnosis of spasmodic dysphonia secondary to underlying essential tremor was applied, and the patient was started on a regimen of 10 mg of oral propranolol (Inderal) three times daily for 1 month; the dosage was then increased to 20 mg three times daily for 1 month.

M.M.'s intelligibility score increased from a baseline level of 48%, 32%, and 57% (average of 46% across three successive AIDS administrations) to 75% and 80% (average of 78%) following 2 months of pharmacotherapy. In conjunction with pharmacotherapy, she was seen for speech therapy for nineteen 50-minute individual biweekly sessions. During this period, M.M. reported using her controls successfully in various situations. She also became increasingly responsive during treatment and more cognizant of her vocal quality in therapy. Voice tremor on sustained phonation was noticeably reduced.

M.M. took a vacation from speech therapy in summer of 1988 to travel, but returned in September. At that time, she revealed that she had discontinued the Inderal due to the inconvenience of returning to Houston for follow-up, and because in her opinion the medication was not responsible for her voice improvement. In September, her baseline intelligibility score was 36% to 59% (average of 44%). In December 1988, following 17 more 50 minute biweekly sessions of speech therapy without medication, her intelligibility score was at 40% to 57% (average of 50%). The patient reported that she was unable to maintain her controls outside of the therapy situation and in the therapy situation only for short periods and with great difficulty.

Spasmodic dysphonia is notoriously variable; however, results of the intelligibility assessment data indicated that M.M.'s intelligibility continued to fluctuate in a range from 36% to 59% without medication when she was not consciously applying therapy controls. The high intelligibility values noted during treatment with Inderal were striking because no instruction to use the therapy controls was employed during those administrations of the AIDS. Further, the generalized ease reported for using controls during that period, within and without the therapy room, is notable. It is likely that speech therapy targeting compensated intelligibility in conjunction with pharmacotherapy to enhance the underlying physiologic substrate for speech was an effective combination for this patient.

Following the original publication of this chapter, M.M. participated in a BOTOX treatment study conducted at the National Institutes of Health in Bethesda, Maryland. Initially, bilateral injections of the vocal folds were employed and yielded highly successful results, with marked improvements in vocal quality and intelligibility. Ten months later, a second bilateral injection was administered with some increase in dosage. Her voice remained improved over preinjection levels, but was somewhat "breathy and quiet." In addition, some dysphagia was noted as a side effect. Ten months later, she received a third treatment, but this was restricted to a unilateral injection of the TA muscle. This yielded good results for voice quality and elimination of swallowing difficulty. Her subsequent injections were unilateral with ongoing adjustment of dosage in pursuit of more optimal voice quality.

The patient recognized that BOTOX was not a "cure" for her voice disorder and continued to actively participate in voice therapy. It was clear that following injections, M.M.'s voice quality, although significantly improved over preinjection levels, did not achieve a normal quality. Following BOTOX injections, single word intelligibility improved to 80% to 85% levels on the AIDS. As voice deteriorated over time, prior to reinjection, it was found to decline to approximately 52% without the use of facilitating techniques and approximately 66% with the use of voice therapy techniques. Later voice therapy activities included the use of slower rate, more precise articulation, reduced intensity, and higher pitch. Ongoing behavioral treatment, in conjunction with BOTOX injection, also successfully incorporated visual feedback using the IBM Speech Viewer system. In addition to speech improvements attained using her therapy techniques during periods between injections, the patient felt that ongoing behavioral therapy provided a valuable "support system" that was helpful in dealing with the multifaceted impact of the voice disorder on her social interaction and routines of everyday life.

Acknowledgments

This chapter is based in part on the author's doctoral dissertation, completed at the University of Texas at Dallas in 1986 and supported by NIH Grant NS 18276. Portions of this chapter have been presented at the Third Biennial Clinical Dysarthria Conference, Tucson, AZ, 1985; the 109th Meeting of the Acoustical Society of America, Austin, TX, 1985; and the 33rd Annual Conference of the Texas Speech and Hearing Association, El Paso, TX, 1989. This author acknowledges Barbara Louera, MS, and David B. Rosenfield, MD, for their contributions to the case study.

References

American Academy of Neurology. (1989). Assessment: EEG brain mapping. *Neurology, 39,* 1100–1101.

Aminoff, M. J., Dedo, H. H., & Izdebski, K. (1978). Clinical aspects of spasmodic dysphonia. *Journal of Neurology, Neurosurgery and Psychiatry, 41,* 361–365.

Aronson, A. E. (1973). *Audio seminars in speech pathology-psychogenic voice disorders*. Philadelphia: Saunders.

Aronson, A. E. (1978). Differential diagnosis of organic and psychogenic voice disorders. In F. L. Darley & D. C. Spriesterbach (Eds.), *Diagnostic methods in speech pathology* (pp. 535–560). New York: Harper & Row.

Aronson, A. E. (1985). *Clinical voice disorders: An interdisciplinary approach* (2nd ed.). New York: Thieme.

Aronson, A. E., Brown, J. R., Litin, M. E., & Pearson, J. S. (1968a). Spastic dysphonia: Part 1. Voice, neurologic, and psychiatric aspects. *Journal of Speech and Hearing Disorders, 33*, 203–218.

Aronson, A. E., Brown, J. R., Litin, M. E., & Pearson, J. S. (1968b). Spastic dysphonia: Part 2. Comparison with essential (voice) tremor and other neurologic and psychogenic dysphonias. *Journal of Speech and Hearing Disorders, 33*, 219–231.

Aronson, A. E., & DeSanto, L. W. (1983). Adductor spastic dysphonia: Three years after recurrent laryngeal nerve section. *Laryngoscope, 93*, 1–8.

Aronson, A. E., & Hartman, D. (1981). Adductor spastic dysphonia as a sign of essential (voice) tremor. *Journal of Speech and Hearing Disorders, 46*, 52–58.

Aronson, A. E., & Lagerlund, T. D. (1991). Neuroimaging studies do not prove the existence of brain abnormalities in spastic dysphonia. *Journal of Speech and Hearing Research, 34*, 801–805.

Axelrod, J. (1974). Neurotransmitters. *Scientific American, 230*, 58–71.

Bender, B., Cannito, M., Matessich, J., Murry, T., & Woodson, G. E. (2000, February). *Speech intelligibility in severe adductor spasmodic dysphonia before and after BOTOX treatment*. Conference on Motor Speech, San Antonio.

Benson, D. F. (1979). *Aphasia, alexia and agraphia*. New York: Churchill Livingstone.

Blitzer, A., Lovelace, R., Brin, M., Fahn, S., & Fink, M. (1985). Electromyographic findings in focal laryngeal dystonia (spastic dysphonia). *Annals of Otology, Rhinology and Laryngology, 94*, 591–594.

Boccino, J. V., & Tucker, H. M. (1978). Recurrent laryngeal nerve pathology in spasmodic dysphonia. *Laryngoscope, 88,* 1274–1280.

Boone, D. R. (1977). *The voice and voice therapy.* Englewood Cliffs, NJ: Prentice Hall.

Botez, M. I., & Barbeau, A. (1971). Role of subcortical structures and particularly of the thalamus, in the mechanisms of speech and language. *International Journal of Neurology, 8,* 300–320.

Boutsen, F., Bakker, K., & Cannito, M. (1998, January). *Mandibular, labial and hand force control in adductor spasmodic dysphonia.* Paper presented at Ninth Biennial Conference on Motor Speech, Tucson, AZ.

Bril, V., Sharpe, J. A., & Ashby, P. (1979). Midbrain asterixis. *Annals of Neurology, 6,* 362–364.

Brodnitz, F. S. (1976). Spastic dysphonia. *Annals of Otorhinolaryngology, 85,* 210–214.

Buder, E. H., Cannito, M. P., Taylor, M., Woodson, G. E., & Murry, T. (1999). Assessment of BOTOX effects on adductor spasmodic dysphonia using LTAS-guided analysis. *Journal of the Acoustical Society of America, 105,* 1247.

Cannito, M. (1986). *Extralaryngeal functions in spasmodic dysphonia: Vocal tract and manual control.* Unpublished doctoral dissertation, University of Texas at Dallas.

Cannito, M. (1989). Vocal tract steadiness in spasmodic dysphonia. In K. Yorkston & D. Beukelman (Eds.), *Recent advances in clinical dysarthria* (pp. 243–262). Austin, TX: PRO-ED.

Cannito, M. (1991). Emotional considerations in spasmodic dysphonia: Psychometric quantification. *Journal of Communication Disorders, 24,* 313–329.

Cannito, M. P., Burch, A. R., Watts, C., Rappold, P. W., Hood, S. B., & Sherrard, K. (1997). Disfluency in spasmodic dysphonia: A multivariate analysis. *Journal of Speech, Language and Hearing Research, 40,* 627–641.

Cannito, M. P., Finitzo, T., Freeman, F. J., & Pool, K. D. (1985). Brain electrical activity mapping in adductor spasmodic dysphonia. *Journal of the Acoustical Society of America, 77*, S87.

Cannito, M. P., Freeman, F. J., Kondraske, G. V., Pool, K. D., Schaefer, S., & Finitzo, T. (1986, October). *Spastic dysphonia: A dysarthria?* Paper presented at the Third Biennial Clinical Dysarthria Conference, Tuscon, AZ.

Cannito, M. P., & Johnson, J. P. (1981). Spastic dysphonia: A continuum disorder. *Journal of Communication Disorders, 14*, 215–223.

Cannito, M. P., & Kondraske, G. V. (1990). Rapid manual abilities in spasmodic dysphonic and normal female subjects. *Journal of Speech and Hearing Research, 33*, 123–133.

Cannito, M. P., Louera, B., & Rosenfield, D. (1989, March). *Neurogenic spasmodic dysphonia: A case for successful intervention.* Paper presented at the annual meeting of the Texas Speech and Hearing Association, El Paso, TX.

Cannito, M. P., Murry, T., & Woodson, G. E. (1994). Attitudes toward communication in adductor spasmodic dysphonia before and after botulinum toxin injection. *Journal of Medical Speech–Language Pathology, 2*, 125–133.

Cannito, M. P., & Woodson, G. E. (2000). The spasmodic dysphonias. In R. D. Kent & M. J. Ball (Eds.), *Voice quality management* (pp. 411–430). San Diego: Singular.

Carpenter, M. B. (1978). *Core text of neuroanatomy.* Baltimore: Williams & Wilkins.

Clark, R. G. (1975). *Essentials of clinical neuroanatomy and neurophysiology.* Philadelphia: Davis.

Cooper, I. S. (1976). Dystonia: Surgical approaches to treatment and physiologic implications. In M. D. Yahr (Ed.), *The basal ganglia* (pp. 369–383). New York: Raven Press.

Crary, M. A., Kotzur, I. M., Gauger, J., Gorham, M., & Burton, S. (1996). Dynamic magnetic resonance imaging in the study of vocal tract configuration. *Journal of Voice, 10*, 378–388.

Critchley, M. (1939). Spastic dysphonia ("inspiratory speech"). *Brain: A Journal of Neurology, 62,* 96–103.

Darley, F. L. (1978). Differential diagnosis of acquired motor speech disorders. In F. L. Darley & D. C. Spriestersbach (Eds.), *Diagnostic methods in speech pathology* (pp. 492–513). New York: Harper & Row.

Darley, F. L., Aronson, A. E., & Brown, J. R. (1975). *Motor speech disorders.* Philadelphia: Saunders.

Dedo, H. H., & Izdebski, K. (1983). Problems with surgical (RLN section) treatment of spastic dysphonia. *Laryngoscope, 93,* 268–271.

Dedo, H. H., Townsend, J. J., & Izdebski, K. (1978). Current evidence for the organic etiology of spastic dysphonia. *Otolaryngology, 86,* 875–880.

Deleyiannis, F. W.-B., Gillespie, M., Bielamowicz, S., Yamashita, T., & Ludlow, C. L. (1999). Laryngeal long latency response conditioning in adductor spasmodic dysphonia. *Annals of Otology, Rhinology and Laryngology, 108,* 612–619.

Devous, M. D., Pool, K. D., Finitzo, T., Freeman, F. J., Schaefer, S. D., Watson, B. C., Kondraske, G. V., & Chapman, S. B. (1990). Evidence for cortical dysfunction in spasmodic dysphonia: Regional cerebral blood flow and quantitative electrophysiology. *Brain and Language, 39,* 331–344.

Diamond, I. T. (1979). The subdivisions of neocortex: A proposal to revise the traditional view of sensory, motor and association areas. *Progress in Psychobiology and Physiological Psychology, 8,* 1–43.

Doody, R. S., & Rosenfield, D. B. (1990). Spasmodic dysphonia associated with palatal myoclonus. *Ear, Nose and Throat Journal, 69,* 829–832.

Dubner, R., Sessle, B. J., & Storey, A. T. (1978). *The neural basis of oral and facial function.* New York: Plenum Press.

Duffy, F. H., Bartels, P. H., & Burchfield, J. L. (1981). Significance probability mapping: An aid in the topographic analysis of brain electrical activity. *Electroencephalography and Clinical Neurophysiology, 51,* 455–462.

Evarts, E. V. (1980). Brain mechanisms in voluntary movement. In D. McFadden (Ed.), *Neural mechanisms in behavior* (pp. 223–252). New York: Springer-Verlag.

Feldman, M., Nixon, J. V., Finitzo-Hieber, T., & Freeman, F. J. (1984). Abnormal parasympathetic vagal function in patients with spasmodic dysphonia. *Annals of Internal Medicine, 100,* 401–495.

Finitzo, T., & Freeman, F. J. (1989). Spasmodic dysphonia, whether and where: Results of seven years of research. *Journal of Speech and Hearing Research, 32,* 541–555.

Finitzo, T., Freeman, F., Devous, M. D., & Watson, B. C. (1991). Whether and wherefore: A response to Aronson and Lagerlund. *Journal of Speech and Hearing Research, 34,* 806–811.

Finitzo-Hieber, T., Freeman, F. J., Gerling, I., Dodson, L., & Schaefer, S. (1981). Auditory brainstem response abnormalities in adductor spasmodic dysphonia. *American Journal of Otolaryngology, 3,* 26–30.

Foltz, E. L., Knopp, L. M., & Ward, A. A. (1959). Experimental spasmodic torticollis. *Journal of Neurosurgery, 16,* 55–72.

Fox, D. (1969). Spastic dysphonia: A case presentation. *Journal of Speech and Hearing Disorders, 34,* 275–279.

Franzen, E. A., & Myers, R. E. (1973). Neural control of social behavior: Prefrontal and anterior temporal cortex. *Neuropsychologia, 11,* 141–157.

Freedman, M., Alexander, M. P., & Naeser, M. A. (1984). Anatomic basis of transcortical motor aphasia. *Neurology, 34,* 409–417.

Freeman, F., Cannito, M., Finitzo, T., & Schaefer, S. (1985). Disordered laryngeal control: Fiberoptic studies of spasmodic dysphonia. *Journal of the Acoustical Society of America, 77,* S87.

Freeman, F. J., Cannito, M. P., & Finitzo-Hieber, T. (1985a). Classification of spasmodic dysphonia by perceptual-acoustic-visual means. In G. Gates (Ed.), *Spasmodic dysphonia: The state of the art, 1984* (pp. 5–18). New York: Voice Foundation.

Freeman, F. J., Cannito, M. P., & Finitzo-Hieber, T. (1985b). Getting to know spasmodic dysphonic patients. *Texas Journal of Audiology and Speech Pathology, 10,* 14–19.

Hall, J. W. (1981). Central auditory function in spasmodic dysphonia. *American Journal of Otolaryngology, 2,* 188–198.

Hall, J. W., & Jerger, J. (1976). Acoustic reflex characteristics in spasmodic dysphonia. *Archives of Otolaryngology, 102,* 411–415.

Hartman, D. E., & Vishwanat, B. (1984). Spasmodic dysphonia [letter to the editor]. *Annals of Internal Medicine, 101,* 403.

Hast, M. H., Fischer, J. M., Wetzel, A. B., & Thompson, V. E. (1974). Cortical motor representation of the laryngeal muscles in macaca mulatta. *Brain Research, 73,* 229–240.

Hast, M. H., & Milojevic, B. (1967). The response of the vocal folds to electrical stimulation of the inferior frontal cortex of the squirrel monkey. *Actaotolaryngologica, 61,* 196–204.

House, E. L., Pansky, B., & Siegal, A. (1979). *A systematic approach to neuroscience.* New York: McGraw-Hill.

Izdebski, K., & Shipp, T. (1985). Model of spastic dysphonia. In G. A. Gates (Ed.), *Spastic dysphonia: The state of the art, 1984* (pp. 44–47). New York: Voice Foundation.

Jankovic, J. (1981). Drug-induced and other orofacial-cervical dyskinesias. *Annals of Internal Medicine, 94,* 788–793.

Jankovic, J. (1983). Brainstem origin of blepharospasm. *Neurology, 33,* 162.

Jankovic, J., & Fahn, S. (1980). Physiologic and pathologic tremors: Diagnosis, mechanisms and management. *Annals of Internal Medicine, 93,* 460–465.

Jankovic, J., & Ford, J. (1982). Blepharospasm and orofacial-cervical dystonia: Clinical and pharmacological findings in 100 patients. *Annals of Neurology, 13,* 402–411.

Jurgens, U. (1976). Projections from the cortical larynx area in the squirrel monkey. *Experimental Brain Research, 25,* 401–411.

Jurgens, U., & Ploog, D. (1970). Cerebral representation of vocalization in the squirrel monkey. *Experimental Brain Research, 10,* 532–554.

Jurgens, U., & Ploog, D. (1981). On the neural control of mammalian vocalization. *Trends in Neuroscience, 4,* 135–137.

Jurgens, U., & Pratt, R. (1979a). The cingular vocalization pathway in the squirrel monkey. *Experimental Brain Research*, *34*, 499–570.

Jurgens, U., & Pratt, R. (1979b). Role of the periaqueductal gray in the vocal expression of emotion. *Brain Research*, *167*, 367–378.

Kelley, A. H., Beaton, L. E., & Magoun, H. W. (1946). A midbrain mechanism for facio-vocal activity. *Journal of Neurophysiology*, *9*, 181–189.

Kelso, J. A. S., & Tuller, B. (1981). Toward a theory of apractic syndromes. *Brain and Language*, *12*, 224–245.

Kiml, P. J. (1965). Recherches experimentales de la dysphonie spastique [Experimental Studies of Spastic dysphonia]. *Folia Phoniatrica*, *17*, 241–301.

Kirzinger, A., & Jurgens, U. (1985). The effects of brainstem lesions on vocalization in the squirrel monkey. *Brain Research*, *358*, 150–162.

Kornhuber, H. H. (1984). Mechanisms of voluntary movement. In W. Prinz & A. F. Sanders (Eds.), *Cognition and motor processes*. New York: Springer-Verlag.

Kuypers, H. A. (1982). A new look at the organization of the motor system. *Progress in Brain Research*, *57*, 381–403.

Lang, A. E., & Marsden, C. D. (1983). Spasmodic dysphonia in Gilles de la Tourette's disease. *Archives of Neurology*, *40*, 51–52.

Liu, C-Y., Yu, J-M., Wang, N-M., Chen, R-S., Chang, H-C., Li, H-Y., Tsai, C-H., Yang, Y-Y., & Lu, C-S. (1998). Emotional symptoms are secondary to the voice disorder in patients with spasmodic dysphonia. *General Hospital Psychiatry*, *20*, 255–259.

Luchsinger, R., & Arnold, G. E. (1965). *Voice-speech-language clinical communicology: Its physiology and pathology*. Belmont, CA: Wadsworth.

Ludlow, C., & Connor, N. (1987). Dynamic aspects of phonatory control in spasmodic dysphonia. *Journal of Speech and Hearing Research*, *30*, 197–206.

Ludlow, C. L., Schulz, G. M., Yamashita, T., & Deleyiannis, F. W.-B. (1995). Abnormalities in long latency responses to superior laryngeal nerve stimulation in adductor spasmodic dysphonia. *Annals of Otology, Rhinology and Laryngology*, *104*, 928–935.

Lundy, D. S., Casiano, R. R., Lu, F.-L., & Xue, J. W. (1996). Abnormal soft palate posturing in patients with laryngeal movement disorders. *Journal of Voice, 10,* 348–353.

Maroun, F. B., Jacob, J. C., & Gowing, P. (1970). Dysphonia associated with cortical neoplasms. *Journal of Neurosurgery, 32,* 671–676.

Marsden, C. D. (1976). Dystonia: The spectrum of the disease. In M. D. Yahr (Ed.), *The basal ganglia.* New York: Raven Press.

Marsden, C. D., & Sheehy, M. P. (1982). Spastic dysphonia, Meige disease, and torsion dystonia [letter to the editor]. *Neurology, 32,* 1202.

McCall, G. N. (1974). Spasmodic dysphonia and the stuttering block: Commonalities or possible connections. In L. M. Webster & L. C. Furst (Eds.), *Vocal tract dynamics and dysfluency* (pp. 124–151). New York: Speech and Hearing Institute.

Merson, R. M., & Ginsberg, A. P. (1979). Spasmodic dysphonia: Adductor type. A clinical report of acoustic, aerodynamic and perceptual characteristics. *Laryngoscope, 89,* 129–139.

Merzenich, M. M., & Kaas, J. H. (1980). Principles of organization of sensory-perceptual systems in mammals. *Progress in Psychobiology and Physiological Psychology, 9,* 1–42.

Meyers, R. (1976). Comparative neurology of vocalization and speech: Proof of a dichotomy. *Annals of New York Academy of Science, 280,* 745–757.

Murphy, A. T. (1964). *Functional voice disorders.* Englewood Cliffs, NJ: Prentice Hall.

Murry, T., Cannito, M. P., & Woodson, G. E. (1994). Spasmodic dysphonia: Emotional status and botulinum toxin treatment. *Archives of Otolaryngology—Head and Neck Surgery, 120,* 310–316.

Murry, T., & Woodson, G. E. (1995). Combined modality treatment of adductor spasmodic dysphonia with botulinum toxin and voice therapy. *Journal of Voice, 9,* 460–465.

Naeser, M. A., & Hayward, R. W. (1978). Lesion localization in aphasia with computed tomography and the Boston Diagnostic Aphasia Exam. *Neurology, 28,* 545–551.

Nash, E. A., & Ludlow, C. L. (1996). Laryngeal muscle activity during speech breaks in adductor spasmodic dysphonia. *Laryngoscope, 106*(4), 484–489.

Pechadre, J. C., Larochelle, L., & Poirier, L. J. (1976). Parkinsonian akinesia, rigidity and tremor in the monkey: Histopathological and neuropharmacological study. *Journal of Neurological Science, 28,* 147–157.

Penfield, W., & Roberts, L. (1976). *Speech and brain mechanisms.* New York: Atheneum.

Ravits, J. M., Aronson, A. E., DeSanto, L. W., & Dyck, P. J. (1979). No morphometric abnormality of recurrent laryngeal nerve in spastic dysphonia. *Neurology, 29,* 1376–1382.

Reich, A., & Till, J. (1983). Phonatory and manual reaction times of women with idiopathic spasmodic dysphonia. *Journal of Speech and Hearing Research, 26,* 10–18.

Robe, E., Brumlik, J., & Moore, P. (1960). A study of spastic dysphonia: Neurologic and electroencephalographic abnormalities. *Laryngoscope, 70,* 219–245.

Rosenbek, J. C. (1985). Treating apraxia of speech. In D. F. Johns (Ed.), *Clinical management of neurogenic communicative disorders* (pp. 267–312). Austin, TX: PRO-ED.

Rosenbek, J. C., & LaPointe, L. L. (1985). The dysarthrias: Description, diagnosis, and treatment. In D. F. Johns (Ed.), *Clinical management of neurogenic communicative disorders* (pp. 97–152). Austin, TX: PRO-ED.

Rosenfield, D. B. (1982). The brain and the stutterer. *Journal of Fluency Disorders, 7,* 81–92.

Rosenfield, D. B. (1984). Stuttering. *CRC Critical Reviews in Clinical Neurobiology, 1,* 117–139.

Rosenfield, D. B. (1988). Spasmodic dysphonia. In J. Jankovic & E. Tolosa (Eds.), *Advances in neurology: Vol. 49. Facial dyskinesias* (pp. 317–327). New York: Raven Press.

Ross, E. D. (1980). Localization of the pyramidal tract in the internal capsule by whole brain dissection. *Neurology, 30,* 59–64.

Ross, E. D. (1981). The aprosodias. *Archives of Neurology, 38*, 561–569.

Rowland, L. P. (1982). Diseases of chemical transmission at the nerve-muscle synapse: Myasthenia gravis and related syndromes. In E. R. Kandel & J. H. Schwartz (Eds.), *Principles of neural science* (pp. 132–137). New York: Elsevier/North Holland.

Rubens, A. B., & Kertesz, A. (1983). The localization of lesions in transcortical aphasias. In A. Kertesz (Ed.), *Localization in neuropsychology* (pp. 245–268). New York: Academic Press.

Sapienza, C. M., Murry, T., & Brown, W. S. (1998). Variations in adductor spasmodic dysphonia: Acoustic evidence. *Journal of Voice, 12,* 214–222.

Sapir, S. (1995). Psychogenic spasmodic dysphonia: A case study with expert opinions. *Journal of Voice, 9,* 270–281.

Schaefer, S. D. (1983). Neuropathology of spasmodic dysphonia. *Laryngoscope, 93,* 1183–1204.

Schaefer, S. D., Finitzo-Hieber, T., Gerling, I. J., & Freeman, F. J. (1983). Brainstem conduction abnormalities in spasmodic dysphonia. *Annals of Otology, Rhinology and Laryngology, 92,* 59–63.

Schaefer, S., Freeman, F., Finitzo, T., Close, L., Cannito, M., Ross, E., Reisch, J., & Marivella, K. (1985). Magnetic resonance imaging findings and correlations in spasmodic dysphonia patients. *Annals of Otology, Rhinology and Laryngology, 94,* 595–601.

Schaefer, S. D., Roark, R. M., Watson, B. C., Kondraske, G. V., Freeman, F. J., Butsch, R. W., & Pohl, J. (1992). Multichannel electromyographic observations in spasmodic dysphonia patients and normal control subjects. *Annals of Otology, Rhinology and Laryngology, 101,* 67–75.

Sharbrough, F. W., Stockard, J. J., & Aronson, A. E. (1978). Brainstem auditory evoked responses in spastic dysphonia. *Transactions of the American Neurology Association, 103,* 198–201.

Shipp, T., Izdebski, K., Reed, C., & Morrissey, P. (1985). Intrinsic laryngeal muscle activity in a spastic dysphonia patient. *Journal of Speech and Hearing Disorders, 50,* 54–59.

Siegel, S. (1956). *Nonparametric statistics.* New York: McGraw-Hill.

Spielberger, C. D., Gorusch, R. L., Lushene, R., Vagg, P. R., & Jacobs, G. A. (1983). *Manual for the state: Trait anxiety inventory.* Palo Alto, CA: Consulting Psychologists Press.

Stillman, R. (1980). Auditory evoked potentials. In P. Levinson & C. Sloan (Eds.), *Auditory processing and language* (pp. 19–34). New York: Grune & Stratton.

Sutton, D., Larson, C., & Lindeman, R. C. (1974). Neocortical and limbic lesion effects on primate phonation. *Brain Research, 71,* 61–75.

Tingley, S., & Dromey, C. (2000). Phonatory-articulatory relationship: Do speakers with spasmodic dysphonia show aberrant lip kinematic profiles? *Journal of Medical Speech–Language Pathology, 8,* 249–252.

Traube, L. (1871). Spastische formder nervoeson heiserkeit [A spastic form of nervous hoarseness]. In L. Traube (Ed.), *Gesammeltbeitrage zur pathalogie und physiologic: Vol. 2* (pp. 674–678). Berlin: Hirschwald.

van Pelt, F., Ludlow, C. L., & Smith, P. J. (1994). A comparison of muscle activation patterns in adductor and abductor spasmodic dysphonia. *Annals of Otology, Rhinology and Laryngology, 103,* 192–200.

Vogel, M., & von Cramon, D. (1982). Dysphonia after traumatic midbrain damage: A follow-up study. *Folia Phoniatrica, 34,* 150–159.

Volpe, B. T., Sidtis, J. J., Holzman, J. D., Wilson, D. H., & Gazzaniga, M. S. (1982). Cortical mechanisms involved in praxis: Observations following partial and complete section of the corpus callosum in man. *Neurology, 32,* 645–650.

von Cramon, D. (1981). Traumatic mutism and the subsequent reorganization of speech functions. *Neuropsychologia, 19,* 801–805.

Watson, B. C., Freeman, F. J., Pool, K. D., Finitzo, T., Chapman, S. B., Mendelsohn, D., Devous, M. D., Schaefer, S. D., Close, L. G., & Kondraske, G. V. (1991). Laryngeal reaction time profiles in spasmodic dysphonia: Relationship to cortical electrophysiologic abnormality. *Journal of Speech and Hearing Research, 34,* 269–278.

Watson, B. C., MacIntire, D., Roark, R., & Schaefer, S. D. (1995). Statistical analyses of electromyographic activity in spasmodic dysphonic and normal control subjects. *Journal of Voice, 9,* 3–15.

Watson, B. C., Schaefer, S. D., Freeman, F. J., Dembowski, J., Kondraske, G., & Roark, R. (1991). Statistical analyses of electromyographic activity in spasmodic dysphonic and normal control subjects. *Journal of Voice, 9,* 3–15.

Wertz, R. T. (1985). Neuropathologics of speech and language: An introduction to patient management. In D. F. Johns (Eds.), *Clinical management of neurogenic communicative disorders* (pp. 1–96). Boston: Little, Brown.

Wolfe, V. I., & Bacon, M. (1976). Spectrographic comparison of two types of spastic dysphonia. *Journal of Speech and Hearing Disorders, 41,* 325–332.

Yorkston, K., & Beukelman, D. (1984). *Assessment of intelligibility of dysarthric speech.* Austin, TX: PRO-ED.

Yorkston, K., Beukelman, D., & Bell, K. (1988). *Clinical management of dysarthric speakers.* Austin, TX: PRO-ED.

Zung, W. W. K. (1967). *The measurement of depression.* Milwaukee, WI: Lakeside Laboratories.

Zwitman, D. (1979). Bilateral cord dysfunctions: Adductor type spastic dysphonia. *Journal of Speech and Hearing Disorders, 44,* 373–378.

Chapter 10

Noninvasive Instrumentation in the Treatment of Stuttering

Ben C. Watson and Peter J. Alfonso

Watson and Alfonso present a rationale for and examples of the clinical use of noninvasive instrumentation to identify and document abnormalities of the respiratory and laryngeal systems as well as aerodynamic irregularities that may be associated with stuttering. Illustrative examples demonstrate the potential value of aerodynamic and kinematic monitoring in identifying physiologic events that may disrupt speech fluency and in facilitating training of therapeutic targets designed to reduce the disruptive impact of these events.

1. *Describe clinical and laboratory evidence that abnormalities in control of the respiratory, laryngeal, and articulatory systems may be associated with stuttering.*

2. *Summarize several practical advantages of incorporating noninvasive instrumentation into therapy procedures.*

3. *How can attainment of therapeutic goals be facilitated through use of noninvasive aerodynamic or kinematic biofeedback?*

❋ ❋ ❋

Rationale for an Instrumented Approach

Williams (1957) suggested that stuttering therapy might be more effective if it focused on evaluating and training appropriate component behaviors of speech production rather than trying to eliminate an "insensible 'something' designated by the word 'stuttering'" (p. 395). Adams and Runyan (1981) concluded that the speech of persons who stutter contains numerous physiologic, aerodynamic, and acoustic abnormalities *in the absence* of perceivable stuttering and that to "continue to direct a narrow focus on just stuttering events, speaking rate and accompanying instrumental or accessory responses cannot be supported" (p. 209). Taken together, these positions argue for systematic exploration of the utility of applying noninvasive instrumentation to the task of identifying and treating—through principles of biofeedback—acoustic, physiologic, and/or aerodynamic abnormalities that may disrupt speech fluency.

Use of biofeedback in the treatment of stuttering is not a new concept. Therapy programs in which output from surface electrodes provided biofeedback representing the level of muscle activity are effective in facilitating relaxation and improving fluency (Guitar, 1975; Hasbrouk, 1992; Hanna, Wifling, & McNeil, 1975; Lanyon, 1977; Moore, 1978, 1984). Goebel, Hillis, and Meyer (1985) and Blood (1995) used visual feedback of chest wall displacement, along with an acoustic intensity display, in therapy programs that targeted gentle phonation onsets and continuous air flow to facilitate speech fluency. Webster (1975), Cronk (1986), and Agnello (1980) used visual feedback of the acoustic signal to help persons who stutter achieve therapy targets, such as gradual phonation onset, sustained phonation, and reduced speaking rate. The approach advocated herein builds on the work of Goebel and others, but adds the ability to select real-time visual feedback from the acoustic signal or from a variety of kinematic and aerodynamic signals as determined by the specific needs of the individual client (Dembowski & Watson, 1991; Watson & Dembowski, 1991). This approach parallels that of biofeedback therapy programs for other forms of motor speech disorder that have incorporated a wide range of laboratory instrumentation (Berry & Goshorn, 1983; Caligiuri & Murry, 1983; Netsell & Daniel, 1979; Rubow & Swift, 1985).

The advocacy of instrumented procedures (i.e., employing instruments traditionally found in a speech laboratory) in the clinical practice in fluency therapy traces its origins to the concept of tenuous fluency described by Adams and Runyan (1981). The concept of tenuous fluency encompasses the belief that abnormal or inefficient subperceptual events (i.e., kinematic, aerodynamic, and other physiologic phenomena not easily characterized without the use of instruments) may or may not co-occur with perceivable (overt) dysfluency. This concept is extended to consider that abnormal and/or inefficient subperceptual events may reflect "core" components of the stuttering disorder or "secondary" struggle reactions to other, undefined "core" components. We are concerned with characterizing respiratory, phonatory, and articulatory events as phenomena in themselves, regardless of whether or not apparent departures from normal function are "core" or "secondary" features of the fluency disorder, and regardless of whether or not they occur in the context of perceivable dysfluency. In short, if the underlying physiology is not consistent with the production of fluency, then instrumented biofeedback can be applied to aid in establishing a physiological base that is, at least, more consistent with fluency.

Several additional assumptions guide this approach. First, it is assumed that certain physiologic events precede the perceived moment of stuttering. Consequently, the associated (and, perhaps, predisposing) physiologic event(s) has passed by the time the moment of stuttering is manifested in the speech acoustic signal. Feedback of the acoustic signal alone is inadequate for developing compensatory strategies designed to avoid or minimize the impact of these antecedent events. Secondly, it is assumed that an instrumented approach to stuttering assessment and treatment provides more sensitive and objective measures of the nature, frequency, and magnitude of physiologic events that may interfere with fluent speech than does an approach based only on descriptions of grossly perceivable, overt, molar dysfluency. Finally, it is assumed that detection and display of abnormal and/or inefficient physiologic events by use of appropriate devices can facilitate the development and implementation of therapeutic strategies for reducing the frequency of occurrence and the magnitude of disrupting events, thereby improving fluency.

Noninvasive instrumentation is appropriate for the treatment of deficits presented in a variety of clinical populations (Barlow & Abbs, 1983; Barlow, Cole, & Abbs, 1983; Forrest, Adams, McNeil, & Southwood, 1991). However, our rationale emerged from research findings and clinical observations that associate disruption of respiratory and laryngeal events with stuttering. An important research application of noninvasive instrumentation in the past has been to identify and characterize physiologic events associated with disruptions of speech motor control in persons who stutter. Results of this research suggest meaningful applications of noninvasive instrumentation in clinical settings. Salient characteristics of these disruptions will be reviewed. In so doing, we can begin to develop a rationale for the selection of appropriate clinical targets for therapeutic intervention. We focus on deficits revealed in movements of the respiratory and laryngeal systems, or as reflected in patterns of airflow through the vocal tract. We do not specifically address direct monitoring of movements of the supralaryngeal articulators because this instrumentation is complex, often invasive, and expensive. Aerodynamic measures are less complex and can be used to infer movements of the supralaryngeal articulators.

Some practical issues regarding clinical applications of instrumentation are also discussed. Our discussion of these issues is not intended to provide a "recipe" for therapy, but rather to highlight specific advantages and disadvantages. Illustrative examples of applications of noninvasive instrumentation in the treatment of stuttering highlight the general applicability of the approach. In sum, the goal of this chapter is to present a rationale for and illustrative examples of the clinical use of noninvasive instrumentation to identify, characterize, and modify certain physiologic events that may interfere with the production of fluent speech.

Respiratory Disruptions

During speech production, the respiratory system provides expiratory airflow and adequate driving pressure to support phonation. This function is realized by a rapid prephonatory increase in lung volume, followed by maintenance of a relatively stable positive pressure across a decreasing lung volume. Maintenance of the relatively stable expiratory driving pressure is accomplished by a balance of nonmuscular forces (i.e., gravity) and forces generated by the contraction of inspiratory and expiratory muscles (Zemlin, 1988). Clinical observations of respiratory abnormalities in stutterers include reduced tidal volume, marked delay between onset of expiratory airflow and onset of phonation, continued speech production at inappropriately low lung volumes, interruption of speech by inspiratory gasps, and speech production on inspiration (van Riper, 1982). These observations suggest that certain stutterers have difficulty coordinating the respiratory events necessary for fluent speech.

Laboratory investigations of respiratory kinematics in stutterers are consistent with clinical observations. For example, Travis (1927) reported both prolonged duration of inspiration relative to duration of expiration and tremor of the abdominal wall. Travis also described pronounced antagonistic movements of the thoracic and abdominal walls. However, oppositional movements of the rib cage and abdominal wall have been observed in normal speakers and reflect the relatively independent contributions of changes in volumes of the thoracic and abdominal cavities to changes in total lung volume (Hixon, Goldman, & Mead, 1973). Oppositional movements alone do not necessarily reflect abnormal respiratory kinematics. Of greater import is the *net* displacement of the entire chest wall. Murray (1932) observed (a) increased variability in both amplitude and duration of inspiratory and expiratory gestures in stutterers relative to nonstutterers during a silent reading task and (b) greater variability in amplitude of stutterers' inspiratory gestures during silent reading than during resting breathing. Nonstutterers showed an opposite pattern; they reduced variability of the inspiratory gesture during the reading task. Stutterers were apparently unable to meet the increased demands for stability of the respiratory system during the reading task. Seth (1934) described respiratory disruption during a stuttering block as characterized by halting, interruption, sudden release, and complete reversal of expiration and inspiration.

The respiratory deficits just noted were observed during the moment of stuttering by all the researchers mentioned except for Murray (1932). Consequently, it is not clear to what extent these phenomena precipitate the stuttering episode or reflect stutterers' attempts to restore control over speech production. Watson and Alfonso (1986) observed several respiratory deficits before and during stutterers' voice onset for production of a perceptually fluent vowel. First, severe stutterers, unlike a mild stutterer and nonstutterers, rarely used prephonatory preparation intervals to execute gestures associated with inflation of the respiratory system. Indeed, analysis of kinematic signals in terms of changes in relative lung volume revealed that significantly lower prephonatory increases in lung volume were achieved by severe stutterers than by the mild stutterer and nonstutterers. Severe stutterers also frequently began respiratory compression (expiratory gestures) for phonation onset well before the moment of vocal fold closure. This pattern suggests inefficient management of the expiratory airstream. Analysis of kinematic data in terms of relative changes in lung volume supports this finding. Severe stutterers showed significantly greater reduction in lung volume before voice onset than did the mild stutterer or nonstutterers. That is, severe stutterers waste pulmonic air before voicing begins.

Taken together, clinical observations and laboratory findings reveal that disruption of normal respiratory function is associated with, and may precipitate, the moment of stuttering. In addition, this review indicates several targets for a therapy program designed to minimize contributions of respiratory disruption to stuttering. For example, therapy might focus on (a) ensuring adequate prephonatory inflation; (b) establishing smooth, uninterrupted expiratory airflow; (c) eliminating attempts to phonate on inspiration; and (d) facilitating efficient airflow management through appropriate organization of respiratory and laryngeal events.

Laryngeal Disruptions

Wingate (1967) noted that smooth transitions between voiced and voiceless segments are critical for fluent speech. An important dimension of laryngeal control during connected speech is rapid onset and offset of vocal fold vibration for the production of contiguous voiced and voiceless segments. Vocal fold vibration is a consequence of the interaction of myoelastic properties of the vocal folds and aerodynamic phenomena (transglottal pressure) (van den Berg, 1958). Consequently, rapid voice onset and offset adjustments require precise regulation of vocal fold tension, medial compression, and position, as well as transglottal pressure (Stevens, 1977). Clinical observations reveal a relation between stuttering and disrupted control of voice onset and offset. Stuttering is more likely to occur in association with voice onset for the initial word of an utterance or phrase (Brown, 1938).

Stutterers' ability to initiate and terminate voicing has been investigated using a variety of experimental paradigms. Some investigations compare frequency of stuttering and/or amount of adaptation on passages containing only voiced segments with passages containing both voiced and voiceless segments (Adams & Reis, 1971, 1974; Adams, Riemenschneider, Metz, & Conture, 1975; Hutchinson & Brown, 1978; Manning & Coufal, 1976). Most of these studies report greater frequency of stuttering and less adaptation for passages containing both voiced and voiceless segments. The interpretation most often applied to this finding is that increased frequency of stuttering, failure to adapt, or both reflects the stutterers' difficulty in executing rapid voice onsets and offsets.

Insights into physiologic events associated with stutterers' apparent difficulty controlling both the laryngeal system and interactions between the respiratory and laryngeal systems derive from studies of laryngeal and respiratory physiology during stutterers' perceptually fluent or dysfluent speech. Conture, McCall, and Brewer (1977), based on fiber-optic filming of the vocal folds during connected speech, describe abnormal positioning of the vocal folds associated with moments of dysfluency. Freeman and Ushijima (1978), recording electromyographic (EMG) signals from intrinsic laryngeal muscles, observed abnormal levels of activity and inappropriate reciprocity in antagonistic laryngeal muscles during dysfluencies. Shapiro (1980) observed similar EMG abnormalities.

Using electroglottography (EGG), Borden, Baer, and Kenney (1985) investigated laryngeal events associated with stutterers' production of perceptually fluent and dysfluent words in a counting task. The EGG signal provides information regarding changes in vocal fold contact area during a cycle of vibration. Analysis of the rise time of the amplitude envelope of the EGG signal yields information corresponding to abruptness of voice onset. Abrupt onset of voicing is associated with a rapid increase in the amplitude of the EGG signal.

Borden et al. (1985) reported several differences between EGG patterns produced by normal speakers and those associated with stutterers' dysfluencies or attempts to recover from a dysfluency. Following a dysfluency, stutterers often demonstrated a gradually increasing amplitude envelope of the EGG signal. This pattern was interpreted as a physiological correlate of perceptual judgments of easy onset of voicing. Indeed, the authors suggest that the EGG signal provides a more reliable index of easy onset than the acoustic signal because it is independent of filtering effects imposed by the supralaryngeal vocal tract. With respect to details of the vibratory cycle after a dysfluency, severe stutterers in particular demonstrated a pattern of rapid glottal opening and an open period of relatively short duration. Borden et al. (1985) suggest that this pattern reflects stiff vocal folds. This suggestion was confirmed by acoustic analyses that showed an increase in fundamental frequency when voicing was initiated after a block. The positive relationship between increases in vocal fold stiffness and increases in fundamental frequency in chest register is well documented (Gay, Hirose, Strome, & Sawashima, 1972). Two aspects of the Borden et al. study are particularly relevant to our goal. First, this study demonstrates that the EGG signal can be a reliable indicator of easy onset of voicing and that changes in the fine structure of the EGG waveform can be used to infer vocal fold stiffness. Second, EGG biofeedback may facilitate establishment of fluency-enhancing techniques (clinical targets) and aid in reducing certain laryngeal abnormalities (such as increased vocal fold tension). These changes may in turn facilitate fluency.

Laboratory studies also reveal stutterers' deficits in organizing laryngeal and respiratory events. Watson and Alfonso (1987) reported abnormal delays in stutterers' onsets of vocal fold abduction and adduction gestures as well as evidence of inappropriate timing of vocal fold closure and onset of expiratory airflow associated with perceptually fluent onsets of isolated, voiced vowels. Peters and Hulstijn (1987), based on an analysis of patterns of prephonatory increases in subglottal pressure, also reported evidence of abnormalities in temporal coordination of respiratory and laryngeal events.

Taken together, studies of laryngeal function in stutterers highlight two classes of abnormality: (a) inappropriate levels of muscle activity that may be associated with increased vocal fold tension and laryngeal resistance to airflow and (b) temporal disruption in the organization of laryngeal opening and closing gestures with respiratory inspiratory and expiratory gestures.

Aerodynamic Disruptions

The consequence of appropriate organization of respiratory and laryngeal events leading to voice onset is the generation of expiratory airflow that is modulated at the level of the larynx and then further modulated and filtered by altering the shape of supralaryngeal cavities. Hutchinson (1974) recorded airflow through the vocal tract and intraoral air pressure in an attempt to characterize aerodynamic patterns produced by stutterers and to relate these patterns to dysfluency type. He identified seven distinct aerodynamic patterns associated with stuttering. Although many of these patterns primarily reflected abnormalities in intraoral air pressure, some of them were characterized by abnormal patterns of airflow. The most frequently observed dysfluency—the *abbreviated vowel element*—was associated with abrupt cessation of airflow. *Prolonged silent blocks* were also associated with an absence of airflow. Hutchinson was able to simulate abnormal patterns associated with abbreviated vowel element dysfluencies by executing a glottal stop gesture. The pattern associated with prolonged silent blocks was simulated by maintaining stable articulatory posturing while not varying respiratory driving force. Further, he reported the sensation being locked into a single articulatory gesture during the simulation. This sensation parallels that reported by stutterers during tonic blocks. The suggestion that specific dysfluency types may be associated with specific aerodynamic patterns implies that monitoring airflow during the production of phonetically specified utterances may be informative in identifying salient aerodynamic characteristics of a stutterer's dysfluencies and may aid in developing a strategy for modifying these patterns to facilitate fluency.

Intraoral air pressure increases during the production of obstruent consonants. Pressure is higher behind oral closure associated with a stop consonant than behind the oral constriction associated with a fricative consonant. That is, the magnitude of the increase in intraoral pressure is related to degree of vocal tract constriction. If respiratory driving pressure is held constant, it is also true that intraoral pressure will increase for stop consonants as the duration of articulatory closure increases. A feature of dysfluency frequently described in the clinical literature is the *hard articulatory contact*. Hard contacts are described as prolonged articulatory closures and are likely associated with excessive increases in intraoral pressure. Consequently, providing visual feedback of the magnitude of intraoral air pressure may aid in reducing the frequency and impact of hard articulatory contacts.

In sum, ample evidence derived from both clinical observation and laboratory investigation permits the conclusion that abnormalities in respiratory and laryngeal function and in patterns of airflow through the vocal tract are associated with stutterers' dysfluencies. Furthermore, the evidence suggests that specific aspects of respiratory and laryngeal function may be amenable to modification by providing clients with biofeedback of kinematic (respiratory and laryngeal) and aerodynamic signals.

Clinical Applications: Advantages and Disadvantages

The next step in the development of our approach for therapeutic application of noninvasive instrumentation is to consider advantages and disadvantages of an instrumented biofeedback approach as an adjunct to traditional approaches. The important consideration here is adjunct. We do not advocate replacing current therapy techniques with a purely instrumented approach. Nor do we assume that all persons who stutter will necessarily benefit from the instrumented feedback, just as not all persons who stutter benefit from the existing behavioral therapies. Instrumental techniques described herein should be considered as yet another tool clinicians can use to develop therapy goals and implement therapy procedures specifically suited to the needs of individual clients. Those caveats notwithstanding, advantages of an instrumented approach include objectivity, quantifiability, real-time visual feedback, and long-term data storage.

Objectivity and quantification are valuable in identification and treatment of deficits associated with any speech disorder. The ability to identify salient characteristics of physiologic deficits, in particular, should aid in focusing therapeutic efforts to match deficits presented by the client. For example, Watson (1983) found that delays in voice onset for a group of stutterers were associated with two different patterns of respiratory-laryngeal organization. The first pattern was characterized by significant delays between the moment of vocal fold closure and the onset of respiratory compression gestures. The second pattern was characterized by significant delays between the onset of compression gestures and the moment of vocal fold closure. Idiosyncratic differences in temporal sequencing of prephonatory respiratory and laryngeal events may be important in developing appropriate therapeutic strategies. Although therapy emphasizing easy voice onset (i.e., onset of exhalation before the moment of vocal fold closure) may be appropriate for a stutterer who demonstrates the first pattern described above, this approach may not be appropriate for a stutterer who demonstrates the second pattern. Instead, this client may benefit from therapy designed to minimize the delay between onset of respiratory compression (i.e., exhalation) and the moment of vocal fold closure.

Apart from the ability to clearly characterize physiologic deficits contributing to an individual's stuttering behavior, quantification of deficits has practical benefits for both clinician and client. In the current atmosphere of increased demands for accountability in health care professions, documentation of both baseline abnormality and changes over time is important in establishing a clear strategy and goals for therapy and in documenting the benefits of therapy.

Real-time visual feedback of kinematic signals is advantageous for other reasons. First, clients can more clearly appreciate the nature of physiologic disruptions and what steps can be taken in therapy to minimize the impact of these disruptions on speech production. This appreciation can increase motivation. Second, the process of minimizing these disruptions is facilitated because both client and clinician receive immediate feedback regarding the success of attempted strategies. Immediate feedback assists the *clinician* in tailoring therapy strategies and assessing their viability. Immediate feedback assists the *client* in mastering these strategies and incorporating them into a new pattern of speech production.

Advantages of long-term data storage parallel those of quantification. The ability to maintain records of baseline measures and periodic assessments of progress during therapy is important in meeting demands for accountability and for providing clients with a tangible chronology of their progress. In addition, periodic review of these data may aid clinicians in identifying the strategies most successful in facilitating improvement for subgroups of clients. This process will in turn assist in the development of more efficient and effective treatment programs.

Disadvantages of an instrumented approach include the obvious (but steadily decreasing) expense of the instrumentation (including monitoring, display, and storage devices), clients' negative reactions to the instrumentation, and generalization difficulties. We recognize that perhaps most clinicians do not have access to the types of instruments we describe. However, we are confident that the technology will become increasingly available and affordable. In the near term, expensive instrumentation is not essential for monitoring certain respiratory and phonatory events. Continuity of exhalation during speech is easily monitored by having the client place a hand on the abdominal wall.

Another limitation arises from the client's interaction with the equipment. Borden and Watson (1987), in their discussion of laboratory use of instrumentation, noted that attaching monitoring devices to subjects seems to produce a decline in the frequency and severity of stuttering behaviors. There is a novelty effect associated with the instrumentation. Clients who experience this effect may not produce overt stuttering behaviors or covert, physiologic phenomena associated with tenuous fluency. As a consequence, certain subtle physiologic deficits may not be identified. However, repeated experience with the instrumentation will lessen the novelty effect. Indeed, in the short term, the novelty effect can be used to great advantage to document physiologic events associated with the "artificial fluency."

Weaning clients from the instruments may be as problematic as weaning clients from delayed auditory feedback. One approach to facilitate generalization is to deprive clients of the visual feedback so as to encourage increased proprioceptive and auditory monitoring. Of course, traditional out-of-clinic transfer exercises are just as important to instrumented therapy as they are to more traditional therapies.

Instrumentation

The following discussion describes noninvasive instrumentation currently used in many speech science laboratories. These devices may be effectively integrated into a biofeedback therapy program designed to address the aspects of respiratory and laryngeal function described earlier. With respect to respiratory kinematics, research and clinical observations suggest that stutterers may benefit from feedback regarding coordination of thoracic and abdominal movements during inspiration and expiration as well as coordination between movements of the respiratory and laryngeal systems. Respiratory kinematics can be evaluated by monitoring changes in the chest wall in several dimensions. For example, Hixon et al. (1973) describe a magnetometer system for monitoring changes in rib cage diameter and in abdominal diameter. Baken (1977) describes a mercury strain-gauge system for monitoring changes in the anterior hemicircumference of the thorax and abdomen. Finally Cohn, Watson, Weisshaut, Stott, and Sackner (1975) describe an inductance coil plethysmograph system (Respitrace®) for monitoring changes in the total circumference of the rib cage and abdomen. Although differing with respect to specific principles of operation, all three systems provide information regarding coordination between the thoracic and abdominal cavities. All three systems can also be calibrated to reveal changes in relative or absolute lung volume.

This review of laryngeal behavior associated with stuttering suggests that certain stutterers may benefit from increased control over several aspects of vocal fold vibration, as well as coordination of laryngeal and respiratory movements. Noninvasive monitoring of vocal fold activity may be achieved using electroglottography (for a comprehensive review of electroglottography, see Childers & Krishnamurthy, 1985). An electroglottograph (EGG) is sensitive to changes in vocal fold contact area. Briefly, this device detects changes in resistance to a high-frequency, low-amplitude signal transmitted between surface electrodes attached superficially to the laminae of the thyroid cartilage (Baken, 1987). Increased vocal fold contact decreases resistance, whereas decreased contact increases resistance.

Resistance changes detected by the EGG reflect changes in contact area during each cycle of vibration. Most commercially available EGG devices provide separate output of both a slow signal (associated with postural adjustments) and a fast signal (associated with vibratory details). However, caution must be used in inferring abductory and adductory vocal fold movements because the slow signal is affected by changes in structures remote from the glottis (e.g., jaw movements or tension in strap muscles), as well as vertical displacement of the larynx. For this reason, the most widely accepted use of EGG is to infer vibratory characteristics of the vocal folds.

Baken (1987) summarizes the primary threats to the validity of the EGG signal. In general, many of these threats are reduced if the electrodes are secured in place at the level of the vocal folds and head movements are kept to a minimum. An additional method of minimizing movement artifacts in the fast EGG signal is to route the EGG output signal through a high-pass filter. This eliminates low-frequency components associated with head movements, contraction of strap muscles, and abduction and adduction movements.

In addition to monitoring respiratory and laryngeal kinematics, treatment of dysfluencies may be aided by use of aerodynamic measures. Airflow is monitored by channeling the expiratory airstream through a flow transducer coupled to a face mask (Baken, 1987). Several transducers (e.g., pneumotachograph) differentiate between egressive and ingressive airflow (Baken, 1987). Thus, an airflow monitoring system may serve as an important supplement to feedback of respiratory kinematic information to document continuity of expiratory airflow during speech. Air pressure increases within the oral cavity during the production of obstruent consonants. Intraoral pressure can be measured by placing a small diameter catheter in the mouth and attaching the distal end of the catheter to a pressure transducer. Elevated intraoral pressure may be observed during prolonged closure of stop consonants and may be indicative of hard articulatory contact.

Clinical Examples

The following examples illustrate the potential value of noninvasive instrumentation in the identification and treatment of respiratory, laryngeal, and aerodynamic abnormalities in persons who stutter. Respiratory kinematics were transduced using a Respitrace inductance plethysmograph (Ambulatory Monitoring Systems, Inc.). In one example, a single inductance coil was placed around the subject's chest wall and provided a gross measure of respiratory system displacement. This is a nonstandard recording procedure as the use of one inductance coil does not permit unambiguous identification of the unique contributions of rib cage and abdominal wall displacements to changes in lung volume during respiration. In many clinical applications, display of separate rib cage and abdominal displacements, or of their net (i.e., summed) displacement, will be more informative. Laryngeal kinematics were transduced using an electroglottograph (Synchrovoice, Inc. or Kay Elemetrics, Inc.). Electroglottographic signals may be routed through a high-pass filter to eliminate low-frequency artifact originating from vertical movements of the larynx. The low-pass filtered signal reveals more clearly changes in vocal fold contact area associated with vocal fold vibration. Oral airflow was detected using a Rothenberg mask (Rothenberg, 1977). Intraoral pressure was detected by attaching an intraoral catheter to a differential pressure transducer in the Rothenberg mask (Rothenberg, 1977).

Identification of Physiological Events That May Compromise Fluency

Respiratory

The first two examples illustrate use of the Respitrace signal to identify respiratory phenomena that may be incompatible with fluent speech. Figure 10.1 shows the acoustic and single Respitrace signals (displacement of the chest wall) recorded from a stutterer during production of a multi-unit syllable repetition. Upward deflection of the Respitrace signal corresponds to expansion of the respiratory system during inhalation, and downward deflection corresponds to compression of the system during exhalation. The dashed line shows the shape

Treatment of Stuttering • 391

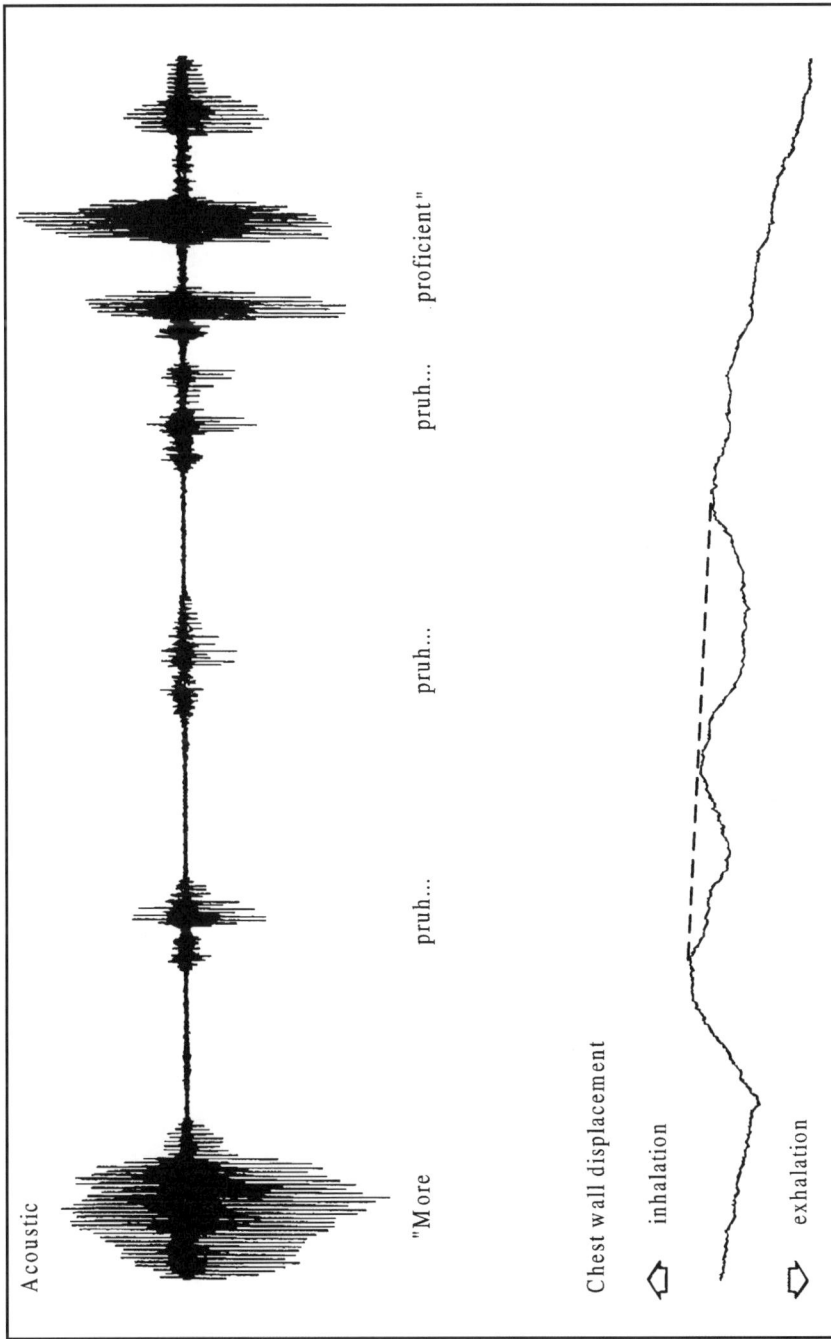

Figure 10.1. Simultaneous acoustic and respiratory kinematic signals recorded during a perceptually dysfluent production of the word *proficient*. The dashed line indicates the predicted, normal respiratory pattern. Repetitions are associated with inspiratory chest wall gestures that interrupt exhalation.

of the predicted, normal respiratory compression gesture for this utterance. In this example, the dysfluency is associated with a disruption in the normal continuity of the compression gesture. Specifically, each repetition unit is preceded by an expansion of the chest wall that interrupts the compression gesture. A goal for therapy should be to stabilize the continuity of expiratory gestures during speech so as to provide appropriate respiratory support for fluency.

Figure 10.2 shows acoustic and summed Respitrace signals (i.e., combined contributions of rib cage and abdominal wall displacements to overall chest wall displacement) recorded during a picture description task. This utterance is 24.5 seconds in duration and contains 27 syllables. There are 10 disfluencies, the longest of which is 2.6 seconds in duration. There are five inspiratory gestures during the utterance, not counting the pre-utterance inhalation. The last inhalation occurs in the middle of the word *toothpaste* (at arrow). This client shows too many inhalations for an utterance of this length, inhalations at linguistically inappropriate times, and inhalations often associated with perceived dysfluencies. A goal for therapy should be to maintain continuous respiratory compression in order to facilitate continuous expiratory air flow and reduce the number of intrusive inhalations.

Laryngeal

The next examples illustrate application of the EGG signal to identify physiological disruption associated with stuttering. Figure 10.3 shows EGG and acoustic signals recorded from an adult male stutterer during two readings of a short passage. Upward deflection of the EGG signal corresponds to increasing vocal fold contact area, or the closing phase of a vibratory cycle. Downward deflection corresponds to decreasing vocal fold contact area, or the opening phase of the cycle. The top set of traces was recorded as the subject produced a double-unit repetition of the initial /s/ in *sister*. The EGG signal shows no changes in vocal fold contact area during the initial period of frication seen in the acoustic signal (corresponding to the initial /s/). Next, the EGG signal shows multiple changes in vocal fold contact area that appear as low-amplitude pulses in the acoustic signal (indicated by the arrow). Finally, the EGG signal shows no change in vocal fold contact area during production of the second /s/. This was perceived as a voiceless repetition, and the acoustic signal shows no obvious evidence of voicing during the repe-

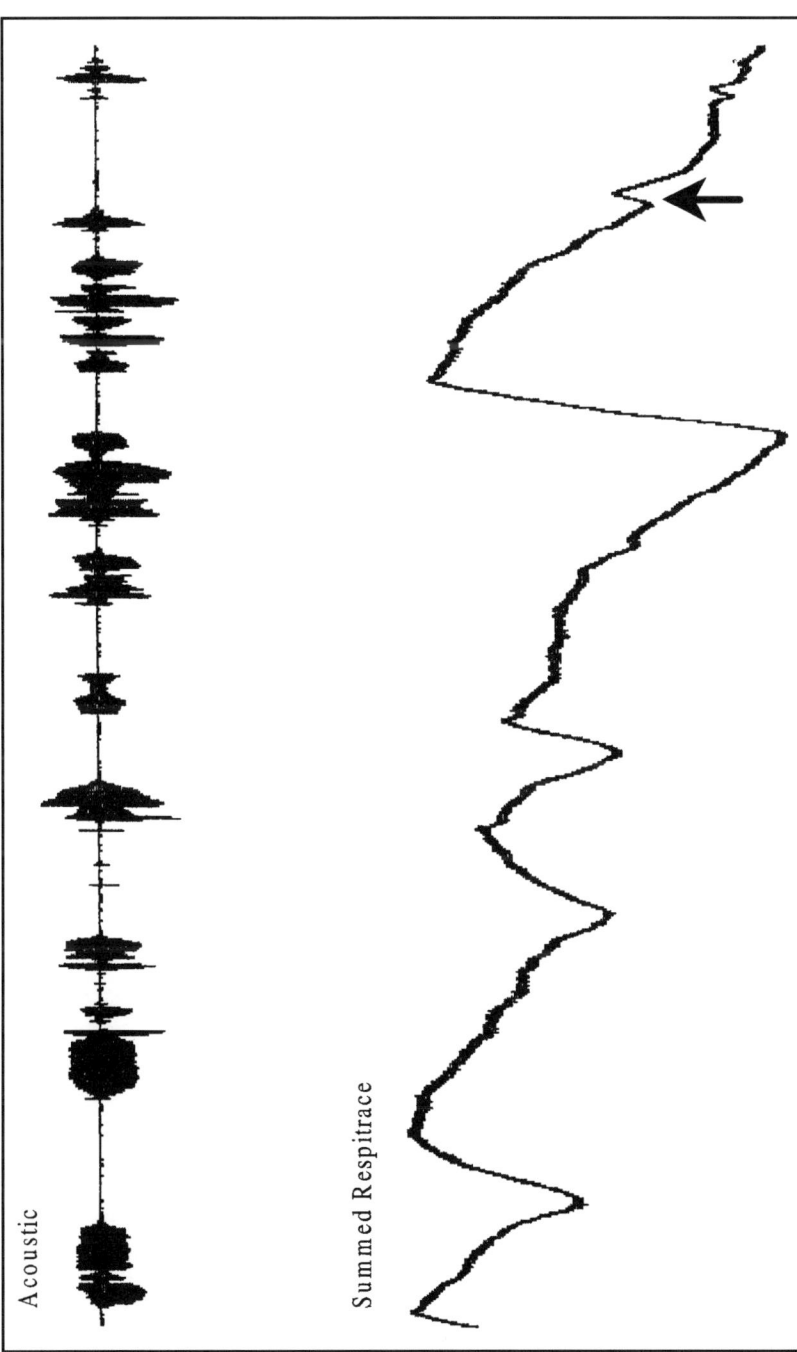

Figure 10.2. Simultaneous acoustic and summed Respitrace signals recorded during a picture description task. Inspiratory gestures occurred at linguistically inappropriate times and were associated with perceived dysfluencies. The arrow indicates an inhalation in the middle of the word *toothpaste*. *Note.* From "Instrumentation in the Evaluation and Modification of Speech Motor Control During Stuttering Therapy," (pp. 503–511), by B. C. Watson and J. Dembowski, in *Speech Motor Control and Stuttering*, edited by H. F. M. Peters, W. Hulstijn, and C. W. Starkweather, 1991, Amsterdam: Excerpta Medica. Copyright 1991 by Elsevier Science. Reprinted with permission.

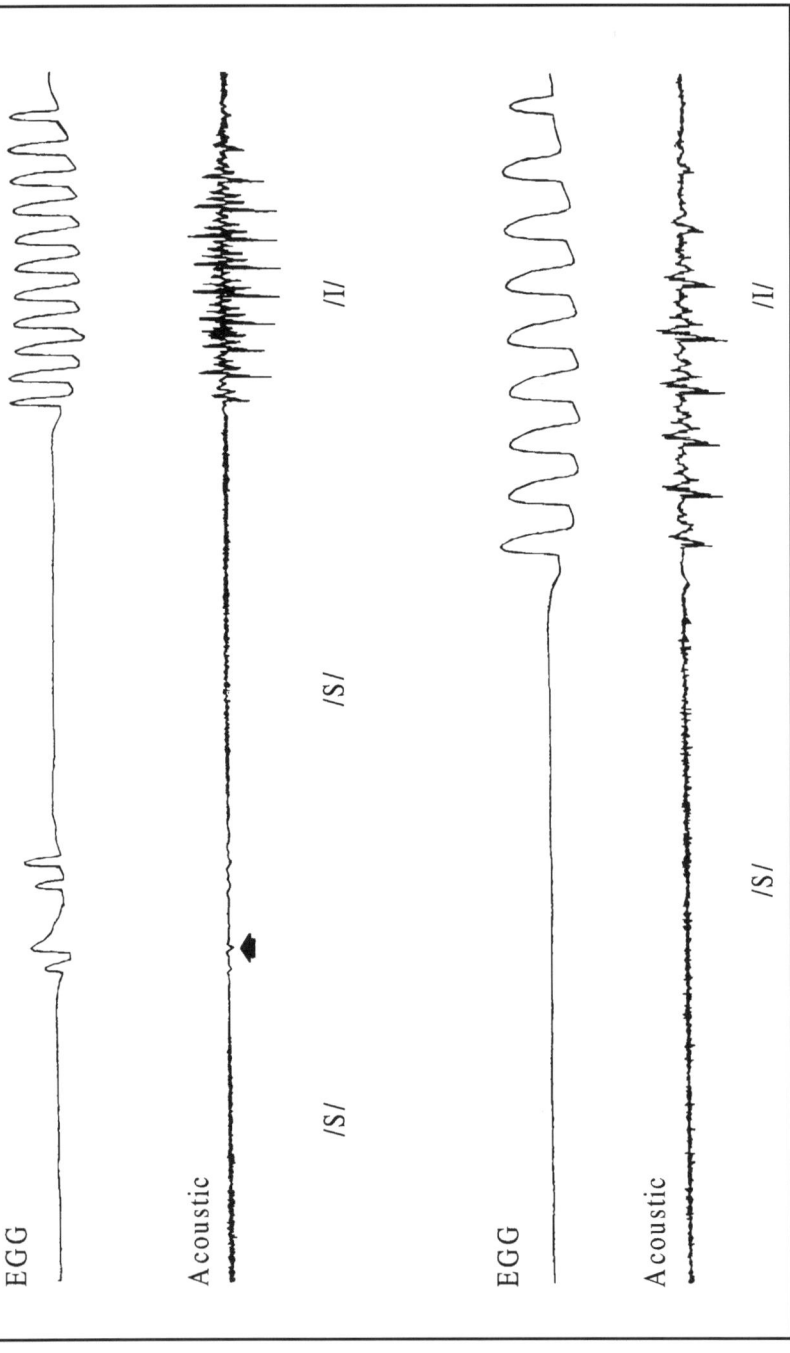

Figure 10.3. Simultaneous acoustic and electroglottographic (EGG) signals recorded during perceptually dysfluent (top) and fluent (bottom) productions of the word *sister*. EGG signal reveals that repetition of the voiceless /s/ in the dysfluent production is associated with inappropriate laryngeal activity that is absent from the fluent production. *Note.* From "Instrumentation in the Evaluation and Modification of Speech Motor Control During Stuttering Therapy," (pp. 503–511), by B. C. Watson and J. Dembowski, in *Speech Motor Control and Stuttering*, edited by H. F. M. Peters, W. Hulstijn, and C. W. Starkweather, 1991, Amsterdam: Excerpta Medica. Copyright 1991 by Elsevier Science. Reprinted with permission.

tition. The EGG signal, however, shows multiple changes in vocal fold contact area during the dysfluency. These changes in contact area appear to represent an aborted attempt to initiate voicing. That is, this perceptually voiceless dysfluency is associated with inappropriate laryngeal activity.

The bottom set of traces was recorded during this client's perceptually fluent production of the same material. Note that the EGG signal shows no changes in vocal fold contact area during fluent production of the voiceless /s/. Apparent differences in fundamental frequency for the vowel /i/ in the two acoustic traces reflect the different time scales used in this figure and do not appear to be related to differences in the fluency of these productions. In this example, the EGG signal permitted identification of an inaudible laryngeal abnormality associated with a voiceless dysfluency.

Inappropriate laryngeal activity during voiceless dysfluencies has been documented in laboratory settings through analysis of electromyographic signals (Freeman & Ushijima, 1978) and fiber-optic films (Conture et al., 1977). This example illustrates, however, that inappropriately organized laryngeal-articulatory activity can be documented in the clinical setting using noninvasive instrumentation. With this information, therapy can focus on eliminating inappropriate laryngeal gestures by instructing the subject to keep the EGG signal at a "neutral," or baseline, position during voiceless consonants.

Figure 10.4 shows acoustic and EGG signals recorded during the transition from the word *either* to the word *a* excerpted from a picture description task. This is an all-voiced phonetic context and should permit uninterrupted vibration. However, the EGG signal shows discontinuities in the amplitude and periodicity of the vocal fold contact at the transition from /r/ to /a/. This observation led to the therapy goal of maintaining continuous amplitude and periodicity of vocal fold contact across voiced-to-voiced phonetic transitions (that is, continuous voicing).

Aerodynamic

The final example illustrates use of aerodynamic information to characterize disruptions in speech fluency. Figure 10.5 shows acoustic and oral airflow signals during a reading of the utterance, "Tommy, pour a kilo of purple paint with care over the tall tapered carton." Negative

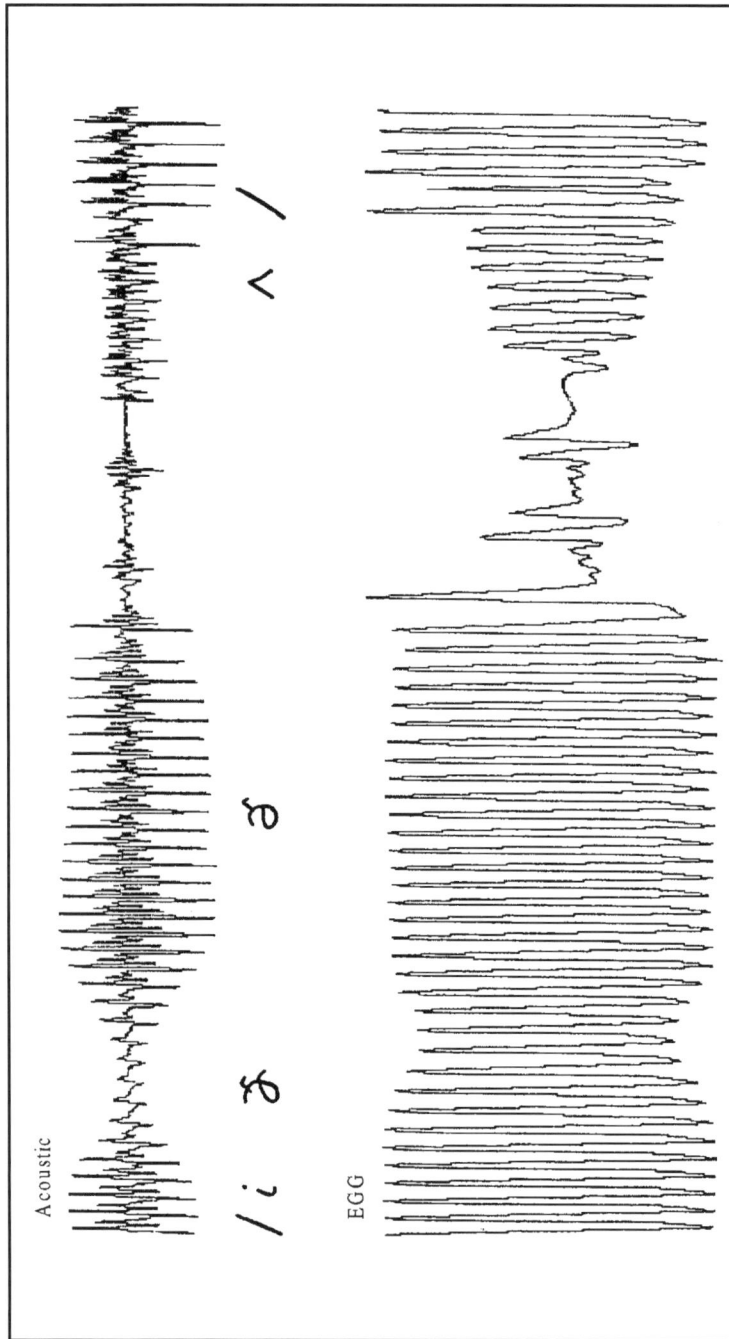

Figure 10.4. Simultaneous acoustic and EGG signals recorded during the transition from *either* to *a* excerpted from a picture description task. The EGG signal shows discontinuities in the amplitude and periodicity of vocal fold vibration during the voiced-to-voiced transition. *Note.* From "Instrumentation in the Evaluation and Modification of Speech Motor Control During Stuttering Therapy," (pp. 503–511), by B. C. Watson and J. Dembowski, in *Speech Motor Control and Stuttering*, edited by H. F. M. Peters, W. Hulstijn, and C. W. Starkweather, 1991, Amsterdam: Excerpta Medica. Copyright 1991 by Elsevier Science. Reprinted with permission.

Treatment of Stuttering 397

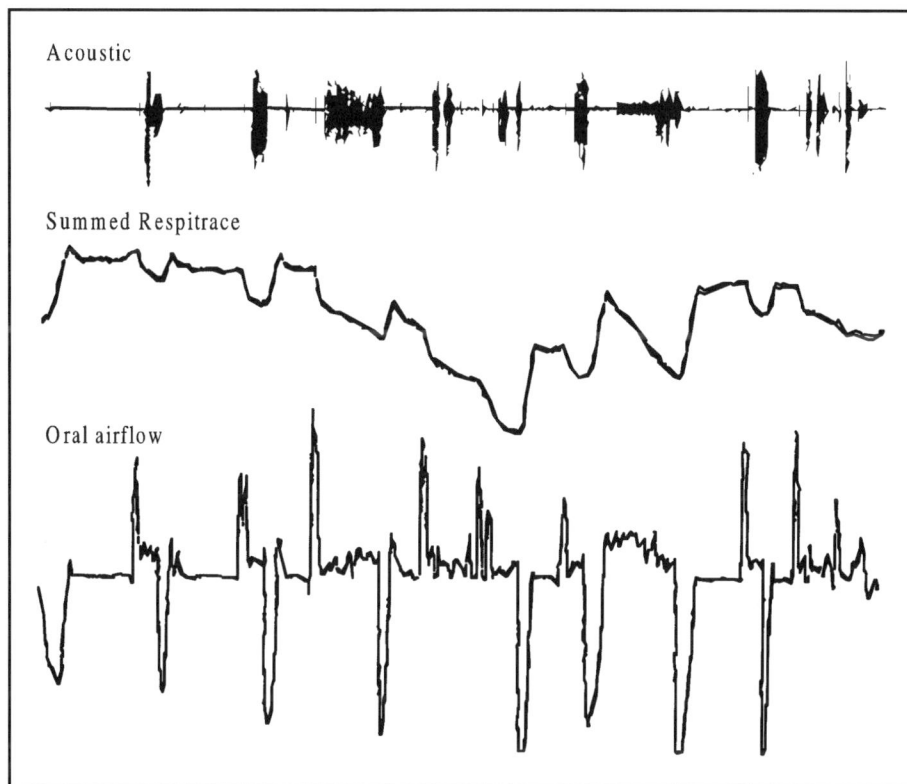

Figure 10.5. Simultaneous acoustic, summed Respitrace®, and oral airflow signals recorded during a reading of the sentence, "Tommy, pour a kilo of purple paint with care over the tall tapered carton." Respitrace® and airflow signals show inappropriate inhalations that interrupt speech fluency. High peak airflow associated with stop consonant releases may be indicative of hard articulatory contacts during consonant closure. *Note.* From "Instrumentation in the Evaluation and Modification of Speech Motor Control During Stuttering Therapy" (pp. 503–511), by B. C. Watson and J. Dembowski, in *Speech Motor Control and Stuttering*, edited by H. F. M. Peters, W. Hulstijn, and C. W. Starkweather, 1991, Amsterdam: Excerpta Medica. Copyright 1991 by Elsevier Science. Reprinted with permission.

peaks in the airflow signal represent inhalation, and positive peaks represent exhalation. The airflow signal shows seven inhalations during this utterance, not counting the pre-utterance inhalation. High peak airflows were associated with releases of the stop consonants. Although an admittedly indirect measure, these high peak flows may reflect hard articulatory contacts during stop consonant closure. As noted earlier, prolonged, or hard, articulatory contacts presumably result in high intraoral pressure and, thus, high peak airflow at consonant release. Average peak airflow for this client ranged from 2.5 to 5.3 standard deviations above the normal mean values for CV syllables reported by Isshiki and Ringel (1964). Goals for therapy were to maintain continuous expiratory airflow during an utterance and to achieve "light" articulatory contacts.

The preceding examples show that certain characteristics of the physiologic disruption associated with a stutterer's dysfluency can be identified when noninvasive instrumentation is used in conjunction with traditional acoustic recordings. These examples also illustrate that much of the clinically valuable information associated with dysfluencies may occur during silent periods. That is, aerodynamic and kinematic records can be important in obtaining sufficiently detailed descriptions of dysfluent speech for the design of appropriate therapy goals.

Treatment of Physiological Events That May Compromise Fluency

The next examples demonstrate therapeutic applications of real-time visual biofeedback. In the various biofeedback protocols (Alamed Corp., Vega, TX) illustrated, the clinician defines the task to be performed, the therapy goal, and the performance criterion. We begin with an example of feedback of the summed Respitrace signal. Recall that analysis of this signal can reveal inappropriate inhalations during speech that disrupt the continuity of respiratory support for speech. Figure 10.6 shows an example of the use of real-time visual feedback of the summed Respitrace signal to establish continuous exhalation during a picture description task. The clinician-defined performance criterion was zero reversals in the exhalation gesture (i.e., no inhalation gestures) during the task. The analysis software detected three reversals during this utterance. All textual information displayed at the top of the

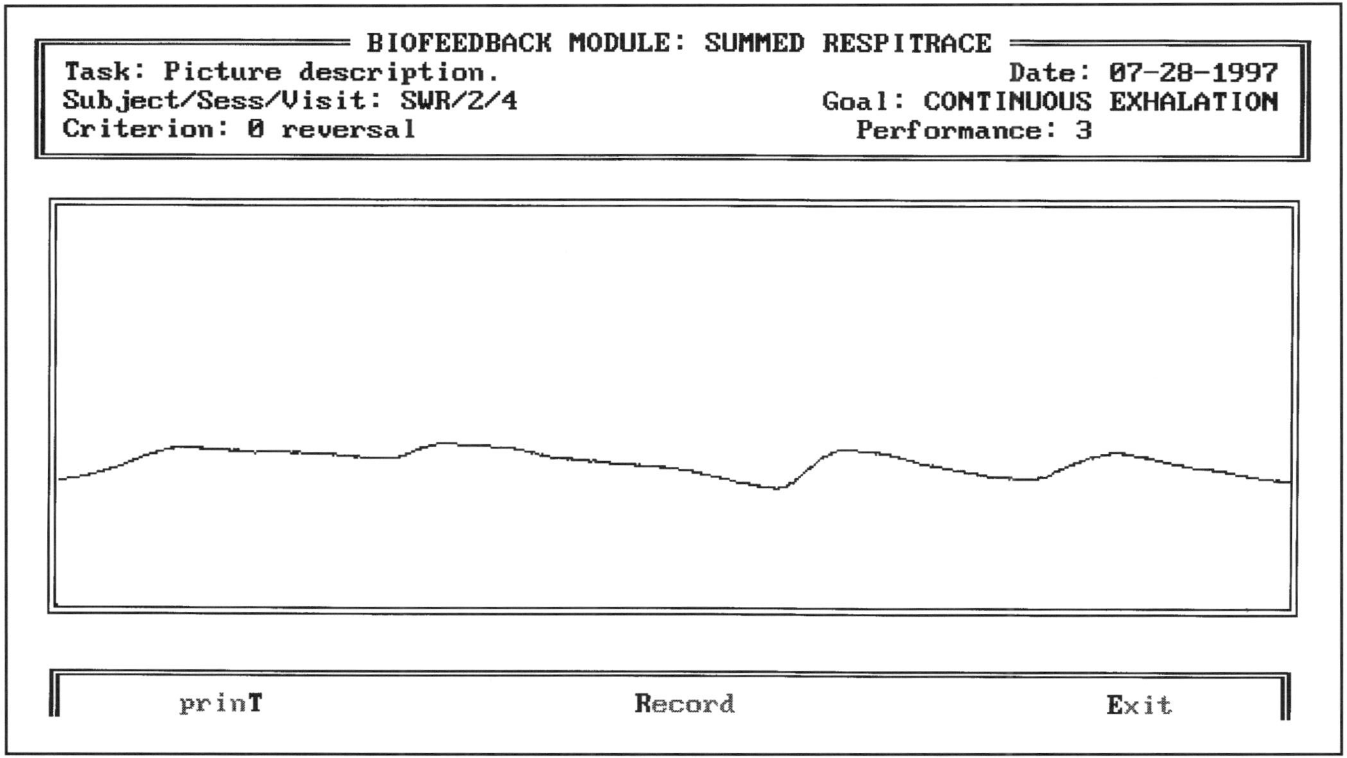

Figure 10.6. Summed Respitrace signal recorded and displayed in real time during a picture description task. Automated evaluation of the trial revealed that performance did not meet the criterion of zero reversals in exhalation during the utterance. Subject, date, task, performance criterion, and actual performance data are stored in an archival text file for documentation of therapeutic progress.

figure can be stored to a text file on the host computer to maintain an archival record of the client's progress in therapy. Once the clinician has established the tasks, goals, and performance criteria and has worked with the client to ensure their understanding of the task, a client can practice unassisted. Later, the clinician can check the permanent record of the client's performance and change the task, goals, and/or performance criterion as needed.

Figure 10.7 shows the EGG signal and acoustic signals recorded as a stutterer used continuous voicing during a picture description task. Recall that analysis of the EGG signal shown in Figure 10.4 revealed discontinuities in the periodicity and amplitude of the EGG signal that reflected instability in the control of voicing. The EGG trace shown in Figure 10.7 is continuous with respect to period and amplitude characteristics for this all-voiced utterance. This figure also illustrates the advantage of using EGG signals as evidence of continuous voicing. Note that amplitude of the acoustic signal is markedly reduced during the period of oral constriction for /ð/ in *either*, whereas the EGG signal displays a constant amplitude, because it is not subjected to damping properties of the vocal tract. The EGG signal provides a more stable and reliable index of the vocal fold vibration than does the acoustic signal.

Figure 10.7 also illustrates a procedural issue regarding visual feedback of kinematic signals. At issue is the duration of the window over which immediate feedback is provided. The temporal window in Figure 10.7 is 400 msec. This window may be too long to provide meaningful feedback to the client. Figure 10.8 shows the effect of decreasing the duration of the window to 168 msec. Clients report little difficulty monitoring the EGG signal when the window is relatively short (i.e., 50–100 msec). However, longer windows (i.e., 2–5 sec) are useful in providing clearer feedback of the continuity of voicing over longer utterances and for slower moving, respiratory kinematic signals.

Figure 10.9 illustrates use of a longer display window for feedback of the EGG signal and the advantage of being able to quantify a client's performance during therapy. The goal was to produce the all-voiced sentence, "Eels ooze all over" using continuous phonation for at least 80% of the utterance. This utterance, constructed of all-voiced continuants, could be produced with 100% continuous phonation. The magnitude of the disruption is quantified by computing the percentage of the utterance for which voicing occurred (i.e., the ratio of the total

(text continues on p. 404)

Treatment of Stuttering 401

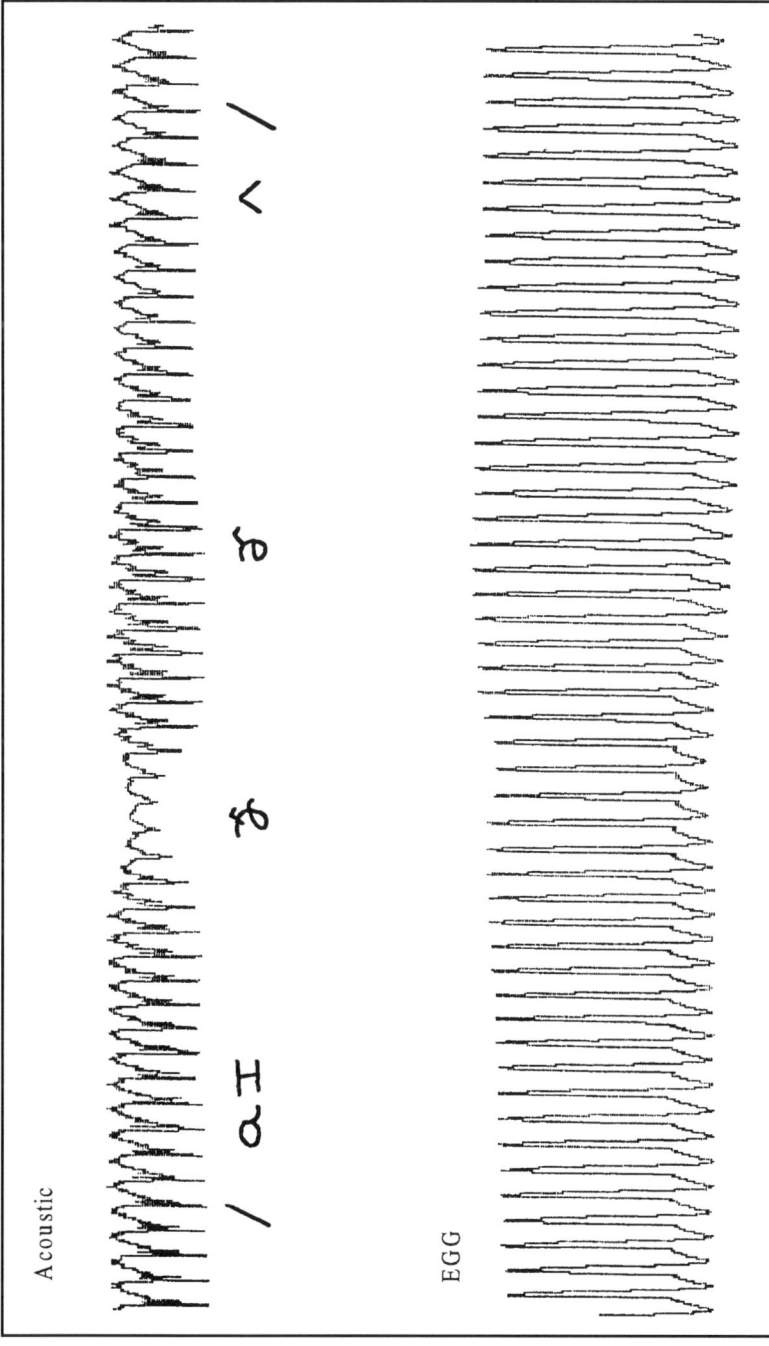

Figure 10.7. Simultaneous acoustic and EGG signals recorded during the perceptually fluent transition from *either* to *a*. The EGG signal shows consistent amplitude and periodicity of vocal fold vibration during the voiced-to-voiced transition.

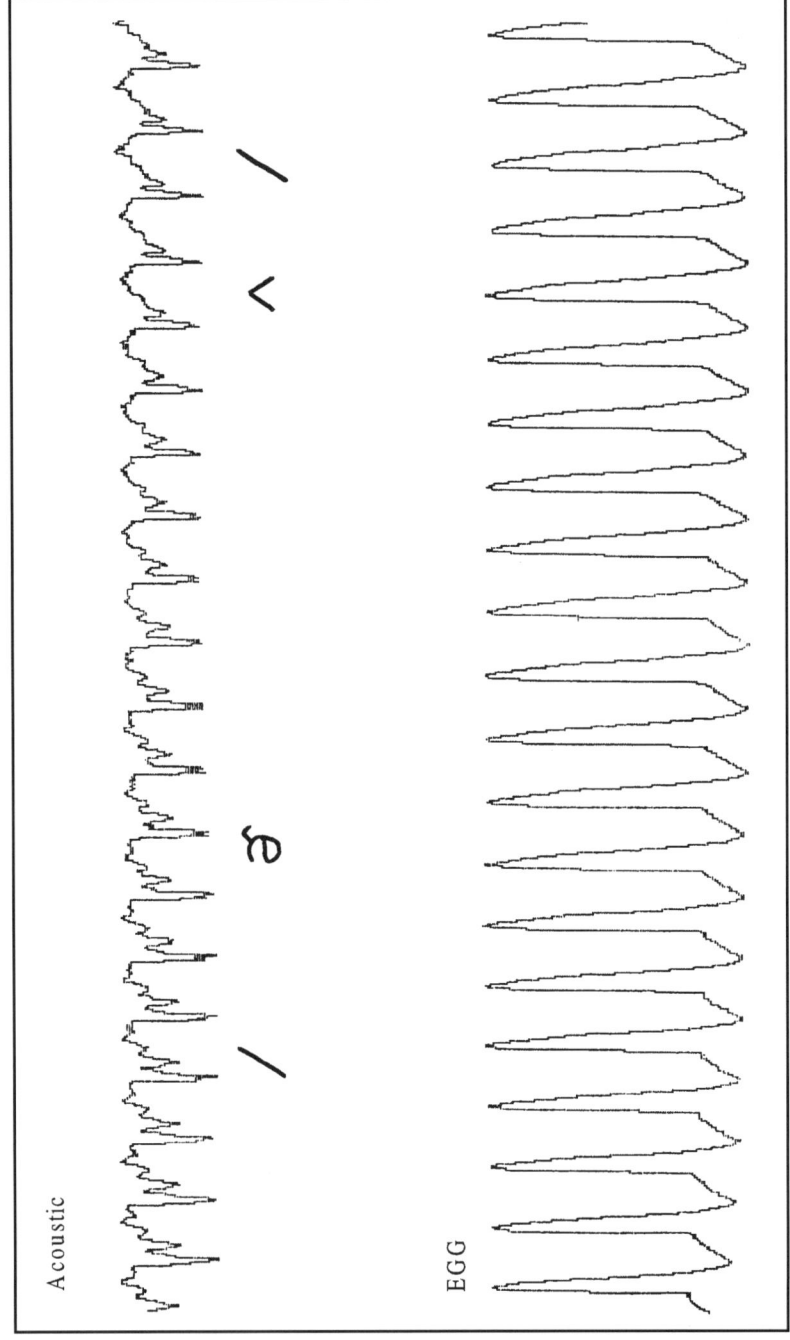

Figure 10.8. Expanded view of the acoustic and EGG signals shown in Figure 10.7. The shorter time window shown here facilitates client use of visual biofeedback under certain circumstances.

Treatment of Stuttering 403

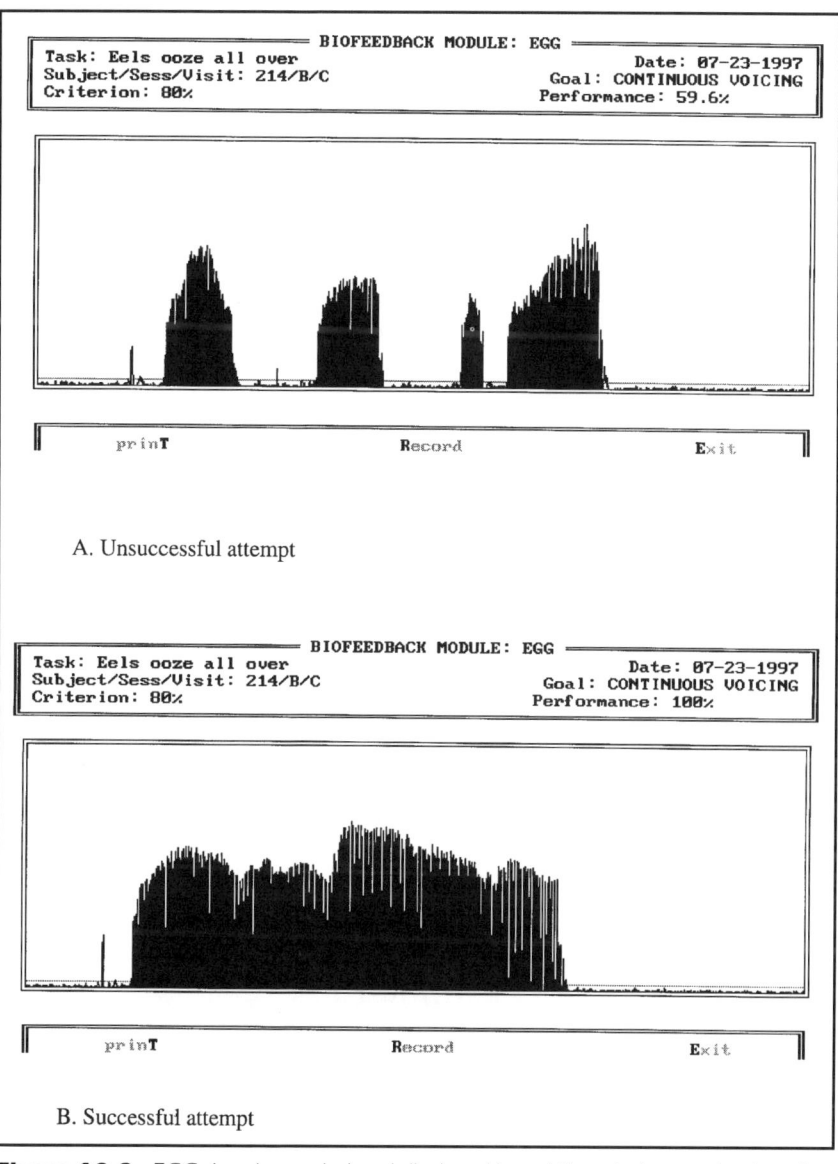

Figure 10.9. EGG signal recorded and displayed in real time during production of an all-voiced sentence. The goal was to produce voicing for at least 80% of the sentence. Figure 10.9A shows an unsuccessful attempt (59.6% voicing). Figure 10.9B shows a successful attempt. Subject, date, task, performance criterion, and actual performance data are stored in an archival text file for documentation of therapeutic progress.

duration of all-voiced intervals to the duration of the entire utterance). Figure 10.9a illustrates an unsuccessful attempt. Note the clear discontinuities in the EGG signal. The analysis software detected voicing during 59.6% of the utterance. Figure 10.9b shows a successful attempt that achieved 100% voicing during the utterance. All of the textual information shown in this figure can be saved to a text file to create an archival record of this client's progress in therapy.

Figure 10.10 illustrates visual feedback and quantitative analysis of the intraoral air pressure signal to reduce the frequency and magnitude of hard articulatory contacts. The goal was to produce the utterance, "Peter Piper picked a peck of pickled peppers" while producing intraoral pressure peaks during the bilabial stop consonant of 50 mm H20 or less. Miller and Daniloff (1977) reported average intraoral air pressure for normally fluent male speakers of 55 mm H20 (range: 42 to 67 mm H20). Figure 10.10a shows that none of the pressure peaks met the 50 mm H20 criterion. Note as well that the second pressure peak shows aerodynamic evidence of a two-unit repetition of the /p/ in *Piper*. Figure 10.10b shows that the 50 mm H20 criterion was met for 87.5% (7 of 8) of the peaks.

These examples illustrate how real-time visual biofeedback can be combined with quantitative analyses to provide a permanent record of a client's performance over the course of therapy. Further, they illustrate how a therapy program can be implemented in such a way that the client can practice therapy exercises independently while the clinician can stay informed of the client's progress and change the therapy program accordingly.

Summary

We have presented a rationale for incorporating noninvasive kinematic and aerodynamic instrumentation in the clinical setting to facilitate identification and treatment of deficits associated with the disordered speech motor control seen in persons who stutter. Several examples illustrated the potential benefits of this approach. To date, we have used visual feedback from noninvasive instrumentation, particularly the EGG signal, to treat vocal symptoms associated with stuttering, spasmodic dysphonia, ideopathic unilateral vocal fold paralysis, and head trauma. Our observations and clients' comments support the

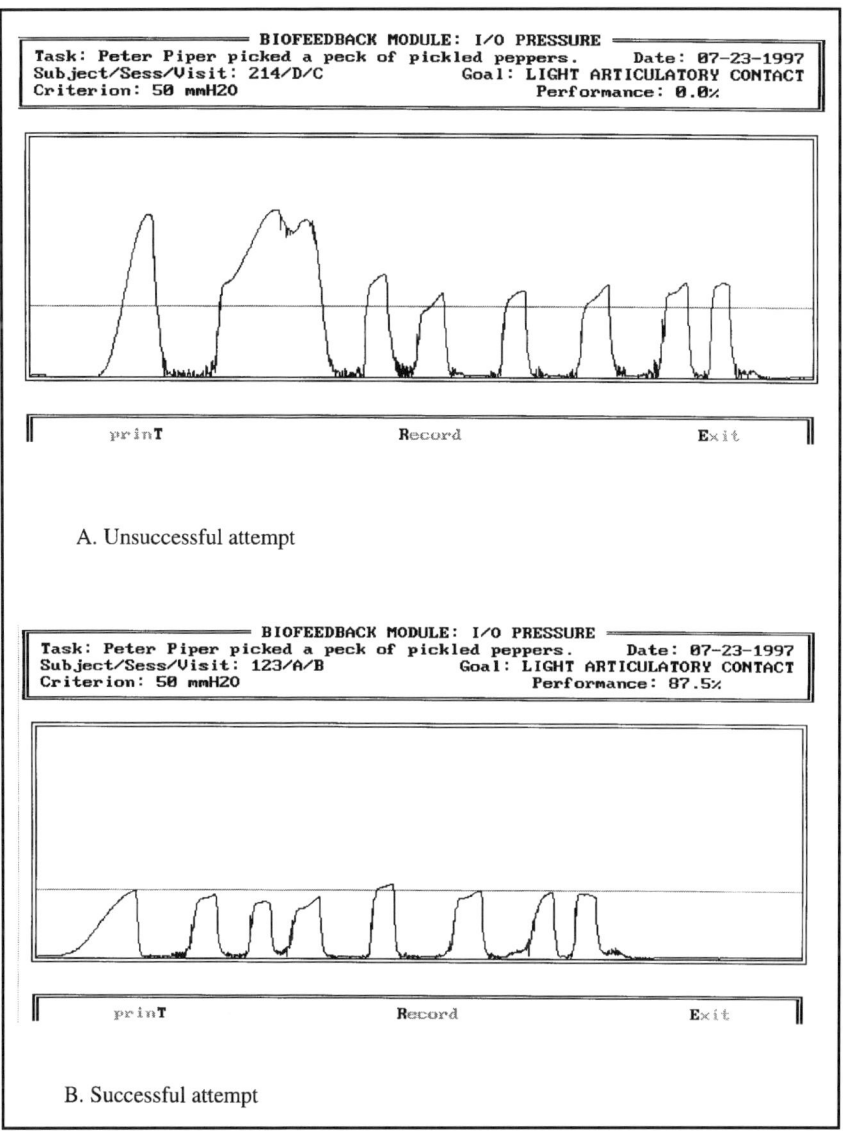

Figure 10.10. Oral air pressure signal recorded and displayed in real time during production of a sentence. The goal was to produce stop consonants using light articulatory contacts so as to generate intraoral air pressures of less than 50 mm H20. Figure 10.10A shows an unsuccessful attempt. Figure 10.10B shows that 87.5% (7 of 8) of the pressure peaks met the 50 mm H20 performance criterion. Subject, date, task, performance criterion, and actual performance data are stored in an archival text file for documentation of therapeutic progress.

potential value of clinical applications of this instrumentation. Insights gained into the nature of physiologic events associated with perceptual symptoms facilitate the development of relevant therapeutic goals. Realization of therapy goals is also facilitated. Clients can "see" the underlying abnormal physiological event and the appropriate event. This information helps clients to understand the rationale for therapy techniques. Finally, the visual display can be explained to clients at different levels of cognitive complexity. Simple descriptions of shapes and patterns may be appropriate for many children and cognitively impaired adults, whereas more complex descriptions of the physiologic mechanisms that underlie the display may be appropriate for other clients. We have successfully applied this approach with a cognitively impaired, post-head-trauma patient and believe programs can be easily modified for use with young children.

Finally, clinical application of noninvasive instrumentation will facilitate an exchange of ideas and information between clinics and laboratories. Often the most interesting and rewarding research has its origins in clinical observations. Increasing the precision and sensitivity of these observations will, no doubt, generate important research questions. On the other hand, clinicians often correctly question the clinical applicability of laboratory findings. A shared technology between clinic and laboratory can facilitate the transfer of laboratory findings to clinical efforts. In the final analysis, the more meaningful interaction between clinic and laboratory permitted by a shared technology will benefit client, clinician, and researcher.

References

Adams, M. R., & Reis, R. (1971). The influence of the onset of phonation on the frequency of stuttering. *Journal of Speech and Hearing Research, 14,* 639–644.

Adams, M. R., & Reis, R. (1974). Influence of the onset of phonation on the frequency of stuttering: A replication and re-evaluation. *Journal of Speech and Hearing Research, 17,* 748–755.

Adams, M. R., Riemenschneider, S., Metz, D., & Conture, E. (1975). Voice onset and articulatory constriction requirements in a speech segment and their relation to the amount of stuttering adaptation. *Journal of Fluency Disorders, 1,* 24–31.

Adams, M. R., & Runyan, C. (1981). Stuttering and fluency: Exclusive events or points on a continuum? *Journal of Fluency Disorders, 6,* 197–218.

Agnello, J. (1980). A comprehensive computer program for facilitating fluency in stutterers. In H. F. M. Peters & W. Hulstijn (Eds.), *Speech motor dynamics in stuttering* (pp. 307–311). New York: Springer-Verlag.

Baken, R. J. (1977). Estimation of lung volume change from torso hemicircumpherences. *Journal of Speech and Hearing Research, 50,* 808–812.

Baken, R. J. (1987). *Clinical measurement of speech and voice.* Boston: College-Hill.

Barlow, S., & Abbs, J. (1983). Force transducers for the evaluation of labial, lingual, and mandibular motor impairments. *Journal of Speech and Hearing Research, 26,* 616–621.

Barlow, S., Cole, K., & Abbs, J. (1983). A new head-mounted lip-jaw movement transduction system for the study of motor speech disorders. *Journal of Speech and Hearing Research, 26,* 283–288.

Berry, W., & Goshorn, E. (1983). Immediate visual feedback in the treatment of ataxic dysarthria: A case study. In W. Berry (Ed.), *Clinical dysarthria* (pp. 253–265). San Diego: College-Hill.

Blood, G. (1995). A behavioral-cognitive therapy program for adults who stutter; computers and counseling. *Journal of Fluency Disorders, 28,* 165–180.

Borden, G. J., Baer, T., & Kenney, M. K. (1985). Onset of voicing in stuttered and fluent utterances. *Journal of Speech and Hearing Research, 58,* 363–372.

Borden, G. J., & Watson, B. C. (1987). Methodological aspects of simultaneous measurements: Limitations and possibilities. In H. F. M. Peters & W. Hulstijn (Eds.), *Speech motor dynamics in stuttering* (pp. 83–96). New York: Springer-Verlag.

Brown, S. (1938). The theoretical importance of certain factors influencing the incidence of stuttering. *Journal of Speech Disorders, 3,* 223–230.

Caligiuri, M., & Murry, T. (1983). The use of visual feedback to enhance prosodic control in dysarthria. In W. Berry (Ed.), *Clinical dysarthria*. San Diego: College-Hill.

Childers, D. G., & Krishnamurthy, A. K. (1985). A critical review of electroglottography. *CRC Critical Reviews in Biomedical Engineering*, *52*, 131–161.

Cohn, M., Watson, H., Weisshaut, R., Stott, F., & Sackner, M. (1975). A transducer for non-invasive monitoring of respiration. In F. Stott, E. Rafferty, P. Sleigh, & L. Gouldring (Eds.), *Proceedings of the second international symposium on ambulatory monitoring* (pp. 119–128). New York: Academic Press.

Conture, E. G., McCall, G. N., & Brewer, D. W. (1977). Laryngeal behavior during stuttering. *Journal of Speech and Hearing Research*, *50*, 661–668.

Cronk, C. (1986). *A clinical application of microcomputer technology in the treatment of stuttering*. Paper presented at the American Speech-Language-Hearing Foundation Computer Conference, Orlando, FL.

Dembowski, J., & Watson, B. C. (1991). An instrumented method for assessment and remediation of stuttering: A single-subject case study. *Journal of Fluency Disorders*, *16*, 241–273.

Forrest, K., Adams, S., McNeil, M., & Southwood, H. (1991). Kinematic, electromyographic, and perceptual evaluation of speech apraxia, conduction aphasia, ataxic dysarthria and normal speech production. In C. Moore, K. Yorkston, & D. Beukelman (Eds.), *Dysarthria and apraxia of speech: Perspectives on management*. Baltimore: Brookes.

Freeman, F. J., & Ushijima, T. (1978). Laryngeal muscle activity during stuttering. *Journal of Speech and Hearing Research*, *25*, 533–562.

Gay, T., Hirose, H., Strome, M., & Sawashima, M. (1972). Electromyography of the intrinsic laryngeal muscles during phonation. *Annals of Otolaryngology*, *85*, 401–409.

Goebel, M., Hillis, J., & Meyer, R. (1985). *The relationship between speech fluency and certain patterns of speech flow*. Paper presented at the national convention of the American Speech-Language-Hearing Association, Washington, DC.

Guitar, B. (1975). Reduction of stuttering frequency using analog electromyographic feedback. *Journal of Speech and Hearing Research, 18,* 672–685.

Hanna, R., Wilfling, F., & McNeil, B. (1975). A biofeedback treatment for stuttering. *Journal of Speech and Hearing Disorders, 40,* 270–273.

Hasbrouk, J. (1992). FAMC intensive stuttering treatment program: Ten years of implementation. *Military Medicine, 157,* 244–247.

Hixon, T. J., Goldman, M. D., & Mead, J. (1973). Kinematics of the chest wall during speech production: Volume displacement of the rib cage, abdomen, and lung. *Journal of Speech and Hearing Research, 16,* 78–115.

Hutchinson, J. M. (1974). Aerodynamic patterns of stuttered speech. In L. M. Webster & L. C. Furst (Eds.), *Vocal tract dynamics and dysfluency: Proceedings of the First Annual Hayes Martin Conference on Vocal Tract Dynamics* (pp. 71–123). New York: Speech and Hearing Institute.

Hutchinson, J. M., & Brown, D. (1978). The Adams and Reis observations revisited. *Journal of Fluency Disorders, 3,* 149–154.

Isshiki, N., & Ringel, R. (1964). Airflow during the production of selected consonants. *Journal of Speech and Hearing Research, 7,* 233–244.

Lanyon, R. (1977). Effects of biofeedback based relaxation on stuttering during reading and spontaneous speech. *Journal of Clinical and Consulting Psychology, 45,* 860–866.

Manning, W. H., & Coufal, K. J. (1976). The frequency of dysfluencies during phonatory transitions in stuttered and nonstuttered speech. *Journal of Communication Disorders, 9,* 75–81.

Miller, C. J., & Daniloff, R. (1977). Aerodynamics of stops in continuous speech. *Journal of Phonetics, 5,* 351–360.

Moore, W. (1978). Some effects of progressively lowering electromyographic levels with feedback procedures on the frequency of stuttered verbal behaviors. *Journal of Fluency Disorders, 3,* 127–138.

Moore, W. (1984). Hemispheric alpha asymmetries during an electromyographic biofeedback procedure for stuttering: A single subject experimental design. *Journal of Fluency Disorders, 14,* 323–350.

Murray, E. (1932). Disintegration of breathing and eye movements in stutterers during silent reading and reasoning. *Psychological Monographs, 43,* 218–275.

Netsell, R., & Daniel, B. (1979). Dysarthria in adults: Physiologic approach to rehabilitation. *Archives of Physical Medicine and Rehabilitation, 60,* 502–508.

Peters, H. F. M., & Hulstijn, W. (1987). Aerodynamic functions in fluent speech utterances of stutterers and nonstutterers in different speech conditions. In H. F. M. Peters & W. Hulstijn (Eds.), *Speech motor dynamics in stuttering* (pp. 229–244). New York: Springer-Verlag.

Rothenberg, M. (1977). Measurement of airflow in speech. *Journal of Speech and Hearing Research, 20,* 155–176.

Rubow, R., & Swift, E. (1985). A microcomputer-based wearable biofeedback device to improve transfer of treatment in parkinsonian dysarthria. *Journal of Speech and Hearing Disorders, 50,* 178–185.

Seth, G. (1934). An experimental study of the control of the mechanism of speech, and in particular of that of respiration, in stuttering subjects. *British Journal of Psychology, 54,* 375–388.

Shapiro, A. (1980). An electromyographic analysis of the fluent and dysfluent utterances of several types of stutterers. *Journal of Fluency Disorders, 5,* 203–231.

Stevens, K. N. (1977). Physics of laryngeal behavior and larynx modes. *Phonetica, 34,* 264–279.

Travis, L. E. (1927). Studies in stuttering. Part 1: Disintegration of the breathing movements during stuttering. *Archives of Neurology and Psychiatry, 18,* 673–690.

van den Berg, J. (1958). Myoelastic-aerodynamic theory of voice production. *Journal of Speech and Hearing Research, 1,* 227–244.

Van Riper, C. (1982). *The nature of stuttering* (2nd ed.). Englewood Cliffs, NJ: Prentice Hall.

Watson, B. C. (1983). *Simultaneous fiberoptic, transillumination, respitrace, and acoustic analysis of laryngeal reaction time in stutterers and nonstutterers.* Unpublished doctoral dissertation, University of Connecticut, Storrs.

Watson, B. C., & Alfonso, P. J. (1986, November). *Prephonatory respiratory activity in stutterers and nonstutterers.* Paper presented at the annual convention of the American Speech-Language-Hearing Association, Detroit, MI.

Watson, B. C., & Alfonso, P. J. (1987). Physiological bases of acoustic LRT in nonstutterers, mild stutterers, and severe stutterers. *Journal of Speech and Hearing Research, 30,* 434–447.

Watson, B. C., & Dembowski, J. (1991). Instrumentation in the evaluation and modification of speech motor control during stuttering therapy. In H. F. M. Peters, W. Hulstijn, & C. W. Starkweather (Eds.), *Speech motor control and stuttering* (pp. 503–512). Amsterdam: Excerpta Medica.

Webster, R. (1975). *Precision fluency shaping program: Clinicians program guide.* Roanoke, VA: Hollins Communications Development Corp.

Williams, D. (1957). A point of view about "stuttering." *Journal of Speech and Hearing Disorders, 22,* 390–397.

Wingate, M. E. (1967). Stuttering as a phonetic transition defect. *Journal of Speech and Hearing Disorders, 34,* 107–108.

Zemlin, W. (1988). *Speech and hearing science: Anatomy and physiology* (3rd ed.). Englewood Cliffs, NJ: Prentice Hall.

Chapter 11

Developmental Apraxia of Speech: Advances in Theory and Practice

Thomas P. Marquardt, Harvey M. Sussman, and Barbara L. Davis

Marquardt, Sussman, and Davis provide a neural dysmorphology theory to account for developmental apraxia of speech and suggest that the model may be helpful in explaining characteristics of the disorder. They note that differential diagnosis of the disorder is difficult due to overlapping characteristics with phonological disorders and specific language impairment, and treatment for the disorder is based primarily on approaches for children with articulation disorders.

1. Why should a theory of neural dysmorphology be employed to account for developmental apraxia of speech? What evidence is available to support this theory?

2. What group of behavioral characteristics serves as the basis for differential diagnosis of the disorder? Is any single feature sufficient for diagnosis?

3. Describe the range of therapy approaches available for treatment of developmental apraxia of speech. Why must treatment for each child be highly individualized?

�֍   �֍   ✯

Developmental apraxia of speech (DAS) is a neurologically based disorder in the ability to carry out coordinative movements of the speech production apparatus for articulation in the absence of impaired neuromuscular function. Although the disorder has been described in similar terms for more than 30 years, there is little agreement about the neurological basis for observed deficits, the characteristics of the disorder, or the most appropriate assessment and treatment regimens. This lack of harmony arises from two major paradoxes. First, neurological insult and maturational dysfunction are the only proposed etiologies, but available data are not sufficient to establish clear evidence of neurological deficits. Evidence for a neurological basis then rests on behavioral symptomatology, and the argument for brain dysfunction becomes tautological: Developmental apraxia is ascribed to neurological origins on the basis of apractic symptoms, which in turn are assigned to the brain dysfunction. Obviously, there will be little advance in our understanding of DAS without a coherent neurological construct to account for the disorder. This will be one of the tasks of this chapter.

A second paradox is the apparent lack of unique characteristics of the disorder. If there are no unique characteristics or valued treatment regimens specific to the disorder, then it can be argued that classification of children with DAS lacks diagnostic legitimacy (Guyette & Diedrich, 1981). This appears to be more a question of definition than of fact. When classifying adult neurological disorders, it has long been the practice to categorize on the basis of the relative prominence of impaired behaviors such as naming, fluency, or agrammatism. No effort is made to search for behaviors that can be found only in a single type of aphasia or dysarthria. For example, adults with anterior left hemisphere damage typically have reduced fluency, but this feature is also common to global aphasia. Individuals with aphasia are uniquely assigned to aphasia categories on the basis of additional criteria, such as the relative involvement of auditory comprehension, naming, and so on. This syndrome-based framework for classification, when applied to DAS children, has produced nomenclature problems because the symptoms used for assignment to a diagnostic category have not been consistently applied. It is not surprising then that the disorder has been variously labeled developmental verbal dyspraxia, childhood verbal dyspraxia, apraxic dysarthria, cortical dysarthria, and developmental apraxia of speech. A second task of this chapter will be to outline, as carefully as possible, the primary features of developmental apraxia and the assessment procedures viewed as requirements for reliable diagnosis.

Given the lack of neurological evidence to establish etiology and the inconsistency of selection criteria for diagnostic assignment, the large variation in approaches to treatment is fully expected. This chapter will review and evaluate the relative merits of these regimens, not because we are able to calibrate their worth fully, but because their relative effectiveness is a necessary prerequisite to the selection of an approach.

Theoretical and Clinical Perspectives

The wide array of speech and language deficits characteristic of DAS has made it difficult to develop a cohesive theoretical construct for describing the disorder. Theoretical accounts of DAS extend from those based on deficits in underlying representations of phonemes, syllables, and suprasegmentals (e.g., Bernhardt & Stoel-Gammon, 1994; Velleman & Strand, 1994) and deficits in premotor organization and sequencing (e.g., Hall, Jordan, & Robin, 1993) to a motor-linguistic perspective that provides a continuum of possible deficits from planning to execution of oral-motor movements (Crary 1984a, 1993). Shriberg, Aram, and Kwiatkowski (1997a) use a heuristic model that includes six linguistic processing stages within the domains of input, organization, and output to provide a schema for viewing the speech and language deficits in DAS. Evidence for DAS as an input deficit includes findings of reduced performance on perception tasks, such as auditory recognition, discrimination, and sequencing (e.g., Bridgeman & Snowling, 1988). Findings of expressive grammatical deficits (e.g., Ekelman & Aram, 1983) implicate organizational processes, whereas phonetic/acoustic analyses of speech errors suggest that DAS is a deficit in speech output processing (Robin, 1992).

Stackhouse (1992) offered four perspectives on DAS: clinical, phonetic, linguistic, and cognitive. Her perspectives included a broad range of factors that encompassed neurological signs, phonetic and phonological features, syntax, intellectual functioning, and reading and spelling. She argued that in DAS, the defining features may depend on the child's level of development and that all four perspectives on the disorder must be considered in the diagnosis of DAS.

Such a large array of possible deficits are encompassed within the theoretical perspectives offered for DAS that we will review the characteristics of DAS with two underlying qualifications. First, not all children will be expected to demonstrate all characteristics of the disorder. Second, with maturation and therapy, it is expected that some of the features of the disorder may no longer be apparent or will be diminished in severity at the time of assessment.

Characteristics

The complex of symptoms indicative of DAS is not universally agreed upon and includes nonspeech, as well as speech, characteristics. Guyette and Diedrich (1981), in a major review of the literature, concluded that there was little agreement on the behaviors or symptoms necessary and sufficient for diagnosis of DAS, that there was little empirical evidence to support conclusions even when agreement was found, and that there was no precise description of how these data could be used as diagnostic indicators. However, it is possible to provide the major characteristics identified from studies of children assigned the DAS diagnostic label. Later, the issue of assessment and diagnostic classification will be examined.

Speech

A key feature of DAS is a severe articulation deficit characterized by a restricted phonemic repertoire (Chappell, 1973; Edwards, 1973); speech sounds are limited to those that occur early in development and contain simple combinations of production features. Crary (1984b), for example, found that the DAS children of his study consistently scored 2 standard deviations below their age level on the *Templin-Darley Screening Test of Articulation* (Templin & Darley, 1969). Stops and nasals are observed, but there is an absence of fricatives and affricates. There is a predominance of omission errors (Rosenbek & Wertz, 1972) and a higher frequency of vowel and diphthong errors than in children with functional articulation deficits (Pollack & Hall, 1991; Rosenbek & Wertz, 1972; Shriberg, Aram, & Kwiatkowski, 1997a; Skinder & Strand, 1998; Smartt, LaLance, Gray, & Hibbett, 1976). Results of feature analyses of consonant errors (Thoonen, Maassen, Gabreels, & Schreuder, 1994) suggest that children with DAS demonstrate a particularly low percentage of place retention in words. That is, when substitutions are compared to their intended targets, children with DAS more frequently retain the features of voicing and manner than the feature of place.

DAS children demonstrate metathetic, perseverative, and anticipatory assimilative errors (Smartt et al., 1976) that may be related to the sequencing of sound elements and to reductions in the complexity of word shapes. There is particular difficulty in the sequencing of phonemic elements (Chappell, 1973; Crary, 1984b; Velleman & Strand, 1994).

In the children we have studied, there appears to be a significant reduction in word shapes with a predominant use of CV, CVC, CVCV, and VC forms. Although not fully explored, restricted use of canonical forms is an expected finding in a child with difficulty in the sequencing of articulatory movements.

Speech production deficits are most obvious on longer units of speech output. DAS children demonstrate difficulty in the production of syllables on diadochokinetic tasks (Nicolosi, Harryman, & Kresheck, 1978). Initiation of utterances is difficult and speech may be accompanied by articulatory groping in the form of sound prolongations, repetitions, or silent posturings preceding or interrupting imitative utterances (Chappell, 1984; Murdoch, Porter, Younger, & Ozanne, 1984). In general, increases in output length are accompanied by increases in errors and reductions in intelligibility.

Rosenbek, Hansen, Baughman, and Lemme (1974) suggest that the errors of DAS children are inconsistent. Inconsistency in terms of speech sound production errors needs to be defined. One would expect to observe variations in speech sound production as a function of phonetic context or length. The increased performance demands associated with particular phonetic contexts and expanded phrase length have the effect of increasing the difficulty of the task. Based on an analysis of phonological process rankings, however, Bowman, Parsons, and Mowis (1984) found that children with DAS use consistent types of phonological processes in the production of spontaneous speech, restricted spontaneous speech (retelling of a story), and word repetition. Phonological process analysis, however, has the effect of obscuring inconsistency by focusing on systematic features of the child's speech output rather than focusing on inconsistencies shown in repeated production of the same words. Inconsistency might best be evaluated by examining repeated productions of the same items.

Shriberg, Aram, and Kwiatkowski (1997b) found that error consistency of children with DAS did not differ from children with developmental phonological disorders. The analysis was based on repeated productions of the same words in a speech sample in which the target was produced incorrectly at least two times. In contrast, Schumacher, McNeil, Vetter, and Yoder (1986) and Skinder and Strand (1998) found increased variability in children with DAS. Smith, Marquardt, Cannito, and Davis (1994), in an acoustic study, reported greater formant frequency variability for a child with DAS compared to that of a normal child and a child with phonological delay. Dodd and McCormack (1995) and Miller (1992) have argued that inconsistency is not limited to children with DAS and have questioned its use as a differential diagnosis marker. The issue of whether greater inconsistency of segmental production is characteristic of DAS is unresolved but appears to be a potentially important diagnostic marker (Davis, Jakielski, & Marquardt, 1998).

Prosody

There are few experimental data on prosody in DAS, and it is not possible to determine whether observed prosodic disturbances are an intrinsic part of the disorder or a compensatory strategy employed in response to motor programming problems. McClumpha and Logue (1972) observed an increase in prosodic disturbances with increasing utterance length, noting longer than normal segmental duration, unsteady pitch, and reduced sound blending. Yoss and Darley (1974a) described an overall reduction in speech rate and a monotony of stress patterning, particularly for older children. Skinder and Strand (1998) found more errors in appropriate stress marking for bisyllabic and multisyllabic words in DAS compared to normally developing children.

In DAS, there is an increase in speech errors with increases in length. A higher incidence of errors coupled with syllable omissions and transpositions have the cumulative effect of altering the intonational contour of the child's utterance. Durational lengthening, monotony of stress, and lack of speech sound blending can be explained as attempts to compensate for severe speech production problems. Shriberg et al. (1997a, 1997b, 1997c), among other findings in a series of studies, concluded that phrasal stress was the only linguistic variable that differentiated 52% of their subjects with suspected DAS from children with phonological delay and that the stress deficit "occurs within linguistic representational levels of phonology, rather than within prearticulatory sequencing" (p. 333). However, stress is marked by specific segmental and suprasegmental phonetic features that also must be programmed and implemented motorically. It is not possible to infer, based on the available data, whether prosodic deficts in DAS are based on impaired processing at a representation or at a motor programming level of operation.

Volitional Nonspeech Movements

Children with DAS demonstrate an impaired ability to produce volitional movements of the speech production structures for nonverbal tasks such as rounding and retraction of the lips and protrusion of the tongue (Bradford & Dodd, 1996; Rosenbek & Wertz, 1972). By contrast, vegetative activities, such as chewing and swallowing, are unimpaired. This feature of DAS is viewed as so pervasive by some investigators (Smartt et al., 1976; Yoss & Darley, 1974a) that impaired ability to volitionally program nonspeech movements has been a primary selection criterion for subjects. This finding, however, is not universal, and Court and Harris (1965) and Morley and Fox (1969) found normal volitional oral movements in some DAS children. Gubbay, Ellis, Walton, and Court (1965) noted fine coordination problems in their sample of children, and Logue and McClumpha (1970) concluded that DAS children may have difficulty in planning sequential movement patterns. Kools and Tweedie (1975), however, did not find a strong relationship within any age interval between articulatory ability and oral and limb praxis in a group of normal children. Similarly Kornse, Manni, Rubenstein, and Graziani (1981) found no significant differences in the manual dexterity of children, although DAS females showed impaired motor skills, but the female control group did not.

The data at this point simply are insufficient to determine whether programmed movements other than of the speech production apparatus are impaired in DAS children. Moreover, there is no clearly established relationship between nonspeech oral movements and speech production in DAS or in normal children. Although reduced nonspeech oral movements may be an expected finding in children with DAS, it is doubtful that it serves as a salient diagnostic criterion.

Cognition

The incidence of DAS, along with a host of other disorders, appears to be higher in children with mental disabilities than in children with intellectual abilities appropriate for their age. DAS has been identified both in children without mental disabilities (Yoss & Darley, 1974a) and children with such disabilities (Ferry, Hall, & Hicks, 1975). In terms of qualitative differences in intellectual abilities, Gubbay et al. (1965) and Walton, Ellis, and Court (1962) found performance IQ scores markedly superior to verbal IQ scores. Decreased intellectual functioning does not appear to be a characteristic distinctive to DAS and may not even serve as a valuable selection criterion for subjects.

Language

Children with apraxia frequently present with delayed development of language (Aram, 1979; Edwards, 1973), particularly for expressive skills (Bowman et al., 1984; Crary, 1984a; Ekelman & Aram, 1983). Rosenbek and Wertz (1972) proposed that the delay is characterized by receptive language skills that are superior to expressive skills. The observations of Rosenbek and Wertz were supported by Snyder, Marquardt, and Peterson (1977), who found significantly higher receptive than expressive scores on the *Northwestern Syntax Screening Test* (Lee, 1971) for DAS children and children with functional articulation disorders but not for normal children.

The effect of a limited repertoire of phonemic elements as found in DAS is the appearance of language deficits at multiple levels. Bowman et al. (1984) found a significant increase in final consonant deletion in the three-syllable words and spontaneous speech of their subjects. Final consonant deletion appeared to be more sensitive to increased word and sentence complexity and had the effect of producing morphological errors—in effect changing the meaning of a word or an entire utterance. Crary (1984a, 1984b) suggested that syntactic deficits observed in DAS children were, for the most part, a result of phonological (phonemic) limitations. Crary and Towne (1984) viewed DAS as an "asynergistic" disorder in which syntactic and phonological systems do not work together, causing specific deficits in expressive syntax and phonology rather than simply a delay in expressive language ability. In effect, they proposed that syntactic errors are a result of phonological limitations. An even broader view was expressed by Panagos and Bobkoff (1984) who argued that DAS, like other phonological disorders, is cognitively based and cannot be separated from language except artificially.

Ekelman and Aram (1983) found that DAS children demonstrated many specific syntactic errors even though mean length of utterance was greater than that associated with Brown's Stage V syntactic development. Subjects in their study demonstrated difficulty with Stage V and more complex markers, and several subjects had difficulty using

Stage II markers. Developmental sentence scores were well below what would be expected for their chronological ages. Phonological limitations could be related to some of the errors observed, such as omission of regular past tense, plural, and present progressive markers and substitutions for irregular past tense. However other errors—such as omission of "in," use of regular and irregular third-person-singular markers, omission of articles, incorrect use of contractible and uncontractible copula and auxillary, and errors in constructing yes–no and "wh" questions—could not be assigned to phonological deficits. Ekelman and Aram concluded that an expressive syntactic disorder, rather than a delay in expressive language, was characteristic of their subjects.

Neurological dysfunction sufficient to preclude the development of the full complement of phonemic elements would be expected to produce a multilevel language deficit characterized by deficits in phonological, morphological, and syntactic organization. Coupled with these language deficits may be other specific grammatical errors secondary to neurological damage or maldevelopment. In general, results from standardized tests of language would show a more prominent deficit in expression compared to comprehension. We would not argue that receptive language skills are necessarily within normal limits in DAS given our proposed theoretical explanation that the disorder is best accounted for on the basis of a lack of neurologically hard-wired phonemic representation. Rather, a significant discrepancy is expected between these two aspects of language processing in children with DAS.

Sensory Deficits

Chappell (1973) and Macaluso-Haynes (1978) included orosensory deficits (2-point discrimination, oral sterognosis) as characteristics of DAS. Aram and Horwitz (1983) found significantly reduced auditory sequencing ability in DAS children on the *Denver Auditory Phoneme Sequencing Test* (Aten, 1979) and the Auditory Sequential subtest of the *Illinois Test of Psycholinguistic Abilities* (Kirk, McCarthy, & Kirk, 1968). However, sensory deficits of this type are common to developmental speech and language disorders and do not appear to be a unique feature of DAS. Crary (1993) has argued, however, that these accompanying auditory deficits may be importantly related to the development of a disorganized phonological representation system in DAS children.

Prognosis

Poor treatment effects cannot be viewed fruitfully as a characteristic of DAS from the standpoint of diagnosis, because prognosis is dependent on the appropriateness of the treatment regimen, the competency of the clinician, and the motivation of the child. However, it has been noted (Blakeley, 1983; Rosenbek et al., 1974; Yoss & Darley, 1973) that DAS children have a poor prognosis for improvement, even with intensive treatment intervention.

There is indirect evidence to support a claim for significant improvement in speech production with treatment and maturation. There are very few descriptions of individuals with a diagnosis of DAS made in childhood who have not developed intelligible speech by the time they reach adulthood. Moreover, older children, but not younger children, with "suspected DAS" are not significantly different on speech severity measures from children with delayed phonological development (Shriberg et al., 1997b). This suggests that speech production has improved *more rapidly* than for the phonologically delayed children. However, the prognosis for improved speech production with intervention and the effectiveness of various approaches to treatment will not be known with confidence until more careful efficacy studies have been completed with consistent differential diagnosis of DAS across studies.

Gender

DAS is more frequently identified in males than females. In a review of 35 studies, Hall et al. (1993) found a ratio of 3:1 for males compared to females. The disorder has an approximate prevalence of 1 to 2 per thousand children and, in some cases, may be heriditary (Shriberg et al., 1997a).

Summary

Both speech and nonspeech characteristics may be used to reach differential diagnostic decisions for DAS. The overlap of DAS features with specific language impairment, phonological disorders, and mental retardation requires that the relative prominence of deficits in speech, language, cognition, and motor and sensory functioning be used to guide diagnosis. There are several potentially salient speech characteristics that may lead to more efficient decision making (e.g., high frequency of vowel errors, inconsistency in repeated production of the same words), but these features have not yet been established as key diagnostic markers. Following a discussion of etiology and the presentation of a neurologically based explanatory construct for DAS, procedures for differential diagnosis of DAS will be examined.

Etiology: Theory and Evidence

An implicit assumption in DAS is that the disorder is the result of brain dysfunction. Two forms of nervous system deficit, not necessarily mutually exclusive, may underlie the disorder. First, there may be diffuse or focal brain damage arising from birth trauma or nervous system pathology incurred early in life. Evidence supportive of this etiology is neural imaging data and historical reports of head trauma accompanied by neurological examination findings. A second possible etiology is a disturbance in normal neurological maturation—perhaps specific to cortical areas responsible for speech and language functions. Supportive data for this etiology are features similar to the first proposed etiology, but with no history of head trauma or frank brain damage. Two studies of DAS will be examined to evaluate these observations.

Rosenbek and Wertz (1972) studied 50 children with DAS selected on the basis of diagnosis by a neurologist and a speech–language pathologist. No other exclusionary criteria were employed. Neurological examinations for 22 of 36 children from the group were normal with the exception of apraxia; the remaining 14 subjects demonstrated apraxia with associated neurological deficits, including muscle weakness, hyperreflexia, spasticity, and hyperkinesis. EEG findings for 15 of 26 children were abnormal with cases of focal and generalized disturbance of the right or left hemispheres or both. Although it cannot be determined from the report what percentage of the children with abnormal EEG findings demonstrated neurological deficits in addition to apraxia, the data can be interpreted as indicating normal EEG results in at least 42% of the children and normal neurological examinations in 61% of the subjects with the exception of apraxia. Data from neural imaging might have increased the number of children diagnosed as having specific brain damage, but the exclusion of children with associated deficits consistent with cerebral palsy or other disorders would have left approximately half with apraxia as the only definitive evidence of nervous system pathology.

Horwitz (1984) investigated 10 children with apraxia who did not have a history of perinatal hypoxia or acquired neurological disease. Diagnosis of apraxia was based on examinations by a pediatric neurologist and a speech–language pathologist following administration of a battery of tests. Results of the neurological examination, an EEG, a CT scan, and amino acid studies were reported. Eight of 10 subjects had abnormal neurological examination findings, but for 4 of the children the findings were restricted to ocular dysfunction. Nine of 10 EEG records were normal with the exception being that of a child with a nonverbal intelligence quotient below 80, who subsequently developed seizures. Similarly, seven of nine CT scans were normal, with the two abnormal scans showing ventricular or cistern enlargement. All seven of the amino acids studies performed were normal. Horwitz observed that the study "failed to demonstrate consistent neurological findings or a specific localizing anatomical basis for the clinical manifestation of DAS" and that "the underlying nervous system abnormalities remain undefined" (pp. 116–117). He concluded by observing that the speech problem might represent a functionally circumscribed component of a larger brain dysfunction not likely to be attributable to isolated biochemical or neurotransmitter defects.

We have undertaken this brief review of two DAS studies to illustrate an obvious fact about the neurological basis of DAS: Of the groups of children selected according to widely differing DAS criteria, each include a large percentage who have no clear-cut evidence of specific neurological impairment. In fact, Williams, Ingham, and Rosenthal (1981), in a partial replication of the Yoss and Darley (1974a) study, found that their two groups of articulation-impaired subjects were not differentiated on the basis of neurological ratings. We would not argue that brain damage in children does not produce significant deficits in speech production because it has been shown (Vargha-Khadem, Watters, & O'Gorman, 1985) that severe bilateral frontal pathology incurred at an early age produces profound speech programming disorders that preclude the development of intelligible speech. Clearly, however, a hypothesis of specific brain damage as the etiological basis for DAS is insufficient for many children with the disorder.

The inability to establish a clear-cut neurological origin for DAS is consistent with efforts to examine the neurological basis for developmental language disorders by auditory evoked response (AER) testing and/or neuroimaging. In a study of three groups of subjects described as developmentally aphasic/dysphasia, motor speech disordered, and neurologically normal (Mason & Millor, 1984), AER recordings showed no consistently significant differences between groups, although smaller amplitudes with the AER were noted for the two groups of children with disorders. Auditory evoked response studies of children described as developmentally aphasic/dysphasic (Roncagliolo, Benitez, & Perez, 1994) and children with a receptive developmental language delay (Akshoomoff, Courchesne, Yeung-Courchesne, & Costello, 1989) have also produced mixed results. Akshoomoff et al. failed to demonstrate abnormal auditory evoked potentials and concluded that the children did not evidence auditory processing difficulties in the initial stages of processing. In contrast, Roncagliolo et al. (1994) presented findings that demonstrated decreased absolute latencies that potentially could account for auditory processing difficulties. These AER studies have been inconclusive in establishing an etiology for developmental speech and language disorders. Although they suggest subtle differences in the filtering abilities and modulatory mechanisms in children with developmental speech and language disorders, the level at which these auditory processing problems emerge has not been established.

Results from neuroimaging of children with developmental communication disorders have been fruitful but inconclusive in establishing the site or type of neurological dysfunction. For example, Knuckey, Apsimon, and Gubbay (1983), using CT scans, found a higher incidence of ventricular enlargement, prominent sulci, and parenchymal brain abnormalities in "clumsy" children compared to normal scans, but the results had little localizing value in determining the type or extent of brain dysfunction. They concluded that the data would support "previously unproven notions that developmental apraxia and agnosia is often associated with anatomical disruption of the brain" (p. 18).

Jernigan, Hesselink, Sowell, and Tallal (1991) employed magnetic resonance imaging to analyze the cerebral structures of 20 children with language and learning impairments and 12 matched control subjects. A primary goal of the study was to define a region that included the posterior perisylvian cortical structures of the temporal and pareital lobes important for the affected language functions. Gross brain stuctures of the disordered group were remarkably normal with only one case demonstrating damage or volume loss. They noted, however, that the disordered group showed asymmetries in the prefrontal region (left greater than right) and pareital region (right greater than left) in direct contrast to the normal subjects. Atypical perisylvian asymmetries have been documented in subsequent studies of children with specific language impairment (Gauger, Lombardino, & Leonard, 1997; Plante, Swisher, Vance, & Rapcsak, 1991). Although these results suggest that there may be some alteration in the course of normal brain development, asymmetry alone would not be expected to be a determining neurophysiological basis for a language disorder because children without a history of specific language impairment (SLI) also may demonstrate asymmetries (Plante, Swisher, Vance, & Rupcsak, 1991). Gauger et al. (1997), in a MRI study of 11 SLI children and 19 matched normal children, concluded from findings of anomalous development of Broca's area and cerebral asymmetries in children with SLI that "language impairment is a consequence of an underlying neurobiological defect in the area of the brain known to subserve language functions" (p. 1278).

Although neuroimaging studies show promise in identifying anatomic differences between children with developmental speech and language disorders and normal children, they have not provided a neurological portrayal of areas of cerebral dysfunction in children with SLI or DAS other than, perhaps, isolating the left cerebral hemisphere as the site of dysfunction. The most parsimonious conclusion based on available data is that there is an anomalous development of brain function and the absence of establishment of neural networks for specific activities such as language (Galaburda, 1989).

Theoretical Framework for Explaining DAS

A major lacuna in DAS research is a viable neurologically based etiological construct to account for the diverse behavioral symptoms of the disorder. To date, generalizations, rather than more highly specified models, have been offered to account for this elusive disorder. Crary (1984b), for example, explained DAS as a "motor linguistic disorder of the developing phonological system with the underlying etiology being deficits in spatial-temporal control of the speech mechanism"

(p. 80). He later defined the disorder as "a group of phonological disorders resulting from disruption of central sensorimotor processes that interfere with motor learning for speech" (Crary, 1993, p. 69) to capture the variability of symptoms in children with this label. Such explanations of DAS fail to capture fully the wide scope of the disorder and the resultant deficiencies in multiple aspects of linguistic development.

Our position is that the two domains of phonological organization—input segmental representation/categorization and articulatory motor output—do not operate in development in a mutually exclusive fashion. Nor can phonological development be dissociated from morphological and syntactic language components. In our view of the neurogenesis of the phonological component of grammar, perceptually established neural substrates isomorphic to phonemic units operate as prerequisites for normal language development. The sine qua non of phonological rule systems for any natural language is the utilization of a finite set of segments (the phonemes) juxtaposed in syllable-bound, phonotactic strings. Without the neurological, hard-wired establishment of phonemic units, lexical construction would be severely compromised. Anomalous or faulty development of brain areas subserving this function would necessitate learning a language without minimal pairs, and, thus, each lexical item would "phonetically be a Gestalt lacking any systematic physical relation to any other" (Lindblom, MacNeilage, & Studdert-Kennedy, 1988, p. 1). Although some form of brain dysfunction is implicitly assumed in DAS, the most likely source appears to lie at a microscopic rather than a gross morphological level (Cohen, Campbell, Elmore, & Yaghmai, 1988; Galaburda, Sherman, Rosen, Aboitiz, & Geschwind, 1985; Gauger et al., 1997; Jernigan, Tallal, & Bellugi, 1988).

Previous work (Sussman, 1986, 1988) based on applications of the *combination-sensitive neuron* found in the auditory cortex of the moustached bat (Suga, O'Neill, Kujirai, & Manabe, 1983) to language acquisition has provided a speculative model of how normal prototypical segmental and syllabic development might form in the child. Substantive contributions to our understanding of what constitutes the hard-wiring underlying the "innateness notion" can be made if findings from animal neurophysiology, especially in species biologically specialized for hearing, are incorporated into human models of language structure. Recent case studies using both postmortem microscopic examination of cerebral tissue and magnetic resonance imaging

(Cohen et al., 1988; Jernigan et al., 1988; Plante, 1988) have revealed cortical anomalies thought to underlie the etiology of developmental dysphasia. As stated by Jernigan et al. (1988), "Preliminary studies suggest that specific cerebral subsystems develop in anomalous ways in these children and that anomalies of development are reflected in gross cerebral dysmorphologies" (p. 19). A child forced to operate with impoverished or deficient neural substrates that are destined, in the normal brain, to derive and signal invariant phonemic categories would be expected to seriously compromise all aspects of language function.

DAS is stereotypically regarded as an output speech disorder, even though language deficits have been reported. Our perspective is that speech perception, speech production, and language will be adversely affected, to some degree, by structurally and operationally deficient neural substrates mediating phonemic identity and categorization. The extent of differential impairment of these interrelated components will not be uniform or linearly predictable, but rather will vary for each individual case.

Speech-related motor and sensory processes develop as early infant sounds and babbling are processed. The motor and sensory systems are intricately interwoven throughout language development so that a level of isomorphism or automatism is created between the two. At the very core of a developing language system, there must exist an internal representation of the phonemic units (i.e., "spectrotopically" mapped fields as described in Sussman, 1989) needed to structure the morphological and lexical output units of language structure. Such internal representations must, by necessity, form from sensory input experience.

Experimental work in the discrimination of nonnative speech contrasts has shown that initial discrimination ability declines during ontogeny in the absence of language experience with phonemic contrasts (Werker, Gilbert, Humphrey, & Tees, 1981; Werker & Tees, 1984). Thus, there is evidence for selective phonological tuning during the first year of life, from an initially broad sensitivity to any natural language stimulus contrast to specific sounds comprising the phonemic system being acquired by the child.

Our position on the underlying etiology of DAS is that the child may not have the basic perceptual processing and internal representation mechanisms that must concurrently develop with speech motor output skills. Deficits in skilled motor articulations can be viewed as stemming from a deficient internal target representation of phonemic elements that are needed to guide or serve as the phonological intent for the motor output algorithms of speech production. The two do not operate as mutually exclusive domains, nor do they function independently from the grammatical rule systems whose syntactic frames must guide phonetic output. Speech production, speech perception, and language will be adversely affected—perhaps to different extents in different speakers—by these structurally and operationally deficient neural substrates mediating phonemic identity and categorization.

Preliminary support for this view comes from studies of rhyming (Marion, Sussman, & Marquardt, 1993) and syllable integrity in DAS (Marquardt, Sussman, & Snow, 1998). Marion et al. (1993) found that DAS children demonstrated a striking inability to recognize and produce rhymes and postulated an impoverished vowel representation system as part of a broader dysmorphology or maldevelopment of neural substrates for encoding phonemic and syllable representations, a deficit that could be coincident with the wide-ranging array of phonetic, phonological, prosodic, and language-based features of the disorder. Marquardt et al. (1998) found that DAS children were impaired—in comparison to a group of children with normal speech production—in their ability to recognize the number of syllables in words, in identifying within-syllable positional differences of segments, and in constructing syllable shapes. The results implicated an impoverished framework for syllabic processing that ultimately affects hierarchical language substrates responsible for lexical structure and syntactic processing.

Though lacking substantial experimental support, we believe the neurogenesis of phonology theory holds promise for providing an explanatory construct for the neurobiological bases of DAS. It provides a guide for further exploration of the disorder, but direct benefits relative to clinical diagnosis and treatment must await further research.

Assessment

There is no single, univerally accepted diagnostic marker for DAS. Shriberg et al. (1997c), based on subjects from several diagnostic clinics, identified inappropriate stress as a possible marker for a subtype of DAS but did not provide a diagnostic framework for identifying children with the disorder. Thoonen, Maassen, Gabreels, Schreuder, and de Swart (1997) suggested that comparison of error rates between real and nonsense words might be important to diagnosis. Stackhouse (1992) argued that DAS is an unfolding developmental disorder whose features would not be expected to be present all of the time and in some cases may not occur at all. Clustering of errors into categories that reflect syllable structure and motor coordination problems may aid in reliable diagnosis because they reflect within- and between-word variability characteristic of DAS (Stackhouse & Snowling, 1992). Other potentially important markers include vowel errors and speech error variability.

Given that a reliable diagnostic marker has not been identified, and recognizing that DAS frequently is overdiagnosed (Davis et al. 1998), the use of a syndrome of speech and language characteristics is the most reasonable means of assigning a diagnosis. We will begin by describing the types of test instruments for determining the level of functioning in each of the major characteristic areas and will follow this description with some comments on differential diagnosis.

Developmental History

Children with DAS typically are quiet babies with poor coordination of sucking, reduced babbling with limited differentiation of consonants and vowels, and limited spontaneous syllable imitation (Velleman & Strand, 1994). The use of spontaneous gestures at an early age due to limited ability in verbal expression is not unexpected. Parents frequently are concerned by the time the child reaches 2 years of age, but establishing a diagnosis of DAS before 3 years of age is very difficult. It is important, as the first step in the diagnostic process, to gather a careful developmental history of motor, social, and communicative development. One useful tool is to ask the parent to complete a profile of language use. A profile of this type asks the parent to indicate what verbal ("Help," "See") and/or nonverbal (positioning, gestures) means are used by the child to acquire help, to obtain objects, to protest, or to direct attention. Also useful is to ask the parent to identify all the words the child consistently uses. For many children with DAS, the total number at age 2 to 3 years may not exceed 20 words.

Screening

The *Screening Test for Developmental Apraxia of Speech* (Blakeley, 1983) has been specifically constructed for differential diagnosis of DAS. Data obtained are not sufficient to detail important features of DAS or to plan therapy, but the measure serves as an initial step in selecting children for additional testing. The eight subtests investigate the discrepancy between expressive and receptive language ability, production of vowels and diphthongs in words, oral motor movements, production of three-syllable sequences, imitation of multisyllabic motorically complex words, production of words presented three at a time, transpositions in the imitation of words, and prosody in connected speech. Weighted scores are used to determine the likelihood of correct assignment to the diagnostic category of DAS. Blakeley's test is not without theoretical and methodological problems (Guyette & Diedrich, 1983), but it has been shown to reliably differentiate children with DAS from children with phonological disorders (Weeks & Madison, 1985). Our experience is that Blakeley's *Screening Test* may be effective for younger children, but after a year or more of treatment focusing on problems in syllable sequencing and speech sound production, the ability of the test to identify children with DAS is markedly diminished.

Additional testing is carried out to explore the most important diagnostic criteria in more detail. A single test seldom will be sufficient in each area of assessment, and the instruments selected are conditioned by the age and developmental level of the child.

Articulation

Tests of articulation are chosen to determine the developmental level of the child, to investigate the frequency and type of speech sound errors, to assess the consistency of production in repeated productions of the same stimuli, and to explore differences in production between single words and connected speech. Typically a norm-based instrument, such as the *Templin-Darley Articulation Test* (Templin & Darley, 1969) or the *Goldman-Fristoe Test of Articulation* (Goldman & Fristoe, 1969), is administered to the older child. Items from the test can be elicited several times in sequence to determine consistency.

A speech sample should be obtained to establish a phonetic inventory and distribution, as well as to carry out analyses of consonant and vowel errors, phonologic process and phonotactic structure use, prosody, intelligibility, and severity (Shriberg & Kwiatowski, 1980). For the younger child who may be hesitant or unable to imitate words, a speech sample may be the only speech output available for analysis.

Language

Two important purposes are served by administration of language measures: (a) examining whether a discrepancy between receptive and expressive language skills is apparent and (b) obtaining a qualitative description of language use. Qualitative expressive language information—such as mean length of utterance, grammatic morphemes used, complex sentence analysis, and structural development—is available from the language sample (Miller, 1981). The choice of additional tests will depend on the age of the child. For young children (less than age 4), it may include the *Sequenced Inventory of Communicative Development* (Hedrick, Prather, & Tobin, 1975). Tests that provide expressive and receptive age scores are particularly helpful for the older child. Regardless of which combination of measures is chosen, the *Peabody Picture Vocabulary Test* (Dunn & Dunn, 1981) should be administered because it is the recommended test for determining a receptive vocabulary score for use on the *Screening Test for Developmental Apraxia of Speech*.

Cognition

Multiple areas of functioning are explored in the psychological examination. A potentially important, but by no means necessary, result for use in the differential diagnosis of DAS is a discrepancy between performance and verbal IQ scores. The *Wechsler Intelligence Scales for Children—Revised* (Wechsler, 1975) provide verbal, performance, and full-scale scores and are perhaps the tests of choice when investigating children from a wide age range. In our experience, DAS children typically demonstrate performance scores at least 10 points higher than verbal scores on tests of intelligence due to their reduced expressive language facility. However, a test of intelligence should be viewed as a single measure; additional testing as the child matures may be necessary before a decision regarding reduced verbal compared to performance abilities can reliably be made.

Sensory and Motor Functioning

Audiometric testing is used to rule out hearing loss as a potential etiology for observed symptomatology. Although verbal sequential deficits are not unique to children with apraxia, use of a measure such as the *Denver Auditory Phoneme Sequencing Test* (Aten, 1979) may provide additional information relative to the verbal sequencing abilities of these children (Aram & Horwitz, 1983). The oral-peripheral examination evaluates the strength, range of motion, and speed of movement of the speech production structures and may be used to determine if a neuromuscular disorder is responsible for observed deficits. Kent, Kent, and Rosenbek (1988) have provided a review of maximum diadochokinetic rates expected for children that can serve as a normative reference in examining the reduced rates for DAS children expected as part of this examination. Both verbal and nonverbal diadochokinetic rates should be determined, but there are, as of yet, no mathematically derived criteria for expected performance by DAS children. However, for children with DAS, diadochokinetic rates are expected to be slow with difficulty maintaining syllable shapes.

Additional testing of volitional oral movements can be obtained by administration of the adaptation (Kools, Williams, Vickers, & Caell, 1971) of the DeRenzi, Pieczuro, and Vignolo (1966) measure for adults with apraxia. We also have found an adaptation of the *Test of Oral and Limb Apraxia* (Helm-Estabrooks, 1992) to be helpful in characterizing the ability to program movements. Finally, fine and gross motor skills also should be examined with age-appropriate assessment tools, such as the *Bruininks-Oseretsky Test of Motor Proficiency* (Bruininks, 1978).

Differential Diagnosis

Determining whether a child demonstrates DAS is dependent upon careful consideration of information obtained from neurologic, psychologic, and communicative assessment. As noted earlier, there is no assurance that the neurologic examination, even when it includes neural imaging, will reveal specific neurologic damage or function. The examination, however, may provide evidence of related symptoms—for example, limb apraxia, delayed motor development, or a significant history of head injury—that can support a diagnosis of neural dysfunction. Co-occurring neuropathology has been reported with sufficient frequency to warrant neurologic referral of DAS children, when possible. The psychological examination is important in determining the presence or absence of mental disabilities, may allow emotional disorders to be ruled out as a causal basis for observed symptoms, and is important in establishing a possible significant discrepancy between performance and verbal intelligence scores.

Neurological and psychological examinations should rule out neuromuscular disorders, emotional disturbance, and auditory impairment as the basis for observed deficits. Evaluation of communicative functioning should further refine the diagnosis to exclude phonological disorders and specific language impairment (SLI). The typical child with DAS will demonstrate auditory language comprehension abilities that are near or within normal limits while expressive language is delayed, which is the key differentiating distinction between DAS and SLI. Children with SLI typically will show language impairment in both comprehension and expression. The presence of a reduced repertoire of phonemes, restricted use of word shapes, inconsistency of production with repetition of the same items, reduced volitional oral movement and verbal diadochokinetic rates, prosodic abnormalities, and very high incidence of omission errors are the key factors or group of factors that will allow DAS to be distinguished from phonological symptoms. However, it must be remembered that apraxia may be evident in other disorders—such as cerebral palsy, mental disability, and hearing impairment—as well as occurring independently, and it is best viewed both as a symptom and as a costellation of deficits. We would argue that when the group of symptoms appears separable from other disorders, it deserves a diagnostic categorization that we have chosen to call developmental apraxia of speech.

Therapy

The suggested treatment regimens for DAS are based primarily on approaches developed for children with phonological disorders (see Table 11.1). These approaches, with modifications, have formed the basis of treatment for DAS because efficacy studies for the disorder have not been completed. Overviews of treatment procedures for DAS, in general, are provided by Pannbacker (1988), Hall et al. (1993), Strand (1995), and Square (1994).

Table 11.1
Therapy Approaches for Phonological and Articulation Disorders

Phonetic Placement (Scripture & Jackson, 1927)	A highly concrete technique that utilizes phonetic placement to correct production of phonemes in error by directions for articulatory points of contact, kinesthetic patterns, airstream dynamics, and so on.
Moto-kinesthetic Speech Training (Young & Hawk, 1955)	Tactual cues and auditory stimulations are used in conjunction with manual manipulation to elicit correct production of target sounds. For example, in the production of /p/, the clinician places the thumb and forefinger on the jaw and moves it upward to contact the lower and upper lips. The jaw is then quickly brought downward to provide the jaw motion and lip abduction requisite for release of the bilabial plosive.
Traditional Articulation Therapy (van Riper, 1978)	This approach is characterized by a sequence of activities for identifying the standard sound, discriminating it from its error, varying and correcting productions until they are produced correctly, and stabilizing and strengthening correct production in various contexts and speaking situations.
Multiple Phoneme Approach (McCabe & Bradley, 1975)	A modification of the traditional approach, multiple phoneme therapy addresses several error sounds at the same time. It is recommended for children who exhibit several sound errors that reflect a common underlying pattern.
Sensory-Motor Approach (McDonald, 1964)	This treatment is based on the rationale that improved articulatory performance can be gained by heightening the auditory, tactile, and proprioceptive feedback of motor patterns. The objectives of treatment are to increase responsiveness to motor productions in connected speech, to reinforce correct production of error sounds, and to facilitate correct production of the sound in systematically varied phonetic contexts. Contexts first are investigated to determine which facilitate correct production of the error sound. Stress and rate then are used as transfer mechanisms to elicit correct production in contexts where the sound previously was produced in error.

(continues)

Table 11.1 *Continued.*

Integral Stimulation (Milisen, 1954)	Auditory, visual, and tactile cues are used to evoke correct production of target sounds. This "watch me and listen" imitative instruction is carried through several levels of complexity (e.g., isolation, syllables) beginning at the highest level at which correct production is achieved.
Contextual Facilitation (Kent, 1982)	The underlying rationale is that certain contexts will facilitate correct production of the target sound and that this is the beginning point for production training. Contextual facilitation is a critical feature of sensory motor training.
Contrast Therapy (Costello & Onstine, 1976)	Treatment to address systematic simplifications of sound classes or word structures is the intent of this approach. Minimal word pairs are presented to the child, who is required to produce correctly the target sound. If the child does not, the resulting communicative breakdown due to uncertainty forces the child to become aware of the error and to change the underlying concept. The approach may be effective in helping children to more readily identify the critical elements to be learned.
Paired Stimuli (Irwin & Weston, 1971)	Like McDonald's sensory motor approach, paired stimuli begin with the identification of a context that facilitates correct production of the target sound. The underlying rationale is that pairing the word in which the target is produced correctly (key word) with another word in which the target appears in the same word position has the effect of transferring correct production to the new context.
Successive Approximation (Nemoy & Davis, 1954)	This is a shaping technique in which the child is guided through a series of transitional movements to the correct production of the target sound.
Speech Pattern Remediation (Hodson & Paden, 1982)	This treatment approach is predicated on the assumption that sound may be within the child's repertoire but is not used correctly. Because phonological processes do not operate at the level of the single sound, the training unit is generally the syllable or word. Other approaches (e.g., contrast therapy, multiple phoneme approach) may be used within this therapy technique to achieve the goal of developing contrasts in the child's phonological system.

Note. Citations are intended to serve as example sources for obtaining information on the treatment approaches described in the table.

A major distinction between DAS and phonological disorders is the prognosis for improved articulation in DAS. Even when intensive stimulation using tactual, kinesthetic, auditory, and visual modalities is employed in conjunction with facilitating contexts, transfer of correct production to other words and linguistic contexts frequently is difficult. The diversity of symptoms in DAS demands that treatment be eclectically developed. Following a discussion of therapy principles and procedures for DAS, we will review treatment approaches adapted specifically for children with the disorder.

Therapy Principles and Procedures for DAS

There is relatively little documentation of the efficacy of treatment for DAS based on investigations of treatment effects or retrospective reviews of progress. Even when this information is available, the diversity of children described makes it difficult to capture the underlying principles of the therapy employed. The following discussion, based on a review of therapy for DAS (Marquardt, Dunn, & Davis, 1985), will look at therapy principles from the standpoint of (a) treatment goals, (b) structure of the treatment sessions, (c) sound stimuli, (d) teaching hierarchy, and (e) treatment strategies.

Goals of Treatment

Primary problems of children with DAS are the failure to develop normally the full repertoire of phonemes of the language and the inability to produce combinations of sounds for words and sentences of increasing length and complexity. Frequently, there is a breakdown between the production of single sounds in isolation and the use of these sounds in longer units of speech output. The primary goals of treatment are to establish the complex, volitional sensorimotor production patterns that the child has failed to develop.

Structure of Treatment Sessions

Children with DAS appear to improve slowly and only after a great expenditure of time and effort. Yoss and Darley (1973), for example, found that only 1 of 10 children enrolled in therapy had been discharged

12 to 16 months later, and then only after 139 hours of intensive treatment. Intensive, systematic, drill-oriented sessions on a daily basis (Blakeley, 1983; Morely & Fox, 1969) are most successful because they provide practice for the motor patterns of the sounds selected for training.

Stimuli

Children with DAS frequently demonstrate vowel errors. If vowels are not produced accurately, it is recommended that correct production of these speech sounds precede work with consonants (Blakeley, 1983; Chappell, 1973). Chappell (1973) recommended beginning with the vowels /o/, /a/, /i/, and /ae/ because they represent highly contrastive tongue positions. It also is apparent that they are acoustically dissimilar and may be easier for the child to distinguish. However, use of an imitation paradigm with isolated vowels is not recommended. Targets should always be incorporated into meaningful CV or VC stimuli.

The consonants selected for treatment should be those that occur early in development (Blakeley, 1983) and that are highly visible (Macaluso-Haynes, 1978; Rosenbek et al., 1974; Smartt et al., 1976; Yoss & Darley, 1974b). Chappell (1973), however, recommended that treatment begin using consonants that offer maximal contrasts in terms of point of articulation and pattern of movement (e.g., /p/, /t/, /k/, /f/, and /s/). His rationale was that these sounds are highly distinguishable and, once established, are available for shaping, modifying, and combining for the production of other consonants.

The emergence of data on babbling may offer insight into the most appropriate stimuli for the young child with limited verbal output. In babbling, low front vowels and labial and alveolar stop consonants and nasals are favored (Davis & MacNeilage, 1995). Within syllable frames there is a high frequency of co-occurence of front vowels with tongue-front consonants and central vowels with labial consonants. Variegation of vowels and consonants typically involves changes in vowel height and consonant manner (Davis & MacNeilage, 1995). In English, monosyllables (e.g., *ball*) predominate over bisyllables, and the first two syllable types are characterized by sequences of the same consonant (e.g., *baby*). The first stimuli to be used for the young apractic child might reasonably include open syllable frames that include stops with vowels selected on the basis of babbling, as well as co-occurence with variegation of the vowel based on height and the consonant based on manner. For example, *daddy* shows co-occurence of an alveolar consonant with a front vowel and includes an expected change in vowel height rather than a change in the vowel front-back dimension. Production of *maybe*, following successful production of *baby*, might be expected because it includes a change in manner rather than in place for the consonant of the second syllable.

In summary, the initial point of treatment is the stabilizing of the consonants and vowels already in the child's repertoire. Selection of additional targets should be based on choosing sounds that occur early in development, are highly visible, offer maximal articulatory and acoustic contrasts, and follow a developmental sequence relative to co-occurence and variegation.

Teaching Hierarchy

The beginning of treatment typically is at a syllable level using simple CV or VC combinations. Gradually reduplicated CVCV combinations are taught followed by monosyllabic words that are salient (meaningful) to the child and that contain the sounds taught at the single syllable level. Chappell (1973) suggested that backward chaining be employed to facilitate the transition from isolated sounds to syllables. This technique involves the production of the new sound at the beginning of the syllable. For example, in the word *cat*, the child is first requested to produce /t/, then /at/, and finally the entire word *cat*. Multisyllabic words are introduced to increase the length and complexity of speech output followed by the production of the trained words in phrases and sentences.

Treatment Strategies

Treatment for the DAS child is marked by the cuing strategies used for establishing movement patterns. In working with children with phonological disorders, the auditory modality is most important for establishing speech sound production. Children with DAS, however, have difficulty learning sensorimotor patterns through auditory cues alone, so visual and tactual inputs must be used as well. Visual cues include visual monitoring in front of a mirror to see articulatory placements and pairing written symbols with the sound. Tactual cues include stimulation of the articulators by application of various textures or pressure and by swabbing or probing the lips and tongue at the site of desired contact.

The use of rhythm, stress, and intonation, paired with movement patterns, has been recommended to facilitate treatment (Rosenbek et al., 1974; Velleman & Strand, 1994). For children who can produce phrases and sentences, rhymes and songs are paired with physical movements, such as beating time with the hand or squeezing a beanbag for each syllable. Children are urged to slow their rate of speech in order to maintain an even stress pattern, which is necessary for maintaining the sounds in the target sequences. For younger children with limited verbal expression, initial treatment sessions may focus on turn-taking activities, because some children with DAS have had very limited experience with turn-taking behaviors in communicative interactions.

A major problem in working with DAS children is the retention of movement patterns so that they can be used in longer and more complex contexts. Chappell (1973) recommended that the time used to practice movement patterns be increased so that accuracy can be maintained for the duration of the task. He also suggested that the time between practice of patterns be gradually increased to aid the child in establishing the memory for particular movement sequences. Finally, he recognized the need to develop self-monitoring skills so that the child can identify and self-correct errors.

Additional Considerations in Treatment

Several other factors may bear on treatment. Rosenbek and Wertz (1972) recommended that for older children, meaningful words, phrases, and sentences be used as stimuli and that self-monitoring and compensatory strategies (e.g., pauses, equal stress on syllables, intrusive schwa in consonant clusters) be taught. Crary (1984b) proposed that differential approaches be used as a function of severity based on the identification of three subgroups of apraxic children. Syllable structure errors were characteristic of the most severely impaired group, sound class errors characterized the middle group, and specific sound errors were the primary feature of the least impaired group. He noted that an increase in sound substitutions corresponded to a decrease in errors related to sequential constraints and syllable shape alterations. This shift occurred not only as a result of the child's replacing omitted segments with substituted phonemes, but also as a result of "grammatical trade-off." By trade-off, he meant incorrect production of previously correct segments as other segments previously produced in error are corrected. Accordingly, he opposed sound-by-sound remediation and instead advocated approaches that facilitated correct production of various syllable shapes at the word level, with careful attention paid to performance load (effects on sound sequencing due to increases in length and grammatical trade-off during intervention). Finally, Ekelman and Aram (1984) documented syntactic deficits in children with DAS and suggested that remediation of syntactic deficits be integrated with therapy procedures directed toward improved motor planning and phonological development.

Therapy principles for DAS clearly are in keeping with the definition of the disorder as an inability to carry out preplanned speech movements in the absence of neuromuscular impairment. Treatment focuses on the production of individual speech sounds in increasingly longer units of output depending on the entry-level skills of the child. Intensive, systematic drill is required because movement sequences are gained through repeated long-term practice using a maximum of speech-related multisensory inputs. If the underlying basis for the disorder is a failure to develop neural substrates for phonemic representation, however, the future direction of treatment relies as much on input types of remedial procedures as it does on the ability to plan and execute speech movements.

For the child with limited oral expression, augmentative communication is a possible intervention option, whether the choice is a gestural or aided system (Hall et al., 1993; Velleman & Strand, 1994). In general, augmentative systems serve as an attractive, albeit limited, option toward the progression to intelligible speech. Augmentative systems, in our view, provide a potentially important bridge for the child to provide an alternative means to expand communicative options. Frequently, parents express concern that the child will default to a nonverbal communication system because speech production is difficult and frustrating. The opposite is more often the case, where the child or parents are not motivated to use a nonverbal communication option. When parents, and most importantly the child, understand the transient purpose of an augmentative system, it serves an important role in allowing for increased communicative success.

Adapted Therapy Approaches for DAS

Several approaches for treating communication disorders have been adapted for use in DAS. To a large extent, they incorporate the therapy principles marked as important to remediation of children with the disorder. Their unique feature is the sequencing of series of tasks within a defined theoretical umbrella. In addition to the treatment programs described in the following sections, gesturally cued procedures for DAS—which rely on gestures provided by the clinician during presentation of the auditory stimulus—have been described by Shelton and Graves (1985) and Klick (1985).

Prompts for Restructuring Oral Muscular Phonetic Targets (PROMPT)

The PROMPT system (Chumpelik, 1984) is constructed to treat DAS as a movement disorder with possible disruptions in planning, sequencing, or executing speech movements. In contrast to other therapy approaches that use imitation or perceptual comparisons, PROMPT imposes a target position or sequence on the child and uses a tactile-based method for reshaping articulatory positions and sequences by providing externally applied cues to the face, the chin, structures associated with voicing and nasality, and jaw opening. A different set of prompts is provided for each English phoneme. The timing of the prompts is important in moving from relatively static segments to transitional coarticulatory movements in phrases and sentences. These transitional effects are facilitated and controlled by the duration of the prompt, the degree of pressure on particular muscle groups, and the tension placed on these muscle groups; they are intended to provide feed-forward information to aid the child in carrying out the preprogrammed sequence as the child is guided toward articulatory targets and transitions. The assumption is that "the system may help provide the lacking and essential kinesthetic feedback (closed-loop) while providing the feed-forward of sequential information (open-loop) that the system needs for transforming conscious motor control into automatic sequences" (p. 152).

The PROMPT system requires that the therapist cue each target or target sequence at a syllable, word, or phrase level. Prompts are strung together in a sequence or administered selectively for specified targets (e.g., final consonant). Timing of prompts for transitive movements and stress is accomplished by altering the duration of individual prompts, the overall speed of combined prompts, and the selection of key prompts over others. Transfer is gained through practice of each phoneme in various contexts.

Touch-Cue Method

This method (Bashir, Grahamjones, & Bostwick, 1984) is an adaptation of cued speech for the deaf and is intended to address phonemic sequencing and patterning deficits in DAS children. Touch cues are the tactile topographic indicators presented in conjunction with auditory and visual cues during initial phases of therapy for consonant sounds. In three discrete stages of treatment, the child progresses from simple CV and CVC syllable shapes to the production of multisyllabic sequences and finally to the production of utterances in spontaneous speech. Stage I uses nonsense syllable drills to teach the topographical cues, to improve sequencing, and to develop self-monitoring accuracy. Bashir et al. indicated that it is critical to the success of the program at this stage that the touch cue elicit the articulatory movements represented by the cue and that accurate self-monitoring of production be established. Stage II is composed of drills that use previously learned sequential movements to produce nonsense and meaningful monosyllabic and polysyllabic words. In Stage III, tasks are employed to carry learned sequencing and self-monitoring skills into elicited utterances and spontaneous speech.

Melodic Intonation Therapy (MIT)

MIT was developed initially to provide a vehicle for establishing propositional phrases in adults with apraxia or Broca's aphasia (e.g., Sparks & Holland, 1976). It uses stereotypical intonation, exaggerated stress, and lengthened tempo in conjunction with hand tapping to capitalize on intact abilities of the nondominant hemisphere in the production of a series of phrases selected on the basis of grammatical simplicity. The program moves through a series of stages from maximum aid from the clinician to increased independence on the child's part for the production of the phrase. MIT was adapted for children with DAS by Helfrich-Miller (1984). Candidacy criteria for MIT include those children 7 to 8 years old with a mean length of utterance of three to four words, poor repetition skills, and an attention span of 15 to 20 minutes. Helfrich-Miller indicated that it takes children who are scheduled for therapy three to four times per week approximately 10 to 12 months to complete the program.

The adapted MIT program includes three stages. Perhaps the major adaptation is the substitution of signed English for the hand tapping that is included for adults. In progressing through the three stages, output length and phonemic complexity are increased, and dependency on the clinician and reliance on intonation are reduced. Phrases in Stage I are two to three words in length, composed of vowels and bilabial stops, and contain a minimum of grammatical morphemes. By Stage III, maximum phonological, morphological, and syntactic complexity is evident in the phrases chosen as stimuli, with high priority given to the functional content of the phrases.

Conclusions

It is not possible to create a fail-safe recipe for providing appropriate and efficient treatment for the child with DAS. What has been offered is a review of techniques for phonological disorders that are adaptable for DAS, along with several organized systems of therapy that have evolved from other disorders but that appear to have value for working with DAS children. What they have in common is a set of principles for treatment including:

1. Use of developmental norms for determining the sequence of speech sounds to be taught

2. Maximum utilization of multimodal inputs (auditory, visual, tactual) to build articulatory movement patterns

3. Recognition of the facilitating effects of context in establishing target productions

4. Early introduction of self-monitoring skills to facilitate self-correction

5. Intensive, systematic drills that provide repetition of sound patterns

6. Emphasis on facilitatory effects of rhythm, stress, intonation, and motor activity in the production of sequences of speech sounds

7. A hierarchical sequence of treatments proceeding from relatively simple, canonical forms to more complex sequences, with greater emphasis on movement sequences and syllabic integrity than on production of individual speech sounds

8. Recognition of the necessity for guiding treatment based on the child's entry-level skills and responsiveness to different treatment approaches

A detailed case history of test findings and treatment for a child with DAS is included in Appendix 11.A. The case study provides a perspective on the ongoing assessment and treatment modifications undertaken for a typical child with DAS.

Summary

Developmental apraxia of speech (DAS) is a severe deficit in the ability to volitionally program speech movements. This disorder has a neurogenic etiology, but evidence of brain damage or dysfunction has not been consistently demonstrated in children diagnosed as having DAS on the basis of widely varying criteria. We have proposed a neurologically based model that potentially accounts for important observed behavioral characteristics of the disorder. Review of speech, language, cognitive, sensory, and motor characteristics provides a framework for appraisal and differential diagnosis of DAS. Evidence relative to the effectiveness of treatment approaches described for DAS is lacking, but case studies and results of efficacy studies may provide more focused direction for therapy intervention.

Appendix 11.A: Case Study

Appraisal and Diagnosis

N. was first evaluated at 3 years of age. Motor developmental milestones were within normal limits, although speech development was characterized as slow. His mother reported that he talked infrequently, was seldom intelligible, and had an oral vocabulary of approximately 35 words. Administration of the *Sequenced Inventory of Communication Development* (Hedrick et al., 1975) yielded a receptive age of 32 months and an expressive age of 16 months. N.'s phonetic inventory was limited to vowels, stops, nasals, and glides (see Table 11.2). Phono logical processes noted included final consonant deletion, cluster reduction, stopping, velar fronting, and unstressed syllable reduction. Although all English vowels were represented in his phonetic repertoire, they frequently did not approximate their phonemic target. Regardless of context, /d/ was typically substituted for target consonants. The most frequently used word shape was CV, which also was used when more complex canonical shapes were attempted.

Conversational speech was severely reduced in intelligibility, and attempted communication was accompanied by a well-developed gestural system. Oral-peripheral examination of the speech mechanism revealed normal structures. However, alternate movement sequences of the tongue and lips and diadochokinetic rates for stop-vowel syllables were performed slowly, and some multisyllabic sequences could not be imitated. Performance on the *Arthur Adaptation of the Leiter Performance Scales* (Arthur, 1952) yielded an intelligence quotient of 123, which was in the high average to superior range. Receptive vocabulary and visual motor integration were within normal limits.

At age 5, additional testing was completed to provide qualitative information on language expression. Results from the *McCarthy Scales of Children's Abilities* (McCarthy, 1972) were within the average range. Frequent omissions of articles, pronouns, verbs, negatives, and conjunctions were found on the *Carrow Elicited Language Inventory* (Carrow, 1974). Adjectives, adverbs, and nouns, however, were almost always retained.

Production of sentences from the *Carrow Inventory* was marked by inconsistent, context-dependent speech sound errors. Variability in sound production was reduced on more complex sentences, with frequent substitution of /d/, /b/, and /w/ for target sounds. Word shapes were primarily CV combinations, and longer utterances were highly unintelligible due to sound and syllable omissions and transpositions. A score of 32 was obtained on the *Templin-Darley Diagnostic Articulation Test* (Templin & Darley, 1969). The mean for male children at this age is 106, indicating a severe delay and a disorder in articulatory development. Phonological process analysis results were similar to performance at age 3. The most frequent processes were consonant deletion, cluster reduction, and stridency deletion. N.'s phonetic inventory was limited to vowels, stops, nasals, glides, and, infrequently, liquids. No frica-

(text continues on p. 454)

Table 11.2
DAS Child N. Test Performance from CA 3-0 to 6-6

Age	Articulation	Language	Motor	Cognition	Other
		Semester 1			
CA 3-0 to 3-4	I. *Goldman Fristoe Test of Articulation* Vowels present [æ, e, i, ɛ, aɪ, I, o, ɔ, u, ʊ, ʌ, ə, aʊ] Consonants present Initial [d, w, n, m] Medial [d, b] Final [t, p] II. Phonological process analysis Process observed: cluster reduction, stopping, velar fronting, final consonant deletion, initial consonant deletion, unstressed syllable deletion	*Sequenced Inventory of Communicative Development* Receptive language age = 32 months Expressive language age = 16 months	Oral-peripheral examination Structures within normal limits but tongue movement limited and speed reduced		Pure tone audiometric screening results within normal limits Normal middle ear function based on impedance testing

(continues)

Table 11.2 Continued.

Age	Articulation	Language	Motor	Cognition	Other
			Semester 2		
CA 3-5 to 3-9	I. Phonetic inventory Initial [d, b, w, h, m] Medial [None] Final [m, t, p, s]	*Peabody Picture Vocabulary Test* Raw score = 40 CA = 3-7 Age score = 3-11 Percentile = 68	I. *Developmental Test of Visual Motor Integration* CA = 3-7 Age score = 3-2 II. Oral-peripheral examination/apraxia measures Difficulty performing more complex oral apraxia tasks (e.g., pucker-up-to-smile sequence, licking lips)	*Leiter Performance Scales* CA = 3-7 MA = 4-5 Ratio IQ = 123	
	II. Syllable shapes CV, VC				
			Semester 3		
CA 3-10 to 4-1	I. Phonetic inventory Initial [m, b, k, h, w] Medial [d, k] Final [m, s]				
	II. Syllable shapes CV, VC, CVCV				

(*continues*)

Table 11.2 Continued.

Age	Articulation	Language	Motor	Cognition	Other
		Semester 4			

CA 4-2 to 4-5	I. *Assessment of Phonological Processes*
	Syllable reduction = 0%
	Cluster reduction = 100%
	Standard deletion = 75%
	Obstruent omissions
	  Prevocalic = 87%
	  Postvocalic = 16%
	Omission of /l/ and /r/ Prevocalic consonants deleted in medial position
	
	II. Phonetic inventory
	Initial [m, pm, b, t, d, k, g, s, t, w, j]
	Medial [None]
	Final [m, n]
	
	III. Syllable shapes
	CV, VC, CVCV, VCVC
		Analysis of speech sample (92 utterances)
		
		MLU = 3.08
			Screening Test for Developmental Apraxia
			Oral Movement subtest: Performed tasks but could not position tongue behind upper teeth. Unable to complete three-syllable sequences.		

(continues)

Table 11.2 Continued.

Age	Articulation	Language	Motor	Cognition	Other
		Semester 5			

CA 4-5 to 4-9	I. *Templin-Darley Test of Articulation*
	             Score Norm
	 Diagnostic 32 106.4
	 Screening 5 34.7
	
	 II. *Assessment of Phonological Processes*
	
	 Syllable reduction 0%
	 Cluster reduction 88%
	 Stridency deletion 89%
	 Velar deviation 62%
	 Obstruent omission
	   Prevocalic 81%
	   Postvocalic 10%
	 Liquid deviation
	   /l/ 54%
	   /r/ 58%
	 Nasal Omissions 58%
	
	 III. Syllable shapes
	     CV, VC, CVCV, CVC
	
	 IV. Conversational speech sample simplifications
	     Cluster reduction
	     Stridency deletion
	     Final consonant deletion
		I. *Test of Auditory Comprehension of Language*
		 Score = 69
		 CA = 4-6
		 Age score = 4-3 to 4-7
		 Percentile rank = 74
		
		 II. *Carrow Elicited Language Inventory*
		 CA = 4-8
		 Total errors = 116
		 Articles = 21
		 Nouns = 5
		 Plurals = 6
		 Pronouns = 18
		 Verbs = 51
		 Negatives = 8
		 Prepositions = 3
		 Demonstratives = 1
		 Conjunctions = 3			

(*continues*)

Table 11.2 Continued.

Age	Articulation	Language	Motor	Cognition	Other
Semester 6					
CA 4-10 to 5-1	I. Assessment of Phonological Processes Cluster reduction = 50% Stridency deletion = 66% Velar deviation = 50% Final obstruent omission = 73% Liquid deviation /l/ = 100% Nasal omissions = 20% II. Phonetic inventory Initial [m, n, p, b, t, d, k, g, f*, r*, w, j, h] Medial [m, n, p, b*, t*, d, k*, w, j, ʔ] Final [m, n, p, t*, d*, r*, f] *newly acquired III. Syllable shapes CV, VC, CVCV, CCV, CVC	Peabody Picture Vocabulary Test Raw score = 68 CA = 5-0 Age score = 5-10 Percentile = 77	I. Bruininks-Oseretsky Test of Motor Proficiency within normal limits II. Modified DeRenzi et al., Tests of Apraxia Limb apraxia 5/10 correct Oral apraxia 5/10 correct III. Boston Diagnostic Aphasia Examination A. Verbal agility = 8/14 B. Nonverbal agility = 6/12	McCarthy Scales of Children's Abilities CA = 5-1 General Cognitive Index = 90 Scale Index Verbal 43 Perceptual-Performance 48 Quantitative 44 Memory 38 Motor 48	Prosody on longer utterances marked by inappropriate use of stress, most noticeably the overemphasis of stressed syllables
Semester 7					
CA 5-2 to 5-4	No testing completed				

(*continues*)

Table 11.2 Continued.

Age	Articulation	Language	Motor	Cognition	Other
		Semester 8			
CA 5-5 to 5-8	I. Assessment of Phonological Processes Final consonant deletion = 63% Cluster reduction = 86% Stridency deletion = 48% Velar deviation = 29% Liquid deviation /l/ = 85% /r/ = 73% Nasal omissions = 5% II. Phonetic inventory Initial [m, p, t, d, k, f, dʒ, w] Medial [m, n, p, t, d, k, ʔ, s, ʃ] Final [m, n, p, t, ʔ, s, ʃ] III. Syllable shapes CV, VC, CVCV, CVC, CCV, CVCC, CVCVC	*Carrow Elicited Language Inventory* CA = 5-6 Total errors = 101 Score Percentile Articles 28 <1 Nouns 3 <1 Pronouns 17 <2 Verbs 38 <1 Negatives 8 <1 Prepositions 1 14 Demonstratives 2 1 Conjunctions 3 1 (Speech characterized by final morpheme deletion as well as word omissions and difficulty with complex sentences)			Pure tone audiometric screening within normal limits bilaterally Impedance testing: middle ear function normal

(continues)

Table 11.2 Continued.

Age	Articulation	Language	Motor	Cognition	Other
Semester 9					
CA 5-9 to 6-1	I. Assessment of Phonological Processes Final consonant deletion = 40% Cluster reduction = 48% Stridency deletion = 36% II. Phonetic inventory Elements missing Initial [ð, z, r, l] Medial [v, θ, ð, z, ʒ, dʒ] Final [v, θ, ð, z, ʒ, l] III. Syllable shapes V, CV, VC, VCV, CVCV, CVC, CCVC, CVCC, CCVCVC	Conversational speech marked by final morpheme deletions (plural, past, present, progressive) and word omissions (articles, verbs, conjunctions, negatives, pronouns)	*Kaufman Assessment Battery for Children* CA = 6.1 Score Percentile Sequential Processing 85 16 Simultaneous Processing 109 73 Mental Processing Composite 100 50 Achievement 97 42		Intelligibility in connected speech increased with reduced rate.
Semester 10					
CA 6-2 to 6-6	I. Assessment of Phonological Processes Final consonant deletion = 35% Cluster reduction = 52% Stridency deletion = 34% II. Phonetic inventory Elements missing Initial [ð, r, l] Medial [v, ð, θ, l, ʒ] Final [v, ð, θ, l, ʒ]	Language sample analysis Problems with grammar (grammatical morphemes and complex sentences). Deletes -ing, plurals, possessives, regular past tense, and irregular third-person singular. Omits articles and contractive forms of "is" and "are" in complex sentences.			

tives or affricates were noted. Avoidance behavior in conversational speech was noted on words containing fricatives, and prosody was characterized by inappropriate loudness dynamics on longer utterances.

Additional measures were used to explore possible limb and oral apraxia. The probability of N.'s correct assignment to an apraxic diagnostic category was greater than 99% based on the results of the *Screening Test of Developmental Apraxia of Speech* (Blakeley, 1980). Perseveration, avoidance, and groping behaviors were noted during testing. On the Boston Verbal Agility subtest (Goodglass & Kaplan, 1972), N.'s productions of multisyllabic stimuli were characterized by transpositions of sounds and syllables and reductions in word complexity. Six of the 10 items of the Kools et al. (1971) adaptation of the DeRenzi et al. (1966) test of oral apraxia were scored as incorrect based on defective amplitude, accuracy, and force. N. also demonstrated difficulty in rapidly producing six of the seven tasks from the Boston Oral Agility subtest (Goodglass & Kaplan, 1972). N. produced only 5 of the 10 items of the Kools et al. (1971) adaptation of the DeRenzi et al. (1966) test of limb apraxia, but nonoral fine and gross motor skills were within normal limits based on the results of the *Bruininks-Oseretsky Test of Motor Proficiency* (Bruininks, 1978).

At 6 years and 5 months of age, a detailed analysis of speech and expressive language functioning was completed. Included in the assessment were the analysis of a speech sample and the administration of the *Carrow Elicited Language Inventory* (Carrow, 1974), the *Assessment of Phonological Processes* (Hodson, 1980), and the *Templin-Darley Diagnostic Test of Articulation* (Templin & Darley, 1969). Results are shown in Table 11.3.

N.'s phonetic inventory contained all sound classes, including vowels. Frequently occurring phonological processes included cluster reduction, liquid simplification, and stridency deletion. Consonants were correct 78% of the time, and vowels were correct 87% of the time. Word and syllable shapes were predominantly simple; however, more difficult canonical shapes were used, including initial, medial, and final clusters. The most frequently used word shapes were V, VC, CV, VCV, CVC, CVCV, and CVCVC.

Analysis of the speech sample and *Carrow Inventory* revealed variable context-dependent errors. As word and sentence length increased, the number of errors increased, whereas word shapes and the complexity of phonemic features were reduced. Intelligibility was reduced due to frequently omitted motorically complex speech sounds, vowel distortions, variable productions of the same word, and the combining of multiword utterances into a single word.

On the *Carrow Inventory*, articles, verbs, and conjunctions frequently were omitted, but not adjectives, adverbs, prepositions, pronouns, and nouns. The spontaneous speech sample analysis yielded a mean length of utterance of 6.4 and a limited number of grammatical morphemes (deVilliers & deVilliers, 1973) and complex sentence types, given N.'s age. Grammatical morphemes observed included *-ing, in, on, a, the*, plurals, and possessives.

In summary, N. demonstrated a severe articulation disorder characterized by vowel errors, inconsistent productions, severely reduced intelligi-

Table 11.3
Summary of Speech and Language Assessment Following
10 Semesters of Treatment for Client N.

	Speech

Sound Classes[a]	Nasals: /m/IM,F,/n/Im,F,/ŋ/F
	Stops: /p/IM,F,/b/IM,F*,/t/IM,F,/d/IM,F,
	  /k/IM,F,/g/IF
	Glides: /j/IM,/w/IM
	Liquids: /l/IM*F,/r/MF
	Fricatives: /f/IF,/v/I*F*,/s/IM,F/z/F,/h/I,
	  /ʃ/I,/ð/I
	Affricates: /tʃ/IF*,/dʒ/I

Consonant error analysis (by %)[b]	n = 12 ŋ = 50 t = 43 d = 20 k = 16 g = 43 w = 10 j = 67 l = 17 r = 44 f = 12 v = 86 s = 19 z = 33
Vowel error analysis (by %)[c]	i = 7 u = 30 I = 10 ɔ = 11 æ = 8 a = 10
Phonological processes (used more than 40% of the time)	Cluster reduction
Templin-Darley Test of Articulation	Raw score = 95 Mean = 117
Predominant word shapes (used more than 10% of the time)	V VC CV CVC VCV CVCV CVCVC
	Language
Mean Length of utterance	6.4
Grammatical morphemes	<50% >50% -ing -plurals -in -possessives -on -the -a
Complex sentences	Conjoined sentences *wh* infinitive clauses Simple infinitive clauses with equivalent subjects Noninfinitive *wh* clause

[a] Asterisks indicate sounds produced two or fewer times.
[b] Total percentage of errors = 22.
[c] Total percentage of errors = 13.

bility, prosodic abnormalities, and reduced use of complex canonical shapes. There also was evidence of oral and limb apraxia in the presence of normal fine and gross motor skills. Although cognitive functioning and receptive language were within normal limits, specific deficits and delays were apparent in expressive language. No evidence of specific neurological damage was reported, but we believe the characteristics demonstrated by N. are consistent with our description of the symptom complex that uniquely sets apart a group categorized as children with DAS.

Treatment

Retrospective views of treatment effects have inherent limitations. They do not allow control over relevant variables such as clinician training and pre- and post-testing instruments. Of greater importance over long periods of treatment is the reduced ability to separate out treatment effects from expected development of articulation skills in children with developmental apraxia. These shortcomings notwithstanding, we will review therapy for N. over a 10-semester period. Because the main thrust of treatment was on phonology and articulation, an estimate of improved performance can be made from a review of assessment results in the articulation category shown in Table 11.2 and from Table 11.3. Treatment approaches for each semester are shown in Table 11.4.

Semesters 1 and 2

Recommendations for management based on initial test results were (a) to establish use of final consonants, beginning with /p/ and /t/; (b) to introduce frication, beginning with /s/ in the final position; (c) to increase use of CVC or CVCV canonical shapes by using target words with these shapes while working on other goals; (d) to establish consistent initial production beginning with /h/ or /w/; and (e) to establish correct vowel production, based on further probing of specific vowels. A modified phonological approach based on Hodson and Paden (1982) was used with several error sounds targeted in each session. Instruction focused on contrast drill in CV and VC syllables and words. A multiple baselines design was implemented because it provided a means of detecting small changes in behavior over time. Clinical techniques included auditory bombardment and auditory-visual stimulation. Every 3 weeks, N.'s parents received a list of one-syllable words containing target phonemes to practice at home. Progress was slow and carryover was seldom observed. Levels of self-monitoring obtained in CV and VC sequences were not demonstrated in connected speech, and performance on sounds previously mastered deteriorated markedly between semester intervals. By the end of Semester 2, N. evidenced only three additional sounds in his phonetic inventory. Contrastive use of sounds was limited. The absence of medial consonants and the reduced number of sounds occurring in final position indicated that N. was unable to maintain syllable structure. His inability to produce sounds in a variety of word structures, variability in production, and reduced ability to perform speech-related movements mandated increased

Table 11.4
Treatment Approaches by Semester for DAS Child N.

Semester	Treatment Approach
1	Hodson's phonological process remediation
2	Hodson's phonological process remediation
3	McDonald's sensory-motor Multiple phoneme approach
4	McDonald's sensory-motor Multiple phoneme approach
5	McDonald's sensory-motor Contrast therapy Traditional approach
6	McDonald's sensory-motor Contrast therapy Melodic intonation
7	McDonald's sensory-motor Contrast therapy Melodic intonation
8	Hodson's phonological process remediation
9	Hodson's phonological process remediation
10	Hodson's phonological process remediation

attention to movement sequences. Only two goals of treatment were achieved at the expected levels of accuracy during these first two semesters of treatment.

Semester 3

Remediation shifted in focus to a modified sensory-motor approach (McDonald, 1964) with utilization of nonsense bisyllabic drills (reduplicated CVCV syllables in which consonants and vowels were the same at first but later systematically varied according to consonant and vowel selection) to teach overlapping sequences of articulatory movements. Imitation of bisyllable combinations, beginning with sounds already established in N.'s repertoire, afforded a transition to more complex canonical shapes emphasizing slow rate, even stress, and careful self-monitoring. Occasional use of meaningful words was incorporated to illustrate the salience of newly learned movement sequences.

Phonological and linguistic elements also were incorporated into the treatment program. Included in the program were (a) selection of CV words at the basic level of production training; (b) acceptance of sound approximations that fell within the same sound class; (c) selection of target sounds (e.g., /k/ as representative of the velar class of sounds); (d) formulation of treatment goals that simultaneously considered phonology and syntax and incorporated structures that were pragmatically useful (e.g., training of sounds at the sentence level using a cloze procedure such as, "Give me the ___ "); and (e) use of an auditory trainer to amplify production of specific target sounds and increase awareness of correct production.

Specific objectives included spontaneous production of the initial /k/ in words and the initials /h/ and /m/ in sentences. Consonants trained in final position included /s/, /d/, and /m/ at the sentence level. Projected goals at a 90% criterion level were not achieved. However, by the end of the semester N. produced six new sounds with greater than 50% accuracy, the velar class of sounds was added to his phonological system, and the /s/ was emerging. Treatment methods appeared successful in accomplishing objectives, although to a lesser degree than expected.

Semester 4

At this point N. produced all consonant manner classes except liquids, but labiodental, interdental, and palatal place features were absent. Six new sounds were added to his phonetic inventory, and a total of 11 sounds appeared in initial position and two in final. Several other phones occurred less than three times in the sample and may have been emerging.

A modified McDonald sensory-motor approach was used to drill on the sequencing of sounds already produced (/s/ and /p/) and to incorporate new sounds (/d/ and /f/) that he appeared to be acquiring. Additional goals in-cluded spontaneous production of monosyllabic words with final /p/, /d/, and /k/. Auditory, visual, and tactile cues were used to establish target production and then were faded to auditory or visual cues or both. The auditory trainer was used to heighten awareness of target phonemes. Chappell's backward chaining procedure was used in the elicitation of final consonants. Only one of the projected therapy goals was achieved. Although 90% accuracy was demonstrated in imitation of /k/ and /p/ in bisyllables with varied vowels, N. was unable to maintain /s/ in CVCV and VCVC sequences. He could not produce /f/ in combination with a vowel. Final consonants were produced with increased accuracy in imitation after training with backward chaining, but levels of accuracy were not maintained in spontaneous speech. Transfer into conversational speech did not occur.

The McDonald sensory-motor approach appeared effective in establishing productions of /k/ and /p/ in initial and medial word positions but was not successful with either /s/ or /f/. Perhaps N. did not have sufficient control over production of these latter sounds to use them in bisyllables. Alternatively, because fricatives first emerge in final position, they should have been targeted in final rather than in initial and medial positions.

Semester 5

A substitution analysis was completed comparing N.'s phonological system with that of an adult. Only seven consonants were produced more often correctly than incorrectly. All were produced in initial position. Stoel-Gammon and Dunn (1985) indicate that 4-year-old children customarily produce 21 consonants. They also list 11 consonants that are correctly produced by 90% of normal 4-year-old children. N. consistently produced only 7 consonants with 80% accuracy in initial position.

A child has eliminated most phonological processes by age 4 (Hodson & Paden, 1982). However inspection of frequency of occurrence of processes (Table 11.2) shows that N.'s consonant production clearly was below age level. Stoel-Gammon and Dunn (1985) indicated that by age 4, errors of normal children occur in isolated sounds and not classes of sounds or word structures. N. had five processes that occurred more than 40% of the time. Finally Templin (1957) noted that many consonant clusters are produced consistently by 4-year-old children in initial and final positions. However N. attempted only two words with clusters—both resulted in substition of /pw/ for /pl/. Obviously N. demonstrated substitution processes that accounted for many of his errors that—with the exception of /d/ and /r/—could be attributed to assimilation processes.

Intervention efforts continued to address imitation of bisyllable structures with systematic variation of consonants N. could produce correctly in combination with varying vowels. Integration of additional sounds (/b/, /d/, /m/, /n/) into the CVCV patterns with varying vowels was accomplished with 90–100% accuracy. Producing transitional patterns with systematic variation of the second consonant was achieved with greater than 50% accuracy for stop-nasal (e.g., p–m) and nasal-stop (e.g., m–k) combinations. A traditional approach was used to establish production of the strident phonemes /f/ and /s/ in the final position of monosyllabic words. Efforts to generalize production of these sounds consisted of activities in which N. used target words in meaningful situations. Greater accuracy was demonstrated in imitation of /s/ and /f/ in CVC words and in spontaneous production. Spontaneous production of final /t/, /k/, /m/, and /p/ in CVC words was not achieved; however, contrast therapy was effective in establishing production in final position of /p/ (100%), /m/ (80%), and /t/ (40%).

By the end of the semester, N. had added six more sounds to his inventory, although these newly acquired phonemes occurred less than three times in the speech sample. He also demonstrated spontaneous use of the first-person pronoun *I* over half the time in conversational speech.

Advances were made during the semester using all three therapy approaches. Contrast therapy afforded a transition to more complex syllable shapes using meaningful linguistic activities with phonemes N. was capable of producing. Phonemes that required more complex articulatory sequencing appeared sensitive to traditional therapy training. Carryover to the following semester was demonstrated on those sounds that received training using contrast therapy and sensory-motor bisyllabic drill. However, success with all three approaches was limited to imitative production.

Semester 6

Drill on CVCV patterns with varied vowels and consonants was continued. Stress patterns were systematically varied in this drill to reduce overemphasis on stressed syllables and to reduce steeper-than-normal intonational contours. Other tasks were directed toward improved rhythmic flow of speech and included (a) the production of two-, three-, and four-syllable words with appropriate stress patterns and (b) practice on simple syllable frames and familiar nursery rhymes accompanied by body movements. The purpose of these drills was to increase awareness of the rhythmic aspects of spoken language. Rhythm was used as a technique to facilitate inclusion of sounds that N. had difficulty producing in connected speech (Blakeley, 1983; Rosenbek et al., 1974). At the beginning of the semester, N. could not clap in rhythm to a nursery rhyme, but this behavior reached 50% accuracy by the end of the 3-month period. Stress patterns were practiced in a hierarchical fashion based on difficulty. Once N. could distinguish between loud and soft auditory stimuli, activities shifted to clapping or tapping out two-part rhythm patterns in imitation. Stimulus words contained consonants that could be produced with the qualification that initially any medial consonant was acceptable. Cues included written stimuli showing the stressed syllables in larger physical movements, such as hitting the table with the appropriate rhythm, and in auditory stimuli distinguishing between loud and soft. Initially N. could not produce a distinction between soft and loud CV syllables, but by the end of the semester he could produce the appropriate stress pattern with 60% accuracy on trisyllables. Prosody seemed more appropriate by the end of the treatment period.

A second major goal was spontaneous production of final stops and nasals in CVC words. Using contrast therapy, 100% accuracy was obtained in imitation of all final consonants, but these sounds were not consistently produced in spontaneous speech. A third goal was spontaneous production of strident phonemes in all word positions to increase intelligibility. An auditory trainer was used to provide auditory stimulation of words with initial /s/ blends and medial fricatives. N. reached the goal on /s/ and /f/ in final position but could not imitate either of these sounds in initial position. Spontaneous production of final /s/ and /f/ was not accomplished.

Semester 7

Therapy activities focused on a more meaningful level as nursery rhyme and bisyllable drills were assigned to a home program. Goals included correct production of final /p/, /t/, /k/, /m/, and /n/ in CVC words, carrier phrases, and sentences. The language master was used along with verbal cuing to increase self-monitoring skills. The /s/ blends also were included for training at the single word and sentence level. Post-testing indicated a 22% increase in final consonant inclusion and improved self-monitoring. In a spontaneous speech sample, nasals and liquids were the most consistently included final consonants, followed by plosives. For the first time, other sound classes in final position—particularly the velar /k/—were noted in spontaneous speech.

Semester 8

The emergence of target sounds was the focus of remediation. Intervention was based on successive cycles (Hodson & Paden, 1982). Goals for cycling included production of the strident phoneme /s/ in final word position and in several final clusters, production of final /ʃ/ and /tʃ/ at the sentence level, and production of velars in words. Activities consisted of minimally paired contrast words, the language master, and card games. An auditory trainer was used to provide stimulation of words ending in final /s/ but was discontinued because N. consistently repeated target words incorrectly. At the end of the semester, imitation of final clusters /ts/ and /ps/ and final production of /ʃ/ and /t/ were improved. However, no progress was demonstrated in spontaneous production. Velar consonants were imitated with 100% accuracy except for /g/. Significant decreases were observed in cluster reduction, final consonant deletion, velar deviation, and liquid deviation, and the phoneme /ʃ/ was added to the phonetic inventory.

The separate cycling of clusters, fricatives, and velars allowed N. to establish these manner classes by focusing attention on representatives from the classes in isolated time periods. (In Semester 4, N. had been confused when several manner classes were targeted in a single session.) The increased spacing between drills produced by the separate cycling periods facilitated production of target sounds.

Semester 9

Informal analysis at this point in treatment revealed spontaneous speech characterized primarily by nasals, stops, and glides. Word shapes were simple, and no instances of abutting consonants were found. Goals were targeted in units lasting for approximately 4 weeks. Included were productions of initial and final /s/ and /f/, initial /s/ clusters, and final /g/. A generalization goal was implemented to provide transfer of targeted sounds to new environments, rhyming activities were continued, and self-monitoring was emphasized.

N. made excellent progress during the semester; he added nine sounds to his phonetic inventory. Phonological processes were substantially reduced and included only cluster reduction, final consonant deletion, and stridency deletion. Canonical forms added included CCVC and CCVCVC. Spontaneous use of correct sound production and generalization to new environments were observed, although continued difficulty was noted in rhyming.

Semester 10

A substitution analysis indicated that many of N.'s errors were related to the substitution of one sound for another (e.g., /w/ for /l/) rather than to classes of sounds. Goals built into 6-week units included production of initial and final /o/ in spontaneous speech and production of /l/. A third goal was the production /s/ and /z/ plural forms. Progress in production of the targeted speech sounds was fair—75% accuracy was obtained in the production of plural markers when pictures containing more than one person or object were described. Rhyming was combined with sound-symbol association and the mastery of 20 sight words in a reading readiness task. Good progress was shown in sound-symbol association and sight words, but poor progress was noted in rhyming. Recommendations for further management included implementation of self-monitoring and carryover activities, continued development of a home program, and increased attention to expressive language and reading skills.

Conclusions

Retrospective reviews of treatment have inherent limitations, as we noted earlier, due to the inability to control relevant variables or to accurately factor treatment effects from developmental progression. However, several observations about treatment for DAS resulted from this in-depth examination.

1. The production phase of the traditional approach to treatment may be effective in dealing with residual error sounds. The traditional approach is less useful in early stages of treatment due to the focus on single consonants.

2. The multiple phoneme approach and auditory bombardment were successful in establishing initial productions of target sounds in CV and VC sequences. The Mcdonald sensory-motor drill helped to establish seven sounds in medial position and to stabilize a number of transitions from varying consonants. Bisyllable drills were effective when used with contrast techniques.

3. Greater progress was demonstrated with minimal pair contrasts when therapy goals were restricted to stabilizing the production of two pairs of sounds containing similar place features such as /m/ and /n/.

4. Semesters during which both bisyllable drill and contrast techniques were used resulted in the greatest number of additional sounds appearing in the child's inventory.

5. Nursery rhymes accompanied by movement; production of two-, three-, and four-syllable words with appropriate stress patterns; and bisyllabic drills with varied stress were successful in reducing prosodic abnormalities.

6. Auditory and visual stimulation, provided in the form of look-and-listen cues related to oral posturing and written stimuli, were more effective than auditory stimuli alone.

Quite obviously, another child with DAS may have required a different series of treatment approaches based on practical considerations. There is no preset idealized series of treatment steps and no treatment approaches so potent that they exclude others from consideration. Only when additional treatment data have been obtained will it be possible to determine which approaches are most efficacious for various aspects of the disorder.

Update

N. subsequently received speech and language services in the public schools. His mother reported that he demonstrated concomitant reading and writing problems that affected academic performance. At age 16, following years of tutoring to improve reading facility, he was able to successfully complete coursework in high school. However, his mother reported he had continued difficulty in learning a foreign language.

References

Akshoomoff, N., Courchesne, E., Yeung-Courchesne, R., & Costello, J. (1989). Brainstem auditory evoked potentials in receptive developmental language disorder. *Brain and Language, 37,* 409–418.

Aram, D. (1979, November). *Developmental apraxia of speech.* Paper presented at the annual convention of the American Speech and Hearing Association, Atlanta, GA.

Aram, D., & Horwitz, S. (1983). Sequential and non-speech praxic abilities in developmental verbal apraxia. *Developmental Medicine and Child Neurology, 25,* 197–206.

Arthur, G. (1952). *The Arthur adaptation of the Leiter International Performance Scale.* Washington, DC: Psychological Service Center.

Aten, J. (1979). *Denver Auditory Phoneme Sequencing Test.* Austin, TX: PRO-ED.

Bashir, A., Grahamjones, F., & Bostwick, R. (1984). A touch-cue method of therapy for developmental verbal apraxia. *Seminars in Speech and Language, 5,* 127–138.

Bernhardt, B., & Stoel-Gammon, C. (1994). Nonlinear phonology: Introduction and clinical application. *Journal of Speech and Hearing Research, 37,* 123–143.

Blakeley, R. (1983). Treatment of developmental apraxia of speech. In W. Perkins (Ed.), *Dysarthria and apraxia* (pp. 23–33). New York: Thieme-Stratton.

Blakeley, R. W. (1980). *Screening Test for Developmental Apraxia of Speech*. Austin, TX: PRO-ED.

Bowman, S. N., Parsons, C. L., & Mowis, D. A. (1984). Inconsistency of phonological errors in developmental verbal dyspraxia children as a factor of linguistic task and performance load. *Australian Journal of Human Communication Disorders, 12*, 109–119.

Bradford, A., & Dodd, B. (1996). Do all speech-disordered children have motor deficits? *Clinical Linguistics & Phonetics, 10*, 77–101.

Bridgeman, E., & Snowling, M. (1988). The perception of phoneme sequence: A comparison of dyspraxic and normal children. *British Journal of Disorders of Communication, 23*, 245–252.

Bruininks, R. (1978). *Bruininks-Oseretsky Test of Motor Proficiency*. Circle Pines, MN: American Guidance Service.

Carrow, E. (1974). *Carrow Elicited Language Inventory*. Lamar, TX: Learning Concepts.

Chappell, G. E. (1973). Childhood verbal apraxia and its treatment. *Journal of Speech and Hearing Disorders, 38*, 362–368.

Chappell, G. E. (1984). Developmental verbal dyspraxia: The expectant pattern. *Australian Journal of Human Communication Disorders, 23*, 15–25.

Chumpelik, D. (1984). The prompt system of therapy: Theoretical framework and applications for developmental apraxia of speech. *Seminars in Speech and Language, 5*, 139–153.

Cohen, M. J., Campbell, L. R., Elmore, J. A., & Yaghmai, F. (1988). Neuropathological abnormalities in developmental dysphasia: A case study. *Journal of Clinical and Experimental Neuropsychology, 10*, 56.

Costello, J., & Onstine, J. (1976). The modification of multiple articulation errors based on distinctive features theory. *Journal of Speech and Hearing Disorders, 42*, 199–215.

Court, D., & Harris, M. (1965). Speech disorders in children: Part 2. *British Medical Journal, 11,* 409–411.

Crary, M. A. (1984a). A neurolinguistic perspective on developmental verbal dyspraxia. *Communicative Disorders, 9,* 33–49.

Crary, M. A. (1984b). Phonological characteristics of developmental verbal dyspraxia. *Seminars in Speech and Language, 5,* 71–83.

Crary, M. A. (1993). *Developmental motor speech disorders.* San Diego, CA: Singular.

Crary, M. A., & Towne, R. L. (1984). The asynergistic nature of developmental verbal dyspraxia. *Australian Journal of Human Communication Disorders, 12,* 27–37.

Davis, B. L., Jakielski, K., & Marquardt, T. P. (1998). Developmental apraxia of speech: Determiners of differential diagnosis. *Clinical Linguistics & Phonetics, 12,* 25–45.

Davis, B. L., & MacNeilage, P. F. (1995). The articulatory basis of babbling. *Journal of Speech and Hearing Research, 38,* 1199–1211.

DeRenzi, E., Pieczuro, A., & Vignolo, L. A. (1966). Oral apraxia and aphasia. *Cortex, 2,* 50–73.

de Villiers, J., & de Villiers, P. (1973). A cross-sectional study of the acquisition of grammatical morphemes in child speech. *Journal of Psycholinguistic Research, 2,* 267–268.

Dodd, B., & McCormack, P. (1995). Differential diagnosis of phonological disorders. In B. Dodd (Ed.), *Differential diagnosis and treatment of children with speech disorder.* London: Whurr.

Dunn, L. M., & Dunn, L. M. (1981). *Peabody Picture Vocabulary Test—Revised.* Circle Pines, MN: American Guidance Service.

Edwards, M. (1973). Developmental verbal dyspraxia. *British Journal of Disorders of Communication, 8,* 64–70.

Ekelman, B. L., & Aram, D. (1984). Spoken syntax in children with developmental verbal apraxia. *Seminars in Speech and Language, 5,* 97–109.

Ekelman, B. L., & Aram, D. M. (1983). Syntactic findings in developmental verbal apraxia. *Journal of Communication Disorders, 16,* 237–250.

Ferry, P., Hall, S., & Hicks, J. (1975). Delapidated speech: Developmental verbal apraxia. *Developmental Medicine and Child Neurology, 17,* 749–756.

Galaburda, A. (1989). Ordinary and extraordinary brain development: Anatomical variation in developmental dyslexia. *Annals of Dyslexia, 39,* 67–79.

Galaburda, A., Sherman, G., Rosen, G., Aboitiz, F., & Geschwind, N. (1985). Developmental dyslexia: Four consecutive patients with cortical anomalies. *Annals of Neurology, 18,* 222–233.

Gauger, L. M., Lombardino, L. J., & Leonard, C. M. (1997). Brain morphology in children with specific language impairment. *Journal of Speech, Language, and Hearing Research, 40,* 1272–1284.

Goldman, R., & Fristoe, M. (1969). *Goldman-Fristoe Test of Articulation.* Circle Pines, MN: American Guidance Service.

Goodglass, H., & Kaplan, E. (1972). *The assessment of aphasia and related disorders.* Philadelphia: Lea & Febiger.

Gubbay, S., Ellis, E., Walton, J., & Court, S. (1965). Clumsy children: A study of apraxic and agnosic defects in 21 children. *Brain, 88,* 295–312.

Guyette, T., & Diedrich, W. (1981). A critical review of developmental apraxia of speech. In N. J. Lass (Ed.), *Speech and language: Advances in basic research and practice: Vol. 5.* (pp. 1–49). New York: Academic Press.

Guyette, T., & Diedrich, W. (1983). A review of Test for Developmental Apraxia of Speech. *Speech, Language, Hearing in Schools, 14,* 202–209.

Hall, P. K., Jordan, L. S., & Robin, D. A. (1993). *Developmental apraxia of speech: Theory and clinical practice.* Austin, TX: PRO-ED.

Hedrick, D., Prather, E., & Tobin, A. (1975). *Sequenced inventory of communication development.* Seattle: University of Washington Press.

Helfrich-Miller, K. R. (1984). Melodic intonation therapy with developmentally apraxic children. *Seminars in Speech and Language, 5,* 119–125.

Helm-Estabrooks, N. (1992). *Test of oral and limb apraxia.* Chicago: Riverside.

Hodson, B. (1980). *The assessment of phonological processes.* Austin, TX: PRO-ED.

Hodson, B., & Paden, E. (1982). *Targeting intelligible speech: A phonological approach to remediation.* Austin, TX: PRO-ED.

Horwitz, S. J. (1984). Neurological findings in developmental verbal apraxia. *Seminars in Speech and Language, 5,* 111–118.

Irwin, J., & Weston, A. (1971). *A manual for the clinical utilization of the paired-stimuli technique.* Memphis, TN: National Education Services.

Jernigan, T. L., Hesselink, J. R., Sowell, E., & Tallal, P. (1991). Cerebral structure on magnetic resonance imaging in language- and learning-impaired children. *Archives of Neurology, 48,* 539–545.

Jernigan, T. L., Tallal, P., & Bellugi, U. (1988). Cerebral morphology on magnetic resonance (MR) in developmental cognitive disorders. *Journal of Clinical and Experimental Neuropsychology, 10,* 19.

Kent, R. (1982). Contextual facilitation of correct production. *Language, Speech and Hearing Services in the Schools, 23,* 66–76.

Kent, R., Kent, J., & Rosenbek, J. C. (1988). Maximum performance tests of speech production. *Journal of Speech and Hearing Disorders, 52,* 367–387.

Kirk, S., McCarthy, J., & Kirk, W. (1968). *Illinois Test of Psycholinguistic Abilities.* Urbana: University of Illinois Press.

Klick, S. L. (1985). Adapted cueing technique for use in treatment of dyspraxia. *Language, Speech, and Hearing Services in Schools, 16,* 256–259.

Knuckey, N. W., Apsimon, T. T., & Gubbay, S. S. (1983). Computerized axial tomography in clumsy children with developmental apraxia and agnosia. *Brain and Development, 5,* 14–19.

Kools, J., Williams, A., Vickers, M., & Caell, A. (1971). Oral and limb apraxia in mentally retarded children with deviant articulation. *Cortex, 7*, 387–400.

Kools, J. A., & Tweedie, D. (1975). Development of praxis in children. *Perceptual and Motor Skills, 40*, 11–19.

Kornse, D. D., Manni, J. L., Rubenstein, H., & Graziani, L. J. (1981). Developmental apraxia of speech and manual dexterity. *Journal of Communication Disorders, 14*, 321–330.

Lee, L. (1971). *Northwestern Syntax Screening Test.* Evanston, IL: Northwestern University Press.

Lindblom, B., MacNeilage, P., & Studdert-Kennedy, M. (1988). *Biological bases of spoken language.* New York: Academic Press.

Logue, R., & McClumpha, S. (1970, November). *Apraxia of speech: A case description.* Paper presented at the annual convention of the American Speech and Hearing Association, New York.

Macaluso-Haynes, S. (1978). Developmental apraxia of speech: Symptoms and treatment. In D. F. Johns (Ed.), *Clinical management of neurogenic communication disorders* (pp. 243–250). Austin, TX: PRO-ED.

Marion, M., Sussman, H. M., & Marquardt, T. P. (1993). The perception and production of rhyme in normal and developmentally apraxic children. *Journal of Communication Disorders, 26*, 129–160.

Marquardt, T., Dunn, C., & Davis, B. (1985). Developmental apraxia of speech. In J. Darby (Ed.), *Speech and language evaluation in neurology: Childhood disorders* (pp. 113–129). New York: Grune & Stratton.

Marquardt, T. P., Sussman, H., & Snow, T. (1998). *The integrity of the syllable in developmental apraxia of speech.* Manuscript submitted for publication.

Mason, S. M., & Millor, D. H. (1984). Brain-stem, middle latency and late cortical evoked potentials in children with speech and language disorders. *Electroencephalography and Clinical Neurophysiology, 59*, 297–309.

McCabe, R., & Bradley, D. (1975). Systematic multiple phonemic approach to articulation therapy. *Acta Symbolica, 6*, 1–18.

McCarthy, D. (1972). *McCarthy Scales of Children's Abilities*. New York: Psychological Corp.

McClumpha, S., & Logue, R. (1972, November). *Approaches to children with motor programming disorders of speech*. Paper presented at the annual convention of the American Speech and Hearing Association, San Francisco.

McDonald, E. (1964). *Articulation testing and treatment: A sensory motor approach*. Pittsburgh: Stanwix House.

Milisen, R. (1954). A rationale for articulation disorders [monograph supplement]. *Journal of Speech and Hearing Disorders, 4*, 5–18.

Miller, J. (1981). *Assessing language production in children*. Austin, TX: PRO-ED.

Miller, N. (1992). Variability in speech dyspraxia. *Clinical Linguistics & Phonetics, 6*, 77–85.

Morley, M. E., & Fox, J. (1969). Disorders of articulation: Theory and therapy. *British Journal of Disorders of Communication, 4*, 151–165.

Murdoch, B. E., Porter, S., Younger, R., & Ozanne, A. (1984). Behaviours identified by south Australian clinicians as differentially diagnostic of developmental articulatory dyspraxia. *Australian Journal of Human Communication Disorders, 12*, 93–107.

Nemoy, E. M., & Davis, S. F. (1954). *The correction of defective consonant sounds*. Magnolia, MA: Expression Co.

Nicolosi, L., Harryman, E., & Kresheck, J. (1978). *Terminology of communication disorders: Speech, language, and hearing*. Baltimore: Williams & Wilkins.

Panagos, J. M., & Bobkoff, K. (1984). Beliefs about developmental apraxia of speech. *Australian Journal of Human Communication Disorders, 12*, 39–54.

Pannbacker, M. (1988). Management strategies for developmental apraxia of speech: A review of literature. *Journal of Communication Disorders, 21*, 363–371.

Plante, E. (1988, November). *MRI findings in children with specific language impairment*. Paper presented at the annual convention of the American Speech-Language-Hearing Association, Boston.

Plante, E., Swisher, L., Vance, R., & Rapcsak, S. (1991). MRI findings in boys with specific language impairment. *Brain and Language, 41*, 52–66.

Pollack, K. E., & Hall, P. K. (1991). An analysis of vowel misarticulations of five children with developmental apraxia of speech. *Clinical Lingusitics & Phonetics, 5*, 207–224.

Robin, D. (1992). Developmental apraxia of speech: Just another motor problem. *American Journal of Speech–Language Pathology, 1*, 119–122.

Roncagliolo, M., Benitez, J., & Perez, M. (1994). Auditory brainstem responses of children with developmental language disorders. *Developmental Medicine and Child Neurology, 36*, 26–33.

Rosenbek, J. C., Hansen, R., Baughman, C. H., & Lemme, M. (1974). Treatment of developmental apraxia of speech: A case study. *Language, Speech and Hearing Services in Schools, 5*, 13–22.

Rosenbek, J. C., & Wertz, R. T. (1972). A review of fifty cases of developmental apraxia of speech. *Language, Speech and Hearing Services in Schools, 3*, 23–33.

Schumacher, J. G., McNeil, M. R., Vetter, D. K., & Yoder, D. E. (1986). *Articulatory consistency and variability in apraxic and non-apraxic children*. Paper presented at the Convention of the American Speech-Language-Hearing Association, New Orleans.

Scripture, M. K., & Jackson, E. (1927). *A manual of exercises for the correction of speech disorders*. Philadelphia: Davis.

Shelton, I. K., & Graves, M. M. (1985). Use of visual techniques in therapy for developmental apraxia of speech. *Language, Speech and Hearing Services in Schools, 16*, 129–131.

Shriberg, L., Aram, D., & Kwiatkowski, J. (1997a). Developmental apraxia of speech: I. Descriptive and theoretical perspectives. *Journal of Speech, Language, and Hearing Research, 40*, 273–285.

Shriberg, L., Aram, D., & Kwiatkowski, J. (1997b). Developmental apraxia of speech: II. Toward a diagnostic marker. *Journal of Speech, Language, and Hearing Research, 40,* 286–312.

Shriberg, L., Aram, D., & Kwiatkowski, J. (1997c). Developmental apraxia of speech: III. A subtype marked by inappropriate stress. *Journal of Speech, Language, and Hearing Research, 40,* 313–337.

Shriberg, L., & Kwiatkowski, J. (1980). *Natural process analysis: A procedure for phonological analysis of continuous speech samples.* New York: Wiley.

Skinder, A., & Strand, E. (1998). *A perceptual and acoustic descriptive study of children with developmental apraxia of speech.* Paper presented at the Motor Speech Conference, Tucson, AZ.

Smartt, J., LaLance, L., Gray, J., & Hibbett, P. (1976). Developmental apraxia: A Tennessee Speech and Hearing Association subcommittee report. *Journal of the Tennessee Speech and Hearing Association, 20,* 21–39.

Smith, B., Marquardt, T., Cannito, M., & Davis, B. (1994). Vowel variability in developmental apraxia of speech. In J. Till, K. Yorkston, & D. Beukelman (Eds.), *Motor speech disorders: Advances in assessment and treatment.* Baltimore: Brookes.

Snyder, D., Marquardt, T., & Peterson, H. (1977). Syntactical aspects of developmental apraxia. *Human Communication, 2,* 151–158.

Sparks, R., & Holland, A. (1976). Method: Melodic intonation therapy. *Journal of Speech and Hearing Disorders, 41,* 287–297.

Square, P. (1994). Treatment approaches for developmental apraxia of speech. *Clinics in Communication Disorders, 4,* 151–161.

Stackhouse, J. (1992). Developmental verbal dyspraxia: I. A review and critique. *European Journal of Disorders of Communication, 27,* 19–34.

Stackhouse, J., & Snowling, M. (1992). Developmental verbal dyspraxia: II. A developmental perspective on two case studies. *European Journal of Disorder of Communication, 27,* 35–54.

Stoel-Gammon, C., & Dunn, C. (1985). *Normal and disordered phonology in children.* Austin, TX: PRO-ED.

Strand, E. (1995). Treatment of motor speech disorders in children. *Seminars in Speech and Language, 16*, 126–139.

Suga, N., O'Neill, W. E., Kujirai, K., & Manabe, T. (1983). Specificity of combination-sensitive neurons for processing of complex biosonar signals in auditory cortex of the moustached bat. *Journal of Neurophysiology, 49*, 1573–1627.

Sussman, H. M. (1986). A neuronal model of vowel normalization and representation. *Brain and Language, 28*, 12–23.

Sussman, H. M. (1988). The neurogenesis of phonology. In H. Whitaker (Ed.), *Phonological processes and brain mechanisms* (pp. 1–23). New York: Springer-Verlag.

Sussman, H. M. (1989). The neural coding of relational invariance in speech: Human language analogs to the barn owl. *Psychological Review, 96*, 631–642.

Templin, M. (1957). *Certain language skills in children*. Minneapolis: University of Minnesota Press.

Templin, M., & Darley, F. (1969). *The Templin-Darley Tests of Articulation* (2nd ed.). Iowa City: University of Iowa.

Thoonen, G., Maassen, B., Gabreels, F., & Schreuder, R. (1994). Feature analyais of singleton consonant errors in developmental verbal dyspraxia (DVD). *Journal of Speech and Hearing Research, 37*, 1424–1440.

Thoonen, G., Maassen, B., Gabreels, F., Schreuder, R., & de Swart, B. (1997). Towards a standardized assessment procedure for developmental apraxia of speech. *European Journal of Disorders of Communication, 32*, 37–60.

Van Riper, C. (1978). *Speech correction: Principles and methods*. Englewood Cliffs, NJ: Prentice Hall.

Vargha-Khadem, F., Watters, G. V., & O'Gorman, A. M. (1985). Development of speech and language following bilateral frontal lesions. *Brain and Language, 25*, 167–183.

Velleman, S. L., & Strand, K. (1994). Developmental verbal dyspraxia. In J. E. Bernthal & N. W. Bankson (Eds.), *Child phonology: Characteristics, assessment, and intervention with special populations* (pp. 110–139). New York: Thieme.

Walton, J., Ellis, E., & Court, S. (1962). Clumsy children: Developmental apraxia and agnosia. *Brain, 85,* 603–612.

Wechsler, D. (1975). *Wechsler Intelligence Scale for Children—Revised.* New York: Psychological Corp.

Weeks, R. A., & Madison, C. L. (1985). Screening test of developmental apraxia of speech: Validity and reliability. *Asha, 27,* 82.

Werker, J. F., Gilbert, J., Humphrey, K., & Tees, R. C. (1981). Developmental aspects of cross-language speech perception. *Child Development, 52,* 349–355.

Werker, J. F., & Tees, R. C. (1984). Cross-language speech perception: Evidence for perceptual reorganization during the first year of life. *Infant Behavior and Development, 7,* 49–63.

Williams, R., Ingham, R. J., & Rosenthal, J. (1981). A further analysis for developmental apraxia of speech. *Journal of Speech and Hearing Research, 24,* 496–505.

Yoss, K. A., & Darley, F. (1973, November). *What happens to children with developmental apraxia of speech? A follow-up of fifteen cases.* Paper presented at the annual convention of the American Speech and Hearing Association, Detroit, MI.

Yoss, K. A., & Darley, F. (1974a). Developmental apraxia of speech in children with defective articulation. *Journal of Speech and Hearing Research, 17,* 399–416.

Yoss, K. A., & Darley, F. (1974b). Therapy in developmental apraxia of speech. *Language, Speech and Hearing Services in Schools, 1,* 23–31.

Young, E., & Hawk, S. (1955). *Moto-kinesthetic speech training.* Stanford, CA: Stanford University Press.

Author Index

Abbs, J. H., 64, 95, 96, 211, 212, 379
Abkarian, G. G., 16, 145, 222
Aboitiz, F., 427
Abramson, A. S., 287
Adams, M. R., 377–378, 382
Adams, S., 101, 105, 211, 219, 379
Aftonomos, L. B., 16
Agnello, J., 378
Ahern, M., 219
Ainsworth, T., 177
Akshoomoff, N., 425
Albert, M., 16, 241
Alexander, M., 208, 210, 241, 336
Alfonso, P. J., 377–406
Alfrey, A. C., 258
Alp, L. A., 92
American Academy of Neurology, 350, 352
Aminoff, M. J., 344
Anderson, J., 210
Andrews, B., 258, 259
Andrews, G., 246, 264
Andy, O. J., 262
Antonak, R., 160, 162
Appelbaum, J. S., 16
Apsimon, T. T., 425
Aram, D., 415, 416, 417, 420, 421, 433, 441
Arend, R., 243, 255
Arnold, G. E., 326
Arnold, R., 242–243
Aronson, A. E., 18, 64, 79, 91, 103, 119–120, 203, 245, 322, 323, 325, 326, 331, 333, 334–335, 339, 340, 344, 354
Arthur, G., 446
Ashby, P., 329
Aten, J., 103, 421, 433
Attanasio, J. S., 251
Avent, J. R., 244
Axelrod, J., 327

Bacon, M., 323
Baer, T., 383
Baird, M., 173
Baken, R. J., 388, 389
Bakker, K., 356
Balan, A., 290
Banzett, R. B., 88
Baran, J. A., 280
Baratz, R., 258, 261
Barbeau, A., 330, 338
Barkmeier, J., 129, 139
Barlow, S. M., 82, 94, 95, 96, 379
Barnes, G. J., 91
Barroso, A. B., 65, 67
Bashir, A., 443
Bassich, C. J., 83, 91
Bauer, R. M., 282
Baughman, C. H., 417
Baumgartner, J., 211, 240, 246, 251–252
Baum, S. R., 280, 282–284, 288–290
Bayles, K., 176
Beaton, L. E., 329
Behrens, S. J., 279, 280–282, 288
Beland, R., 199
Bell, K., 80, 120, 359

Bellugi, U., 427
Bender, B., 360
Benitez, J., 425
Bennett, R., 176, 177
Benson, D. F., 243, 336
Berkman, L., 172
Bernard, J., 174
Bernhardt, B., 415
Bernstein-Ellis, E., 16
Berry, M. F., 278
Berry, W., 105, 126, 378
Beukleman, D. R., 80, 83, 86, 93, 100, 105, 120, 131, 138, 144, 145, 221, 359, 361
Bhatnagar, S. C., 262
Bielamowicz, S., 354
Binnie, C. A., 129
Blakely, R., 422, 431, 438, 454, 460
Bless, D. M., 101
Blitzer, A., 332
Blonder, L. X., 280, 281, 282
Blonsky, E. R., 95
Blood, G., 378
Bloodstein, O., 67, 68, 70
Bloomer, H. H., 103
Blumstein, S. E., 281, 290
Bobkoff, K., 420
Boccino, J. V., 325
Boller, F., 67
Bollier, B., 219
Bombardier, C., 108, 130
Bonitati, C., 100, 120
Boone, D. R., 322
Borden, G., 212, 383, 387
Boshes, B., 95
Boss, P., 170

475

Bostwick, R., 443
Botez, M. I., 330, 338
Boutsen, F., 356
Bowers, D., 280, 282, 286
Bowman, S. N., 417, 420
Boyczuk, J. P., 290
Boyle, M., 225
Boysen, A. E., 79
Bradford, A., 419
Bradley, D., 435
Bradley, W. G., 50
Bradvik, B., 282, 286
Brady, J. P., 68
Bray, G., 168, 169
Breckenridge, J., 292
Brennen, T., 198
Brewer, D., 383
Brewer, R. P., 63
Brickman, P., 165
Bridgeman, E., 415
Bril, V., 329
Brin, M., 332
Brodnitz, F. S., 323
Brookshire, R. H., 8
Brown, D., 382
Brown, J. R., 18, 64, 79, 119–120, 203, 245, 322, 323, 334, 344
Brown, S., 382
Brown, W. S., 333
Bruininks, R., 433, 454
Brumlik, J., 334
Bryan, K. L., 280–282, 288
Bryan, W., 162, 185
Bryant, F., 165
Buckingham, H., 198, 199, 203
Buder, E. H., 91, 95, 356
Buffalo, M. D., 249–250
Burns, M., 210
Burton, M. K., 96
Burton, S., 355
Butler, I. J., 52
Butler, R. B., 243, 263
Butler, S. M., 280
Butterworth, B., 196, 198, 199, 200, 202, 208

Caell, A., 433
Caldognetto, E. M., 282
Califiuri, M., 378
Callaway, E. A., 252
Calne, D. B., 47
Cambell-Taylor, I., 176
Campbell, L. R., 427
Cancelliere, A. E. B., 280, 282, 283, 286
Candy, S., 176
Cannito, M. P., 16, 126–129, 131, 138, 139, 144, 212, 239–269, 321–363, 417
Canter, G. J., 69, 91, 210, 214, 215, 216, 243, 245, 249
Caplan, D., 199, 210
Caplan, G., 160
Caplan, L., 254
Caramazza, A., 198, 206
Cariski, D., 219
Carpeggiani, P., 243
Carpenter, M. B., 326, 329
Carrow, E., 446, 454
Carter, C. R., 128, 131
Carter, J. E., 31
Carter, P. B., 31
Casiano, R. R., 355
Casper, J. K., 91, 101
Cedarbaum, J. M., 45–48, 51–57, 59–61, 63–64
Chappell, G. E., 416, 417, 421, 438, 439, 440
Chesselet, M. F., 43, 46
Childers, D. G., 389
Chumpelik, D., 219, 220, 442
Clark, R. G., 326
Cohen, M. J., 427, 428
Cohen, R., 285
Cohn, M., 388
Cole, K., 95, 379
Coleman, J., 198, 210
Collins, M., 219, 222, 254
Colsher, P. L., 283
Committee on Aging, 174

Connor, N., 346
Conture, E., 382, 383, 395
Cooper, I. S., 331
Cooper, J. R., 40, 41, 42, 48
Cooper, W. E., 279, 281–286, 288, 290, 296, 297, 306, 308, 309
Corey, G., 184
Coslett, B., 290
Coslett, H. B., 280, 282
Costello, J., 425, 436
Cotelingam, M., 68
Coufal, K. J., 382
Coulton, R. H., 91, 101
Countryman, S., 100, 120
Couper-Kuhlen, E., 279, 285, 288
Courchesne, E., 425
Court, D., 419
Court, S., 419–420
Crary, M. A., 355, 415, 416, 420, 421, 426, 427, 440
Critchley, M., 245, 331, 344
Cronk, C., 378
Crow, E., 105, 138
Cruttenden, A., 285
Cullata, R., 240, 241
Curlee, R. F., 248

Dabul, B., 216, 217, 218, 219
Dagenais, P. A., 127, 129, 138, 216
Dalby, M., 282, 286
Dalton, P., 248
Damasio, A., 210
Damasio, H., 210, 283
Daniel, B., 82, 378
Daniloff, K. J., 288
Daniloff, R., 288, 404
Danly, M., 280–282, 284–286, 288, 290
Dardaranada, R., 287, 288, 290
Darley, F., 18, 64, 79–81, 83, 85, 104,

119–120, 203, 244, 245, 323, 334, 340, 359, 416, 418–419, 422, 431, 446, 454
Daroff, R. B., 50
David, D., 198
Davis, B. L., 413–463
Davis, S. F., 436
Deal, J., 219, 239–269
DeBito, M. A., 71
Dechongkit, S., 280
Deck, J., 221
Dedo, H. H., 322, 325, 331, 335, 339, 344
DeLacoste-Utamsing, C., 290
Deleyiannis, F. W. B., 354
Delfs, J. M., 43, 46
Dell, G., 196, 198–205, 207
Dembowski, J., 378, 393, 394, 396, 397
Dempsey, G. L., 240
Denes, G., 282
DeNil, L. F., 247–248
DeRenzi, E., 433, 454
DeSanto, L. W., 322, 325
De Swart, B., 430
Devereaux, F., 252
De Villiers, J., 285, 454
De Villiers, P., 454
Devous, M. D., 246–247, 353, 354
De Vresse, L., 282
Diamond, I. T., 337
Diedrich, W., 414, 416, 431
Dietrich, S., 250
DiLollo, A., 69, 239–269
Dodd, B., 418, 419
Dodson, L., 326
Dogali, M., 63
Doherty, W., 173
Dongilli, P., Jr., 126–127, 131
Donnan, G. A., 254, 255, 262
Doody, R. S., 355
Doro, J. M., 240, 251

Dowden, P., 131
Downie, A. W., 105, 264
Doyle, P., 213, 222
Driver, L. E., 252
Dromey, C., 93, 100, 120, 356
Drummond, S. S., 249–250
Dubner, R., 327
DuBois, A. B., 94
Duffy, J. R., 8, 80, 86, 87, 104, 211, 212, 214, 240, 246, 251–252, 259, 351
Dunham, M., 221
Dunn, C., 459
Dunn, L., 227, 432, 437
Dunn, M., 163
Dworkin, J. P., 16, 102, 104, 145, 222
Dyck, P. J., 325

Eady, S. J., 279, 286, 297
Edmonston, J. A., 280
Edwards, M., 416, 420
Ehlers, L., 282, 286
Ekelman, B. L., 415, 420, 441
Ekman, P., 138
Elliot, R. L., 259
Elliott, L. L., 126
Ellis, E., 419–420
Elman, R. J., 16
Elmore, J. A., 427
Emmorey, K. D., 280, 288–289
Enderby, P., 88, 105, 138
Eng, N., 287
Erber, N. P., 129
Evans, R., 170
Evarts, E. V., 357
Ewan, W. G., 310

Fahn, S., 47, 332, 333
Fairbanks, G., 248
Farmer, R., 183, 185
Feldman, L., 281
Feldman, M., 323, 326

Ferry, P., 419
Feyereisen, P., 282
Filstead, W., 179
Finichel, G. M., 50
Finitzo-Hieber, T., 322, 323, 326
Finitzo, T., 246–247, 323, 347, 349, 353, 354
Fink, M., 332
Fischer, J. M., 336
Fisher, B., 225
Fisher, H. B., 95
Fleet, W. S., 256
Florance, C., 219
Flowers, C. R., 280, 282
Fluchaire, I., 198
Fok, A. Y.-Y., 287
Folkins, J., 212
Foltz, E. L., 329
Ford, C. N., 101
Ford, J., 331
Forrest, K., 96, 379
Fox, D., 322
Fox, J., 419, 438
Fox, P. T., 247
Franzen, E. A., 335
Frazier, K., 220
Freed, D., 220
Freedman, M., 336, 348
Freeman, F., 69, 246–248, 322, 323, 326, 331, 339, 347, 349, 353, 354, 395
Freund, H., 240
Friedrich, F., 210
Friesen, W. V., 138
Fristoe, M., 431
Fukusako, Y., 214

Gabreels, F., 416, 430
Gacek, P. R., 71
Gagnon, D., 196, 204
Galaburda, A., 426, 427
Gandour, J., 280, 287–290
Garcia, J., 119–150, 216, 299
Garrett, K., 221

Gauger, J., 355
Gauger, L. M., 426, 427
Gay, T., 383
Gazzaniga, M. S., 348
Gearing, M., 63
Gerber, K., 165
Gerling, I., 326
Gerratt, B. R., 79
Gertsman, L. J., 282
Geschwind, N., 427
Gibbons, P., 103
Gilbert, J., 428
Gillespie, M., 354
Ginsberg, A. P., 323, 339
Gintautus, J., 244
Glaser, L., 220
Glenn, C., 210
Goebel, M., 378
Goetz, C. J., 54, 55, 64
Goffman, E., 176, 177, 180
Goldberg, S. A., 240
Goldman, M., 179, 381
Goldman, R., 431
Goldstein, J. A., 70
Goloskie, S., 282
Gonzalez, J., 103
Goodglass, H., 223, 227, 241, 284, 454
Goodglass, J., 198
Goodstein, R., 160
Gordon, C. D., 68
Gorelick, P. B., 281
Gorham, M., 355
Gorusch, R. L., 346
Goshorn, E. L., 105, 126, 378
Gottesman, L., 179
Gowing, P., 335
Gracco, L. C., 92
Gracco, V. L., 92, 211, 212
Graff-Radford, N. R., 283, 288, 306, 308, 309
Grahamjones, F., 443
Granich, M., 240
Graves, M. M., 442
Gray, J., 416
Graziani, L., 419
Greenberg, S., 164, 183

Greenwald, B., 259
Grela, B., 288–290
Gubbay, S., 419, 425
Guitar, B., 265, 266, 378
Gutierrez, R., 103
Guyette, T., 414, 416, 431

Hall, J. W., 326
Hall, P. K., 415, 416, 422, 434, 441
Hall, S., 419
Hallett, M., 51, 72
Hamby, S., 285
Hammen, V. L., 79–109, 128, 130, 131
Handzel, L., 243
Hanna, R., 378
Hansen, R., 417
Hanson, W., 105, 263–264
Hardcastle, W. J., 248
Hardman, J. G., 31, 34
Hardy, J., 98, 103
Harley, T., 200, 201, 204, 205
Harney, J. H., 290
Harris, E., 219
Harris, K. S., 287
Harris, M., 419
Harryman, E., 417
Hartman, D. E., 64, 333, 356
Hasbrouk, J., 378
Hashi, M., 216
Hast, M. H., 336
Hawk, S., 435
Hawley, J., 99
Hays, P., 70
Hayward, R. W., 348
Head, H., 242
Heath, R. L., 280
Hedrick, D., 432, 446
Heilman, K. M., 256, 280, 282, 283, 286, 290
Hekeler, R., 183
Helfrich-Miller, K. R., 444
Helm, N. A., 105, 145, 241, 243, 245, 255–256, 258, 262

Helm-Estabrooks, N. A., 146, 240, 245, 246, 249–251, 253, 257–261, 263, 266, 267, 269, 433
Henderson, G., 162, 185
Hesselink, J. R., 425–426
Heuer, R. J., 267
Hibbett, P., 416
Hicks, J., 419
Hickson, M. L., 138
Hill, A. B., 29
Hill, R., 170
Hillel, A. D., 90
Hillis, A., 198, 206
Hillis, J., 378
Hinkel, K., 102
Hinton, V. A., 94
Hireose, H., 383
Hixon, T., 92, 99, 381, 388
Hodge, M., 83
Hodson, B., 436, 454, 461
Hoehn, M., 120
Hoit, J. D., 88
Holland, A., 221, 223, 443
Holtzapple, P., 221
Holzman, J. D., 348
Homan, R. W., 280
Honsinger, M. J., 93
Horii, Y., 100, 120
Horner, J., 227, 245, 246, 256
Horwitz, S., 421, 424, 433
Hoskins, B., 133, 141
Hotz, G., 240, 251
Hough, M., 213–216
Houle, S., 248
House, E. L., 328, 329, 330
Hubbard, D. J., 129
Hudson, A., 176
Hughes, O., 211
Hulstijn, W., 384
Humphrey, K., 428
Hunker, C. H., 96
Hunter, L., 213, 215, 216
Hutchinson, J. M., 382
Hux, K., 221
Hyland, J., 221

Imber-Black, E., 172
Ingelfinger, J. A., 30
Ingham, R. J., 247, 424
Ireland, J., 215
Irwin, J., 436
Itoh, M., 214
Izdebski, K., 322, 325, 326, 327, 344, 356

Jackson, 277
Jackson, E., 435
Jackson, P. L., 129
Jackson, S., 184
Jacob, J. C., 335
Jacobs, G. A., 346
Jakielski, K., 418
Jankovic, J., 48, 51, 53, 62, 69, 71, 72, 330, 331, 333
Jenkins, J. J., 242–243
Jerger, J., 326
Jernigan, T. L., 425–428
Jimenez-Pabon, E., 242–243
Joanette, Y., 210, 281
Johns, D. F., 16, 103, 145, 222, 244
Johnson, A. B., 100, 120
Johnson, J. P., 321, 323, 339
Jones, K., 170, 173
Jongman, A., 285
Jordan, L. S., 139, 278, 415
Jurgens, U., 66–67, 327, 329–330, 335, 336, 338

Kaas, J. H., 337
Kahana, E., 177
Kaiser, G., 258
Kalikow, D. N., 126
Kalinyak-Fliszar, M., 221
Kalotkin, M., 68
Kaplan, E., 223, 227, 284, 454
Kapur, S., 248
Karnell, M. P., 94

Kastenbaum, R., 176
Kaszniak, A., 176
Katz, W., 285
Kebabian, J. W., 41
Keller, E., 211
Kelley, A. H., 329, 337
Kelso, J. A. S., 337
Kennedy, M. R. T., 132
Kenney, M. K., 383
Kent, J. F., 83, 433
Kent, R., 81, 82, 83, 87, 93, 95, 211, 216, 245, 248, 280, 290, 291, 433, 436
Kertesz, A., 280, 283, 284, 286, 336
Khunadorn, F., 280
Kiml, P. J., 328, 334
Kirk, S., 521
Kirk, W., 421
Kirzinger, A., 327, 335
Klawans, H. L., 54, 55, 64
Klich, R., 213–216
Klick, S. L., 442
Klouda, G. V., 285, 288, 290–291, 293, 296, 304, 306, 308, 309
Knopp, L. M., 329
Knuckey, N. W., 425
Koch-Weser, J., 31
Kohn, S., 196, 199, 200, 202–204, 206, 208–210
Koller, W. C., 53, 245, 258
Kondraske, G. V., 346
Kools, J. A., 419, 433, 454
Kornhuber, H. H., 357
Kornse, D. D., 419
Kotzur, I. M., 355
Koury, L. N., 178, 180
Kramer, L., 280
Kresheck, J., 417
Krishnamurthy, A. K., 389
Kroll, R. M., 248
Kuehn, D. P., 102, 211
Kujirai, K., 427
Kushner-Vogel, D., 129
Kuypers, H. A., 337

Kwiatkowski, J., 415–417, 432

Lagerlund, T. D., 354
LaLance, L., 416
Lang, A. E., 43–47, 52–55, 59–61, 63–64, 331–332
Lanyon, R., 378
LaPointe, L. L., 99, 101, 103, 104, 120, 217, 227, 245, 264, 298, 300, 358
Larochelle, L., 329
Larsen, J., 280
Larson, C., 335
Lea, W. A., 279
Lebrun, Y., 246, 252–254, 258–259, 282, 286
Lecours, A., 210
Lee, L., 420
Leeper, L., 241
Leleux, C., 246, 252–254, 259, 282
Lemkau, J., 165
Lemke, J. H., 100, 120
Lemme, M., 211, 219, 258, 417
Leonard, C. M., 426
Lessines, A., 282
Lester, G., 170
Levelt, W., 196, 198, 199, 200, 202
Lewis, J., 288
Lieberman, M., 177
Lieberman, P., 285, 292
Limbird, L. E., 31, 34
Lindblom, B., 427
Lindeman, R. C., 335
Lindsay, D. D., 105, 264
Linebaugh, C., 104
Liss, J. M., 82, 102, 103, 144, 290
Litin, M. E., 322, 323, 344
Liu, C.-Y., 359
Livneh, H., 160, 162
Lofqvist, A., 92, 211, 212
Logemann, J. A., 95

Logue, R., 418, 419
Lombardino, L. J., 426
Longstretch, D., 219
Lorell, D. M., 96
Lotts, D. W., 296
Lotz, W. K., 82
Louera, B., 360
Lovelace, R., 332
Low, J. M., 105, 264
Lozano, R., 1–24
Lubinski, R., 157–189
Luchsinger, R., 242–243, 326
Ludlow, C. L., 68, 83, 91, 332, 346, 354
Lu, F.-L., 355
Lundy, D. S, 355
Luschei, E. S., 82, 96
Lushene, R., 346
Luterman, D., 169
Lyon, J. G., 146

Maassen, B., 416, 430
Macaluso-Haynes, S., 421, 438
MacAndrew, S., 204, 205
MacIntire, D., 323
MacNeilage, P., 427, 438
Madison, C. L., 431
Magoun, H. W., 329
Maitz, E., 170
Mallory, A., 129
Malmgren, L. T., 71
Manabe, T., 427
Mandel, S., 267
Manni, J. L., 419
Manning, W. H., 382
Marek, K. P., 92
Marin, O., 210
Marion, M., 429
Market, K. E., 249–250, 265–266, 269
Maroun, F. B., 335, 336
Marquardt, T., 16, 212, 413–463
Marsden, C. D., 47, 50, 331–333
Marshall, R., 220, 221, 225, 226, 265, 269

Martinez, A., 222
Martin, N., 196, 204–207
Martin, R., 83, 176, 211, 214
Maslach, C., 183–185
Mason, S. M., 425
Massaro, D. W., 129
Massey, E. W., 245, 246, 256
Mateer, C. A., 279, 280, 292
Matessich, J., 360
Max, J. E., 96
Mazzuchi, A., 243, 254, 258
McCabe, R., 435
McCall, G. N., 323, 326, 332, 337, 383
McCarthy, D., 446
McCarthy, J., 421
McClean, A. J., 259
McClean, M. D., 259
McClumpha, S., 418, 419
McCormack, P., 418
McCubbin, H., 170, 171
McDonald, A., 103
McDonald, E., 435, 457
McDowell, F. H., 45–48, 51–57, 59–61, 63–64
McHenry, M. A., 97
McKeehan, A., 247
McNeil, B., 378
McNeil, D., 213–217
McNeil, M., 221, 222, 258, 290, 379, 417
McNeill, D., 138
Mead, J., 381
Meghji, C., 259
Merson, R. M., 323, 339
Merzenich, M. M., 337
Messert, B., 254
Mesulam, M. M., 258, 261, 280–282
Metter, E. J., 105, 263–264
Metz, D., 129, 382
Meyer, A., 199, 200
Meyer, R., 378
Meyers, R., 338
Michelow, D., 282
Milenkovic, P. H., 295

Milisen, R., 436
Miller, C. J., 404
Miller, J., 432
Miller, L., 119–150, 299
Miller, M., 182, 285
Miller, N., 418
Miller, R. M., 90
Miller, S., 216
Millor, D., 425
Milojevic, B., 336
Minifie, F. D., 105
Minton, J. J., 97
Mirra, S. S., 63
Monahan, L., 183
Monoi, H., 214, 215
Monrad-Krohn, G. H., 277–279
Monsen, R., 131
Montague, J. C., Jr., 249–250
Montgomery, A. A., 129
Moore, P., 334, 344
Moore, W., 378
Morely, M. E., 438
Moretti, G., 243
Morley, M. E., 419
Morningstar, E., 219
Morris, H., 103
Morrison, E., 177
Morrissey, P., 326
Mosteller, F., 30
Mowis, D., 417
Mueller, P. R., 279, 296
Murdoch, B. E., 92, 417
Murgatroyd, S., 182
Murphy, A. T., 323
Murray, E., 381
Murry, T., 91, 333, 356, 359, 360, 378
Myers, P. S., 278, 298, 299
Myers, R. E., 335

Naeser, M., 210, 336, 348
Nagel, H. N., 286
Nash, E. A., 332
Nawy, R., 286
Nekemikis, A., 165
Nemoy, E. M., 436

Nespoulous, J., 199, 210, 215
Netsell, R., 79, 82, 99, 103, 104, 378
Netter, F. H., 36, 39
Neuberger, S. I., 265–266, 269
Newhoff, M., 221
Nicol, J., 282
Nicolosi, L., 417
Niemi, J., 288
Nies, A. S., 31
Nixon, J. V., 323
Noll, J. D., 102
Nowack, W. J., 251–253, 256, 262, 266–267
Nudelman, H. B., 67
Nurnberg, H. G., 259

Obler, L. K., 287
O'Brien, C., 120
Odell, K., 213, 215–216
O'Gorman, A. M., 424
Ohala, J. J., 285, 310
O'Neill, W. E., 427
Onstine, J., 436
Orpwood, L., 198
O'Seaghdha, P., 198–201
O'Shaughnessy, D., 286
Ouellette, G., 289
Owens, R. E., Jr., 125
Oxman, T., 172
Ozanne, A., 417

Packard, J. L., 287, 288
Paden, E., 436, 461
Paini, P., 243
Palumbo, C., 210
Panagos, J., 420
Pannbacker, M., 434
Pansky, B., 328
Parma, M., 243
Parsons, C. L., 417
Patterson, J., 171
Pawlas, A. A., 100
Pearl Solomon, N., 96
Pearson, J. S., 322, 323, 344
Pechadre, J. C., 329
Pellat, J., 198

Pell, M. D., 280, 282–284, 286
Penfield, W., 335
Perez, K. E., 93
Perez, M., 425
Perkins, J. M., 280, 283
Perkins, W. H., 248
Peters, H. F. M., 384
Peterson, H., 420
Petty, H. S., 287
Pick, 277
Pick, C. G., 262
Pickering, J. E., 280
Pieczuro, A., 433
Pierce, R., 195–227, 214
Pike, K. L., 285
Pines, A., 184, 185
Plante, E., 426, 428
Ploog, D., 66–67, 329–330, 337, 338
Poirier, L. J., 329
Pollack, K. E., 416
Ponglorpisit, S., 280
Pool, K. D., 246–247, 349
Porfert, A. R., 67
Porter, S., 417
Potter, R., 182
Power, P., 168
Prather, E., 432
Pratt, R., 329–330, 337, 338
Prescott, T. E., 258
Proctor, J., 247
Purdy, P. D., 290
Purves, D., 41, 42
Putnam-Rochet, A., 94

Quader, S. E., 259
Quinn, P. T., 246, 258, 259

Raines, S., 173
Ramig, L. A., 91
Ramig, L. L., 100
Ramig, L. O., 16, 91, 93, 100, 120
Rao, P., 221
Rapcsak, S., 426
Rappoport, J. L., 68
Rasmussen, T., 281
Rauth, T., 174

Ravits, J. M., 325
Raymer, A., 222
Read, C., 95
Reed, C., 326
Reich, A., 346
Reis, R., 382
Remits, A., 282
Rentschler, G. J., 252, 259
Retif, J., 258
Riemenschneider, S., 382
Rigrodski, S., 177
Riley, D. E., 43–47, 52–55, 59–61, 63–64
Ringel, S. P., 91
Ringo, C. C., 250
Roark, R., 323
Robe, E., 334, 344
Roberts, L., 335
Robey, R. R., 16
Robin, D., 96, 139, 214, 277–311, 415
Rodnitzky, R. L., 96, 278
Rogers, C., 182
Rogers, M., 215, 216, 222
Roncagliolo, M., 425
Rosen, G., 427
Rosenbek, J. C., 79, 80, 83, 99, 101, 103, 104, 120, 213, 215–219, 222, 244–245, 254, 255, 256, 258, 264, 265, 267, 269, 280, 290, 291, 298, 300, 358, 359, 416, 417, 419, 420, 422, 423, 433, 438, 440, 460
Rosenberger, P. B., 68
Rosenfield, D. B., 27–73, 254, 331, 339, 344, 355, 358, 360, 361
Rosenstock, R., 179
Rosenthal, J., 424
Ross, E. D., 280–283, 285–286, 290, 348, 352
Rossi, J., 179
Rothenberg, M., 390
Rothenberg, R., 179
Rousseau, J. J., 252
Rowland, L. P., 325

Rubens, A. B., 241, 336
Rubenstein, H., 419
Rubow, R., 101, 378
Rudensey, K., 182
Runyan, C., 377–378
Ryalls, J. H., 279, 281, 284–285

Sackner, M., 388
Saffran, E., 196, 204, 205, 207
Safilios-Rothchild, C., 162
Salvatore, A., 16
Samandari, R., 93
Sapienza, C. M., 333
Sapir, S., 323
Sasanuma, S., 214
Sataloff, R. T., 267
Saunders, W. B., 341
Sawashima, M., 383
Schaefer, S., 323, 326–328, 332, 338, 339, 347, 355
Schecter, J., 160
Scherer, K. R., 279
Scherer, R. C., 91
Schiavetti, N., 129
Schiller, F., 246
Schlanger, B. B., 282–283, 286
Schlanger, P., 282
Schmidt, R., 214
Schneider, J. A., 63
Schnell, H., 224
Scholes, R., 282
Schreiber, S., 262
Schreuder, R., 416, 430
Schuell, H., 242–243, 264
Schulz, G. M., 354
Schumacher, J. G., 417
Schum, R. L., 139
Schwartz, M., 196, 204, 207
Schweiger, J., 103
Scott, C. M., 141
Scripture, M. K., 435
Seddoh, S., 213, 214, 216, 277–311
Seibert, G. B., 280
Selkirk, E. O., 279

Seman, T., 172
Semenza, C., 282
Seron, X., 282–283, 286
Sessle, B. J., 327
Seth, G., 381
Shapiro, A., 383
Shapiro, B., 280–282, 284–286, 288, 290
Shapiro, D. A., 240, 245, 257, 258, 261
Shapiro, L. P., 286
Sharbrough, F. W., 326
Sharpe, J. A., 329
Shattuck-Hufnagel, S., 199, 200, 202
Shea, S. A., 88
Sheehy, M. P., 331
Sheldon, S., 247
Shelton, I. K., 442
Sherman, G., 427
Shipp, T., 326, 327, 332, 356
Shriberg, L., 415–418, 422, 429–430, 432
Sidtis, J. J., 280, 282, 283, 286, 289, 291, 348
Siegal, A., 328
Siegel, S., 340
Silber, S. R., 91
Simmons-Mackie, N., 226
Simmons, N., 219, 222
Simpson, M., 103
Sitler, R. W., 129
Ska, B., 210
Skelly, M., 221
Skinder, A., 416, 417, 418
Smartt, J., 416, 419, 438
Smith, B., 417
Smith, C. D., 280
Smith, K., 196, 199, 200, 202–204, 206, 208–209
Smith, M. E., 93
Smith, P. J., 332
Smitheran, J., 92
Snowling, M., 415, 430
Snyder, D., 420
Soares, C., 282
Solomon, N. P., 96

Sorby, W. A., 246
Sorensen, J. M., 279, 288, 297
Southwood, H., 216, 379
Sowell, E., 425–426
Sparks, R., 221, 443
Speedie, L., 280, 282, 290
Spielberg, S. T., 31
Spielberger, C. D., 346, 359
Square, P., 176, 211, 214, 219, 434
Square-Storer, P., 220
Stackhouse, J., 415, 430
Stacks, D. W., 138
Stager, S. V., 68
Starch, S. A., 265
Steele, R. D., 16
Stevens, E., 220
Stevens, K. N., 126, 279, 382
Stierwalt, J. A. G., 96, 104
Stillman, R., 329
Stockard, J. J., 326
Stoel-Gammon, C., 415, 459
Stone, R. E., 251–253, 256, 262, 266–267
Stoof, J. C., 41
Storey, A. T., 327
Storkel, H., 216
Stott, F., 388
Strand, E., 80, 91, 120, 128, 132, 213–216, 416, 417, 418, 434, 440, 441
Strand, K., 415, 416, 430
Strome, M., 383
Studdert-Kennedy, M., 427
Stump, D., 247
Suga, N., 427
Sullivan, M., 225
Summerfield, Q., 129
Sundberg, J., 310
Sussman, H. M., 413–463
Sussman, M., 162
Sutphin, S., 216
Sutton, D., 335, 337
Swift, E., 378
Swisher, L., 426

Tallal, P., 425–427
Taylor, M., 356
Tees, R. C., 428
Templin, M., 416, 431, 446, 454
Terrell, P., 129
T'Hart, J., 285
Theodoros, D. G., 92
Thibodeau, I. A., 30
Thomas, B. J., 259
Thompson, C., 222
Thompson, L., 100, 120, 174
Thompson, R. D., 280
Thompson, V. E., 336
Thoonen, G., 416, 430
Tice, R. L., 105
Till, J., 79, 92, 346
Tingley, S., 356
Titze, I. R., 91
Tjaden, K., 144
Tobin, A., 432
Tompkins, C. A., 279, 280, 282
Towne, R. L., 420
Townsend, J. J., 325
Tranel, D., 210, 283
Traube, L., 323
Travers, N., 267
Travis, L. E., 380–381
Traynor, C. D., 86, 105, 145
Trost, J., 210, 244
Tseng, C. H., 290
Tucker, D. M., 282
Tucker, H. M., 325
Tuller, B., 337
Turner, G., 96, 211
Tweedie, D., 419

U.S. Department of Commerce, 176
Ushijima, T., 395

Vagges, K., 282
Vagg, P. R., 346
Vaissiere, J., 285
Valletutti, P., 164, 183
Vance, R., 426
Van Cramon, D, 216

Van den Berg, J., 382
Van der Kaa, M. A., 282
Van der Linden, , M., 282
Van Kleeck, A., 121, 137
Van Lancker, D., 280–283, 286, 289, 291
Van Pelt, F., 332
Van Riper, C., 239, 244, 269, 380, 435
Vargha-Khadem, F., 424
Velleman, S. L., 415, 416, 430, 440, 441
Vetter, D. K., 417
Vickers, M., 433
Vignolo, L. A., 433
Vishwanat, B., 356
Vogel, D., 16, 31, 42, 119–150, 299
Vogel, M., 330, 338
Volpe, B. T., 348
Von Cramon, D., 330, 338–339

Waaland, P., 172–173
Wachtel, J. M., 102
Wada, J., 281
Wahrborg, P., 162
Wallach, G. P., 121–122, 137, 141
Wallen, V., 240
Walton, J., 419–420
Wambaugh, J., 213, 221, 222
Ward, A. A., 329
Ward, S., 198
Ware, J. H., 30
Warren, D. W., 94
Warrington, E., 198
Waters, G., 199
Watkins, C., 172
Watson, B. C., 246–248, 323, 336, 354, 377–406
Watson, H., 388
Watson, R. T., 282, 290
Watters, G., 424
Watts, R. L., 63
Waugh, P., 221
Webster, R., 378

Wechsler, D., 432
Weeks, R. A., 431
Weidner, W., 215
Weiner, A. E., 240
Weintraub, S., 227, 280–282, 288
Weisiger, B. E., 81
Weismer, G., 79, 82, 83, 95, 96
Weiss, A. L., 96
Weiss, D., 243
Weisshaut, R., 388
Werker, J. F., 428
Wertz, R. T., 16, 79, 217, 219–222, 245, 254, 298, 416, 419, 420, 423, 440
Westby, C. E., 141
West, J., 213, 222
Weston, A., 436
Wetzel, A. B., 336
Wheelden, L. A., 68, 198, 199, 200
Wifling, F., 378
Williams, A., 433
Williams, C. E., 279
Williams, R., 424
Wilson, D. H., 348
Wilson, J., 99
Wilson, L., 170
Wilson, R. L., 97
Wingate, M. E., 382
Wingfield, A., 198
Winholtz, W. S., 91
Wolfe, V. I., 323
Wood, F., 247
Wood, P. H. N., 83, 84, 107
Woodson, G. E., 91, 356, 359, 360
Wu, J. C., 247

Xue, J. W., 355

Yaghmai, F., 427
Yairi, E., 244
Yamashita, T., 354
Yenkosky, J., 280
Yeung-Courchesne, R., 425

Yoder, D. E., 417
Yorkston, K. M., 80, 86, 90, 91, 92, 93, 97, 99, 100, 101, 103–106, 108, 120, 128, 130–133, 138, 144, 145, 221, 359, 361
Yoss, K. A., 418–419, 422, 424
Young, E., 435
Younger, R., 417
Yui, E. M. L., 287

Zemlin, W., 380
Zeplin, J., 81
Zettin, M., 282
Ziegler, W., 216
Zimmerman, R., 285
Zung, W. W. K., 359
Zwirner, P., 91
Zwitman, D., 323
Zyski, B. J., 81

Subject Index

Abbreviated vowel element, 384–385
ABCX model of family stress, 170–174
Abductor type of spasmodic dysphonia (ABSD), 323, 355
Aberdeen Speech Aid, 263–264
ABR. *See* Auditory brainstem responses (ABR)
ABSD. *See* Abductor type of spasmodic dysphonia (ABSD)
Acetylcholine (ACh), 33–35, 38, 39
Acoustic evaluations, 83, 278, 293, 295–296
Acquired neurogenic dysfluency
　delayed auditory feedback (DAF) and, 265–266
　developmental stuttering differentiated from, 248–251
　differential diagnosis of, 248–253, 269
　fluency-modification therapies for, 265–268
　management of, 239–269
　neural substrate for fluency and, 246–248
　neurogenic dysfluency, 240–253
　occult stuttering and, 239–240
　pharmacotherapy for, 261–262
　prosthetic devices for, 261–264
　psychogenic dysfluency and, 240, 251–253
　surgery for, 261–262
　terminology for, 240–242
　treatment for, 261–267
　types of, 253–259
Acquired stuttering, 240. *See also* Stuttering
Adaptability, 173, 177
Adductor type of spasmodic dysphonia (ADSD), 322–323, 355
Aerodynamic characteristics of speech, 92, 384–385, 389, 395–398

Aerophone, 92
AER. *See* Auditory evoked response
Age, 163, 164
AIDS. *See* Assessment of the Intelligibility of Dysarthric Speech
Alcohol, 71, 187, 188
"Alien hand sign," 63
ALS. *See* Amyotrophic lateral sclerosis (ALS)
Alzheimer's disease, 10, 245, 258
American Indian Sign, 221
American Speech-Language-Hearing Association (ASHA), 2, 3
Amplitude, 278
Amyotrophic lateral sclerosis (ALS), 10, 13, 21–22, 98, 341, 342, 343
Anger, 160, 161
Anomia, 254
Anomic aphasia, 19
Anticonvulsant medication, 261–262
Anxiety, 160, 161, 177, 269, 346. *See also* Depression; Emotional disorders
Aphasia. *See also* Broca's aphasia; Wernicke's aphasia
　classifications of, 19
　evaluation for, 16, 17–18, 267–268, 425
　fundamental frequency (F0) and, 284–285, 287–288
　global aphasia, 414
　intonation and, 286
　neurogenic dysfluency and, 241–244, 246
　nonfluent aphasia, 289–290
　nonverbal communication and, 221
　patient reactions to, 162
　speech therapy for, 264
　stroke causing, 241, 253–254
Aphasia Diagnostic Profiles, 260
Aphasic symptomatology, 241–242

485

Aphonia, 330
Apraxia Battery for Adults, 216–217, 217
Apraxia of speech. *See also* Developmental apraxia of speech (DAS)
  Broca's aphasia and, 212
  case study on, 223
  description of, 212, 214–216
  diagnosis of, 216–218
  imitation therapy, 218–219
  neurogenic dysfluency and, 244–245, 246, 254
  nonverbal communication and, 221
  phonological encoding and, 212–223
  prosody and, 290, 298
  speech programming and, 212–223
  speech rate and, 222–223
  speech therapy for, 264
  stuttering as, 244–245
  treatment of, 218–223, 264, 359–360, 443–444
Apraxic dysarthria, 414
Aprosody, 279
Arthur Adaptation of the Leiter Performance Scales, 446, 448
Articulatory system
  evaluation of, 89, 94–98
  treatment for, 98, 103–106, 435
ASHA. *See* American Speech-Language-Hearing Association
Assessment of the Intelligibility of Dysarthric Speech (AIDS), 86, 361
Assessment of Phonological Processes, 449, 451, 452, 453
Assimilative errors, 416
Ataxic dysarthria, 2, 22–23
Athetosis, 42, 45
Attending, 130
Auditory brainstem responses (ABR), 326
Auditory evoked response (AER), 425
Auditory inputs, 198

Babinski reflex, 8
Ballismus, 45
Bargaining, 168
Basal ganglia
  acquired dysfluency and, 246
  description of, 43

dystonia and, 47
extrapyramidal diseases and, 42, 330–333
neurogenic stuttering and, 253
spasmodic dysphonia (SD) and, 324, 330–333, 356–357
BDAE. *See* Boston Diagnostic Aphasia Examination (BDAE)
BEAM. *See* Brain electrical activity mapping (BEAM)
Belladonna, 57
Bilateral vascular episodes, 255–256
Biofeedback therapies, 98, 266–267, 378
Blepharoplasm, 331
Blood-brain barrier, 58, 60
Boston Diagnostic Aphasia Examination (BDAE), 223, 224, 451
Boston Naming Test, 227
BOTOX. *See* Botulinum toxin (BOTOX) treatment
Bottom-up approach to dysarthria, 121–122, 147–148
Botulinum toxin (BOTOX) treatment, 354–356, 358–359
Bradykinesia, 46
Brain
  basal ganglia, 42, 43, 47, 246, 253, 324, 330–333, 356–357
  blood-brain barrier, 58, 60
  brainstem, 246, 253
  cerebellum, 10, 246, 253
  cerebral cortex, 246, 247, 253, 324, 334–337
  corpus callosum, 290–291, 304–307, 348
  left-hemisphere, 282, 284–290, 307–310, 414
  medulla, 324, 326–329
  midbrain, 324, 329–330, 338
  nervous system and, 32–34, 40–41
  neuromotor control system of speech and, 32, 66–67
  right hemisphere, 280–284, 286, 289, 290–292, 298, 301–304
  spasmodic dysphonia loci in, 324, 325–339
Brain electrical activity mapping (BEAM), 347, 349–351, 353
Brainstem, 246, 253

Broca's aphasia, 19, 212, 223–224. *See also* Aphasia; Wernicke's aphasia
  apraxia of speech and, 212
  in case study, 223–224
  fundamental frequency (F0) and, 284–285, 288
  left frontal premotor cortex lesions and, 336
  linquistic planning and, 286
  phonemic stress contrasts and, 289
  symptoms of, 19
  treatment for, 443–444
Bruegel's syndrome, 331
Bruininks–Oseretsky Test of Motor Proficiency, 433, 451, 454
Buccolingual dyskinesia, 331
Bulbar palsy, 340, 341, 342, 343

CADL. *See Communicative Abilities in Daily Living* (CADL)
CAIDS. *See Computerized Assessment of the Intelligibility of Dysarthric Speech* (CAIDS)
Carrow Elicited Language Inventory, 446, 452, 454
CA. *See* Conduction aphasia (CA)
Catecholamines, 40–41
Central noradrenergic system, 40
Cerebellar ataxia, 340, 341, 342, 343
Cerebellum, 10, 246, 247, 253
Cerebral cortex, 246, 247, 253, 324, 334–337
Cerebral palsy, 10, 49, 98
Childhood verbal dyspraxia, 414
Choline, 38
Cholinesterase inhibitors, 39, 40
Chorea
  classifications of, 49
  description of, 44–45
  drug-induced chorea, 51, 54
  as extrapyramidal disease, 42
  hereditary chorea, 47–49
  spasmodic dysphonia (SD) symptoms and, 343
Choreiform dyskinesia, 55
Cognition, 419–420, 432
Coma, 330
Combination errors, 208

Combination-sensitive neuron, 427
Communication. *See also* Language
  assumptions about listeners and, 139–140
  attending and, 130
  bottom-up aspects of, 122–123
  communication-impaired environments, 177–178
  connotative meanings and, 134
  cooperation in, 140–141
  denotative meanings and, 134
  directness of intention in, 139
  discourse knowledge and, 141–145
  everyday discourse, 142–143
  familiarity in, 144–145
  indirect communication, 139
  interactive aspects of, 123
  job-related discourse, 143–144
  listener's perspective in, 136–137
  metalinguistic processing and, 133
  metapragmatics and, 121, 137–141
  Model of Interactive Processing and, 148–150
  morpho-syntax and, 127–128
  nonverbal communication, 123, 132, 134, 138, 180, 221
  phonology and, 128–130, 159–160
  positive communication environments, 179–181
  predictive message content in, 126–127
  primary-level pragmatics and, 130–133
  prosody and, 141
  reactions to communication problems, 161–164
  semantics and, 125–127
  speech rate and, 132, 138
  top-down aspects of, 121–123
  topics and, 131
  turn-taking and, 131–133
  word-referent relationships and, 133–137
Communicative Abilities in Daily Living (CADL), 223
Computerized Assessment of the Intelligibility of Dysarthric Speech (CAIDS), 85, 86, 106
Computerized tomography (CT) scans, 12, 347, 425

Conduction aphasia (CA), 19, 203, 209–210, 225
Connotative meanings, 134
Contextual facilitation, 436
Continuous positive airway pressure (CPAP), 98, 102–103
Contrast therapy, 436
Coprolalia, 52
Corpus callosum, 290–291, 304–307, 348
Cortical dysarthria, 414
Cortical stuttering, 240
Counseling, 299, 358, 359
CPAP. *See* Continuous positive airway pressure (CPAP)
Cranial nerve examinations, 6
Cspeech software, 295, 296
CT. *See* Computerized tomography (CT)

DAF. *See* Delayed auditory feedback (DAF)
DA. *See* Dopamine (DA)
Declarative sentences, 288
Declination, 285
Deductive thinking, 121
Deep dysphasia, 204
Delayed auditory feedback (DAF), 105, 263–264, 265–266
Delayed motor development, 433
Dementia, 59, 258
Denial, 160, 161, 168
Denotative meanings, 134
Denver Auditory Phoneme Sequencing Test, 433
Depression. *See also* Anxiety; Emotional disorders
  dysarthria and, 160, 161, 168–169
  Parkinson's disease and, 62–63
  spasmodic disorder and, 323, 346
Developmental apraxia of speech (DAS). *See also* Apraxia of speech
  articulation and, 431–432
  assimilative errors and, 416
  case study on, 446–463
  characteristics of, 414, 416–423
  clinical perspectives on, 415
  cognition and, 419–420, 432
  conceptual framework for, 426–429
  developmental history and, 430
  diagnosis of, 424, 429–430, 433–434

  etiology of, 423–426, 445
  evaluation for, 424, 429–434
  gender and, 422
  impairment levels of, 440–441
  input deficits and, 415
  intonation and, 440
  language development and, 420–421, 432
  neuroimaging and, 423–426
  neurological deficits and, 414–415, 423–425, 445
  neuromuscular disorders and, 433
  omission errors and, 416
  output deficits and, 415, 428
  phonological disorders distinguished from, 437
  prognosis for, 422
  Prompts for Restructuring Oral Muscular Phonetic Targets (PROMPT) and, 442–443
  prosody in, 418
  rhyming inabilities and, 429
  rhythm and, 440
  screening for, 432
  sensory deficits and, 421
  sensory and motor functioning with, 433
  speech errors and, 416–418
  speech rate and, 418
  stress patterning and, 418
  syntactic deficits and, 420–421
  teaching hierarchy in treatment, 439
  theories on, 413–463
  treatment of, 434–446
  vocal stress and, 440
  volitional nonspeech movements and, 419
Developmental Test of Visual Motor Integration, 448
Development dysphasia, 428
Dialysis dementia, 258
Disability, definition of, 84
Discourse knowledge, 141–145
Dopamine (DA), 40, 42, 57–58, 61, 64
Dysarthria
  acoustic evaluation for, 83
  activation decay rate and, 204
  articulatory system and, 89, 94–98
  ataxic dysarthria, 2, 22–23

bottom-up approach to dysarthria, 121–122, 147–148
case studies on, 106–109, 145–147
characteristics of, 81, 83–84, 85, 86, 106, 212
chronic disorder model of evaluation for, 83–85
deep dysphasia, 204
employment and, 160
evaluation tools for, 85–88
hypernasality and, 93, 102, 106
as impairment, 83–85
institutionalization of dysarthric individual, 174–181
kinematic analysis of, 95–96
laryngeal system and, 89, 90–93, 98
neurogenic dysfluency and, 245, 246
oral-motor evaluation for, 85–86
pacing boards and, 263
palatal lift and, 98, 103, 107
perceptual evaluation for, 80–81
physiologic evaluation for, 82
prosody and, 298
prosthetic devices, 101, 103
pseudobulbar dysarthria, 338, 341
psychosocial impact of, 157–189
respiratory system and, 88–90, 98–100
spasmodic dysphonia (SD) compared with, 339–343
spastic dysarthria, 334
speech intelligibility testing and, 85, 86–87
speech production subcomponent assessment for, 88–97
as stress, 164–165
symptoms of, 18, 120
top-down treatment approach for, 119–150
treatment for, 97–150, 264
velopharyngeal system and, 89, 93–94, 98
Wilson's disease and, 12
Dysarthria therapy. *See* Speech therapy
Dysdiadochokinesis of tongue, 334
Dysfluency. *See* Acquired neurogenic dysfluency; Neurogenic dysfluency; Stuttering
Dysmetria, 2
Dysphasia, 428

Dysphonia, 334
Dyspraxia, 348
Dysprosody, 279
Dystonia. *See also* Spasmodic dystonia
  description of, 45, 46–47
  differentiated from other diseases, 342
  drug-induced dystonia, 54
  as extrapyramidal disease, 42
  idiopathic torsion dystonia, 331
  neurologic disturbance and, 71
  oral-facial-cervical dystonia, 331
  oral-mandibular dystonia, 331
  torsion dystonia, 331
  vocal symptoms, 341
Dystonic writer's cramp, 332

Eaton–Lambert syndrome, 10
Echolalia, 198
Electroencephalograph (EEG), 334, 349, 423–424
Electroglottography (EGG), 383–384, 388–389, 392, 394, 400–404
Electromyography (EMG), 12, 266, 332, 355
Emotional disorders, 434. *See also* Anxiety; Depression
Employment, 160
Encaphalopathies, 10
Encephalitis, 10
Epinephrine, 33, 35
Essential tremor, 331, 333
Ethics, 29
Evaluation
  acoustic evaluations, 83, 278, 293, 295–296
  for aphasia, 16, 17–18, 267–268
  of articulatory system, 89, 94–97
  auditory-perceptual measures, 79, 425
  chronic disorder model of evaluation, 83–85
  for depression, 346
  for developmental apraxia of speech, 424, 429–434
  of dysarthria, 80–97
  evaluation tools, 85–88
  fluoroscopic assessments, 332
  Frenchay Dysarthria Assessment, 85, 87–88
  laboratory tests, 9, 11–13

of laryngeal system, 89, 90–93
misdiagnosis, 30–31
motor system evaluations, 6
of neurogenic dysfluency, 259–261
neurological evaluation, 6–13
oral-motor evaluation, 85–86
perceptual evaluations, 80–81, 293, 295
Phonetic Intelligibility Test, 87
physiologic evaluation, 82
of prosodic disorders, 292–298
pulmonary function testing, 90
ramp-and-hold maneuver and, 96–97
of respiratory system, 88–90
of speech production, 85, 88–97, 377–380
of velopharyngeal system, 89, 93–94
Everyday discourse, 142–143
Extrapyramidal diseases, 42, 43–45, 258
Extrapyramidal motor cortex, 343–344

F0. *See* Fundamental frequency (F0)
Family
  adaptability of, 173
  "inner language," 172
  probe questions for, 174, 175–176
  psychosocial impact of dysarthria on, 166–174
  sources and support for, 172–173
  as system, 170–174
FDA. *See* Food and Drug Administration (FDA)
Fear, 168, 177
Figurative language, 125
Fisher–Logemann Test of Articulation Competence, 95
Fisher's *t* test, 342
Fluoroscopic assessments, 332
Food and Drug Administration (FDA), 14, 32
FORCE software program, 96
Formal (phonic verbal) paraphasia, 203–206
Frenchay Dysarthria Assessment, 85, 87–88
Frustration, 169, 181
Functional limitation, 83–84

Fundamental frequency (F0)
  as acoustic property of speech waveform, 278
  aphasia and, 284–285, 288
  corpus callosum and, 291
  intonation and, 280, 287
  measures for, 296–297
  speech timing and, 287–288

Gender, 322, 422
Gilles de la Tourette syndrome. *See* Tourette's syndrome
Global aphasia, 19, 414
Goldman–Fristoe Test of Articulation, 431
Goodman and Gillman's "The Pharmacological Basis of Therapeutics", 31

Hallucinations, 59
Hard articulatory contact, 385
Head trauma-induced dysfluency, 258
Hemiballismus, 42
Hostility, 160, 161
Humming, 219
Huntington's disease, 10, 47–51, 341
Hyperkinesia, 43–45, 423
Hyperlexia, 198
Hypernasality, 93, 102, 106
Hyperprosody, 279
Hyperreflexia, 334, 423
Hyperthyroidism, 44
Hypokinesia, 45–46

Ideopathic unilateral vocal fold paralysis, 404
Idiopathic cerebral calcinosis, 245
Idiopathic torsion dystonia, 331
Imitation, 218–219, 417
Impairment, definition of, 84
Indirect communication, 139
Inductance coil plethysmograph system, 388
Inductive learning, 122
Institutionalization of dysarthric individual
  communication-impaired environment and, 177–178
  effects of, 176–177

family and, 174–176
positive communication environment
  and, 179–181
Instrumentation treatment of stuttering
  aerodynamic disruptions and,
    384–385, 395–398
  applications of, 385–387, 398–404
  instruments used in, 388–389
  laryngeal disruptions and, 382–384,
    392–395
  rational for, 377–380
  respiratory disruptions and, 380–382,
    390–398
Integral stimulation, 436
Interactive processing, 123
Interiorized stuttering, 239–240
Interrogative sentences, 288
Intonation
  Broca's aphasia and, 284–285
  in declarative sentences, 288
  fundamental frequency (FO) and, 280, 287
  in interrogative sentences, 288
  left-hemisphere and, 282, 288–289
  prosody and, 279
  right-hemisphere and, 281–284, 286, 289, 290
  speech timing and, 290
  vocal stress and, 279, 288–289, 293, 295, 300–301
IOPI. *See* Iowa Oral Performance Instrument (IOPI)
Iowa Oral Performance Instrument (IOPI), 96
Ischemia, 10

Jacob–Creutzfeldt disease, 10
Jaw, 85, 104, 329
Job-related discourse, 143–144
Joint attending, 130

Kaufman Assessment Battery for Children, 453

Language
  bottom-up processing and, 122
  brain loci for impairments of, 426
  developmental apraxia of speech
    (DAS) and, 420–421, 432
  development of, 122
  figurative language, 125
  inductive learning and, 122
  "inner language" of family, 172
  interactive processing and, 123
  joint attending and, 130
  levels of meaning in, 134–136
  metalinguistic processing and, 133
  metapragmatic functions in, 121, 137–141
  morpho-syntax and, 127–128
  phonology and, 128–130, 159–160
  primary-level pragmatics and, 130–133, 136–137
  primary level top-down characteristics of language processing, 124–133
  prosody disorders, 277–311
  rhyming, 429
  Rhythm Rule, 289
  semantics and, 125–127
  syntactic forms, 125–126
  tonal languages, 287–288
  word/referent relationships and, 133–137
  word specificity, 125
  word substitution, 125
Laryngeal system
  evaluation of, 89, 90–93
  laryngeal dyskinesias, 354
  stuttering and, 379, 382–384, 392–395
  thyroplasty and, 101
  treatment for, 98, 100–102
  videostroboscopy and, 93
Laryngeal tremor, 333
Lee Silverman Voice Therapy program, 100
Left hemisphere of brain, 282, 284–292, 307–310, 414
Lemma, 196, 198, 209
Lesions, 8, 210, 241
  lesion loci for spasmodic dysphonia (SD), 324, 325–339
  neural imaging and, 347–348, 354

prosodic disorders and, 280–284, 307–311
vascular lesions, 254–257
Limb apraxia, 433
Limbic system, 324, 337–339
Lips, 85, 96, 104
Listener's perspective, 136–137, 139–140
Lithium, 259
Loudness, 91
LSD, 41
Lues, 10

McCarthy Scales of Children's Abilities, 446, 451
Magnetic resonance imaging (MRI), 12, 247, 347, 353–354, 425–426
Mann-Whitney *U* test, 342
Mapping of phoneme segments, 199–200, 208, 209
Mayo Clinic, 340
Medulla, 324, 326–329
Meige's syndrome, 47, 71, 331
Melodic Intonation Therapy (MIT), 220–221
Meningitis, 10
Mental disabilities, 419–420, 434
Mental status examinations, 6
Metacommunicative functions, 121
Metalinguistic functions, 121, 133
Metapragmatic functions, 121, 137–141
Midbrain, 324, 329–330, 338
Minnesota Test for the Differential Diagnosis of Aphasia, 224
MIT. *See* Melodic Intonation Therapy (MIT)
Mixed transcortical aphasia, 19
Model of Interactive Processing, 148–150
Morphemes, 198
Moto-kinesthetic speech training, 435
Motor speech disorders. *See* Speech motor disorders
Mourning, 169
Movement disorders. *See also* specific diseases
  athetosis, 42, 45
  ballismus, 45
  chorea, 42, 44–45, 47–51
  cures for, 72

drug-induced movement disorders, 51, 54–55, 64
dystonia, 42, 45, 46–47
extrapyramidal diseases, 42
hemiballismus, 42
hyperkinesia and, 43–55
hyperthyroidism and, 44
hypokinesia and, 45–46, 55–66
rigidity, 46
spasticity, 46
speech compromise and, 64–65
tics, 44, 51–52
Tourette's syndrome, 51–52
tremors, 43–44, 53, 71, 72
MRI. *See* Magnetic resonance imaging (MRI)
Multiple infarct dementia, 245
Multiple Input Phoneme Therapy, 220, 435
Multiple sclerosis, 10, 339
Muscle weakness, 423
Mutual attending, 130
Myasthenia gravis, 10, 65

Nasometer, 93
NCV. *See* Nerve conduction velocities (NCV)
Neologisms, 203, 206–208, 209
Nerve conduction velocities (NCV), 12
Nervous system, 32–34, 40–41
Neurogenic dysfluency. *See also* Acquired neurogenic dysfluency
  aphasia and, 241–244, 246
  apraxia of speech and, 244–245, 246
  clinical syndromes of, 242, 246
  definition of, 239
  developmental stuttering differentiated from, 248–251
  as drug induced, 259
  dysarthria and, 245, 246
  evaluation for, 259–261
  extrapyramidal disease with, 258
  head trauma-induced dysfluency, 258
  interiorized stuttering and, 239–240
  management of, 239–269
  nonvascular etiologies, 258–259
  occult stuttering and, 239–240
  palilalia, 245

psychogenic dysfluency and, 240, 251–253
as speech motor disorder component, 244–246
strokes and, 253–254, 257
terminology of, 240–242
vascular lesions with and without aphasia and, 254–257
Neurogenic stuttering, 240
Neurological evaluation. *See also* Assessment and evaluation
differential diagnoses, 9
electrophysiologic studies for, 12–13
imaging techniques for, 12
laboratory tests, 9, 11–13
neuroimaging, 12, 247, 247–248, 347–354, 353–354, 423–426, 425–426
neurologic diagnosis, 9
neurologic examination and, 6–8
patient history and, 6
Neurologists
"disease-state" orientation of, 19–20
disordered speech motor control and, 1–24
patient management approach of, 5–17
Neuromuscular junction, 34, 37–39
Neurotransmitters
acetylcholine and, 33, 34, 35, 37, 39
catecholamines and, 40–41
cholinergic and adrenergic nerves, 32–34
dopamine, 40–41, 42
epinephrine and, 33, 34
neuromuscular junction and, 34, 37–39
norepinephrine and, 33, 35
serotonin, 41–42
Nonfluent aphasia, 289–290
Nonverbal communication, 123, 132, 134, 138, 180, 221
Norepinephrine, 33, 35
Northwestern Syntax Screening Test, 420
Nursing homes, 181

Occult stuttering, 239–240
Olivopontocerebellar degeneration, 10
Omission errors, 416
On-off phenomenon, 61
Oral-facial-cervical dystonia, 331

Oral-mandibular dystonia, 331
Oral-motor evaluations, 85–88

Pacing boards, 104–105, 263
Paired stimuli, 436
Palatal lift, 98, 103, 107
Palilalia, 245, 262–263
Paraphasias
anatomy of, 210
auditory comprehension and, 225
case study on, 226–227
combination errors and, 208
conduction aphasia (CA) and, 225
description of, 202, 225
evolution of, 208–209
flowchart of spreading activation, 205
formal (phonic verbal) paraphasia, 203–206
imitation and, 225
mapping difficulties with, 208, 209
neologisms, 206–208
phonemic paraphasias, 202–203, 208
phonological encoding and, 196–210
semantic paraphasias, 206
spreading activation theory and, 204, 207
treatment for, 224–226
verbal paraphasia, 203
Wernicke's aphasia (WA) and, 203, 225
Parathyroid disease, 10
Parkinsonism, 54, 64, 343
Parkinsonism-plus syndromes, 63
Parkinson's disease
aerodynamic characteristics of speech and, 92
articulation error patterns and, 95
classifications of, 56
depression and, 62–63
description of, 55
disordered speech motor control and, 10
dopamine and, 40
drug-induced Parkinson's disease, 51
dysarthria and, 83
as extrapyramidal disease, 42
impact on family, 166
laryngeal abnormalities and, 93
midbrain and, 329

palilalia and, 245, 262–263
rigidity and, 83
spasmodic dysphonia vocal symptoms and, 341
speech rate control and, 105
stuttering and, 69, 245
tongue strength and, 96
treatment for, 57–63
tremors and, 43, 83
PASS. *See* Phonological assembly subsystem (PASS)
Peabody Picture Vocabulary Test–Revised (PPVT–R), 227, 432, 448, 451
PERCI-SARS, 94
Peripheral nerve, 324, 325–326, 356
PET. *See* Position emission tomography (PET)
Pharmacology. *See also* Treatment
abbreviations for dosages, 33
for acquired neurogenic dysfluency, 261–262
of autonomic nervous system, 35–36
clinical trials and, 29
dosage and, 30–31
for dystonia, 48
ethics and, 29
fundamental concepts of, 29–31
information resources for, 31–32
medication errors, 31
movement disorders and, 42–66
of neuromuscular junction, 34, 37–39
neurotransmitters, 32–42
on-off phenomenon and, 61
of Parkinson's disease, 58
patient compliance and, 30–31
side effects of, 28, 30, 51, 54–55, 64–66, 259
for spasmodic dysphonia, 70–72, 358–359
speech motor disorders and, 27–73
for stuttering, 28, 67–70
wearing-off effect, 61
Pharyngeal flap surgery, 98
Phoneme segment mapping, 199–200, 208, 209
Phonemic paraphasias, 202–203, 209
Phonetic derivation, 219

Phonetic Intelligibility Test, 87
Phonetic placement, 435
Phonological assembly subsystem (PASS), 200
Phonological disorders, 437
Phonological encoding
auditory inputs and, 198
definition of, 196
flowchart of, 197
language production system and, 196
lemma and, 196, 198
mapping of phoneme segments and, 199–200, 208
paraphasias and, 196–210
phonological assembly subsystem (PASS) and, 200
phonological lexicon, 200–202
process of, 196–200
speech motor control and, 211–212
spreading activation theory for, 201–202, 204–207
verbal production stages, 210–212
visual inputs and, 198
Physician's Desk Reference (PDR), 31–32
Pitch, 91
Polysystemic central nervous system degeneration, 258
Position emission tomography (PET), 247
Post-encephalitic parkinsonism, 63–64
Postural changes, 98
Postural tremor, 331, 333
PPVT–R. *See Peabody Picture Vocabulary Test–Revised* (PPVT–R)
Pragmatics, 130–133, 136–137
Predictive message content, 126–127
Primary-level pragmatics, 130–133
Progressive supranuclear palsy, 10
Prolonged silent blocks, 384–385
Prompts for Restructuring Oral Muscular Phonetic Targets (PROMPT), 219–220, 442–443
Prosodic disorders
apraxia of speech and, 290, 298
aprosody, 279
assessment of, 292–298
case study on, 301–304, 307–310
cerebral injury causing, 279–292

Subject Index   495

corpus callosum damage causing, 290–291, 304–307
counseling for, 299
dysarthria and, 298
dysprosody, 279
hyperprosody, 279
left-hemisphere damage causing, 282, 284–292
prosodic perception disorder treatment, 299–300
prosodic production deficit treatment, 300–301
right hemispheric damage causing, 280–284, 289, 291–292, 298, 301–304
treatment for, 298–301
Prosody
communicative functions of, 279
declination and, 285
definition of, 278–279
in developmental apraxia of speech (DAS), 418
intonation and, 141
neurogenic disorders of, 277–311
Rhythm Rule and, 289
syntactic juncture and, 293
vocal stress and, 279, 288–289, 293, 295, 300–301
Prosthetic devices, 101, 103, 261–264
Pseudobulbar dysarthria, 338, 341
Pseudobulbar palsy, 245, 338, 342
Psychogenic dysfluency, 240, 251–253
Psychosocial impact of dysarthria
ABCX model of family stress, 170–174
age and, 163, 164
case studies, 186–189
coping mechanisms, 162
depression, 160, 161, 168–169
on family, 166–174
institutionalization of dysarthric individual and, 174–181
overview of, 157–159
patient reactions to disability, 160–164
phonology and, 159–160
stress, 164–165
therapy compliance and, 165–166
vocational limitations, 160

Pulmonary function testing, 90
Puns, 135

Rapprochement, 169
RCBA. *See* Reading Comprehension Battery for Aphasia (RCBA)
rCBF. *See* Regional cerebral blood flow (rCBF)
Reading Comprehension Battery for Aphasia (RCBA), 227
Referral, 15–17
Regional cerebral blood flow (rCBF), 246
Regression, 183
Relaxation-breathing techniques, 267
Repetition, 206, 245, 417
Respiratory system
"5 for 5" rule, 99
evaluation of, 88–90
respiratory patterning, 90
stuttering and, 379, 380–382, 388, 390–392
treatment for, 98–100
Respitrace, 388, 390, 398, 399
Rhyming, 429
Rhythm, 440
Rhythm Rule, 289
Riddles, 134
Right hemisphere of brain, 280–284, 286, 289, 290–292, 298, 301–304
Right-sided vascular episodes, 256–257
Rigidity, 46, 83

Scan copier, 200
Schizophrenia, 51, 68
Screening Test for Development Apraxia of Speech, 431, 432, 449, 454
SD. *See* Spasmodic dysphonia (SD)
See-Scape, 94, 102
Self-Rating of Depression Scale, 359
Semantic paraphasias, 206, 207
Semantics, 125–127
Senile chorea, 49
Sensory-motor approach therapy, 435
Sensory system testing, 6, 8
Sequenced Inventory of Communicative Development, 432, 446
Serotonis, 41–42

Side effects, 28, 30
Single photon emission computerized tomography (SPECT), 246
Sound spectrograph, 295
Spasmodic blinking, 330
Spasmodic dysphonia (SD)
  abductor type (ABSD) of, 323
  abnormal auditory brainstem responses (ABR) and, 326
  adductor type (ADSD), 322–323
  articulatory abnormalities and, 339
  basal ganglia and, 324, 330–333, 356
  case studies, 360–363
  cerebral cortex and, 334–337
  as continuum disorder, 323
  counseling for, 358, 359
  depression and, 323
  description of, 70, 321–322
  dysarthrias compared with, 339–343
  extralaryngeal motor functions in, 343–347
  high brain activity and, 351
  instrumentational treatment of, 404
  lesion loci for, 324, 325–339, 357
  limbic system and, 324, 337–339
  medulla and, 324, 326–329
  midbrain and, 324, 329–330, 338
  neuroimaging and, 347–354
  onset of, 322, 351
  peripheral nerve and, 324, 325–326, 356
  pharmacology for, 70–72, 358–359
  prevalence of, 322
  pyramidal motor dysfunctions with, 334
  recent developments for, 354–356
  symptomological imitation of, 335
  treatment for, 354–356, 358–360
Spasmodic torticollus, 331
Spastic dysarthria, 334
Spasticity, description of, 46
Spastic paralysis, 334
SPECT. *See* Single photon emission computerized tomography (SPECT)
Speech intelligibility testing, 85, 86–87
Speech–language pathologists
  academic preparation for, 3
  assessment of speech disorders, 17–18
  burnout of, 182, 184–185
  clinical fellowship year (CFY) and, 4
  clinical preparation for, 4–5
  disordered speech motor control and, 1–24
  family and, 169–170, 173–174, 181–182
  frustration of, 181
  health care and, 28–29
  nursing homes and, 181
  patient management approach of, 17–20
  patient stress and, 164–165, 181
  personal stress and, 182–186
  pharmacology and, 28
  probe questions for stress levels of, 185–186
  relationship with patient, 182–183
Speech motor disorders. *See also* specific disorders
  apraxia of speech as, 214–216
  case studies of, 20–23
  common underlying neurologic causes of, 10
  cranial nerves involved in, 7
  as drug-induced, 64–65
  evaluation for, 425
  lesions and, 8, 9
  misconceptions about, 27–28
  neurogenic dysfluency as, 244–246
  neurological evaluations, 6–13
  neurologic evaluation for, 6–13
  neurons and, 66–67
  normal speech output, 66–67
  pharmacologic approaches to, 27–73
  phonatory tremors and, 71, 72
  phonological encoding and, 211–212
  referral to speech–language pathologist, 15–17
  stress affecting, 67
  treatment for, 13–15
Speech pattern remediation, 436
Speech Perception in Noise (SPIN), 126
Speech rate
  apraxia of speech and, 222–223
  breathing modification and, 106
  communication ability and, 132, 138
  DAS and, 418
  delayed auditory feedback (DAF) and, 105

dysarthria and, 263–264
nonverbal communication and, 138
pacing board and, 104–105, 263
visual feedback and, 105–106
Speech therapy. *See also* Speech–language pathologists; Treatment
 for acquired neurogenic dysfluency, 264
 for aphasia, 264
 for apraxia of speech, 218–219, 264, 359–360, 434–444
 articulatory system and, 98, 103–106
 contextual facilitation, 436
 contrast therapy, 436
 delayed auditory feedback (DAF) and, 265–266
 for developmental apraxia of speech, 434–444
 for dysarthria, 264
 fluency-modification therapies, 265–268
 humming as, 219
 imitation and, 218–219
 integral stimulation, 436
 laryngeal system and, 98, 100–102
 Melodic Intonation Therapy (MIT), 220–221, 443–444
 moto-kinesthetic speech training, 435
 Multiple Input Phoneme Therapy, 220
 multiple phoneme approach therapy, 435
 paired stimuli, 436
 patient compliance and, 165–166
 phoneme placement, 435
 probe questions for, 166, 167
 PROMPT system and, 219–220, 442–443
 regression and, 183
 respiratory system and, 98–100
 sensory-motor approach therapy, 435
 speech pattern remediation, 436
 stress of, 181–186
 stuttering modification therapy, 265
 successive approximation, 436
 top-down approach, 119–150
 touch-cue method, 443
 traditional articulation therapy, 435
Speech Viewer, 101

SPIN. *See* Speech Perception in Noise (SPIN)
Spreading activation theory, 201–202, 204–207
State–Trait Anxiety Scale, 359
Steele–Richardson–Olszewski syndrome, 63
Steroids, 65–66
Strengthening exercises, 103–104
Stress
 ABCX model of family stress, 170–174
 coping with, 184–185
 of individual with dysarthria, 164–165, 181
 speech–language pathologist and, 182–184
 stuttering and, 67, 251
 vocal intonation, 279, 288–289, 293, 295, 418, 440
Strokes, 10, 241, 253–254, 257
Stuttering
 abbreviated vowel element and, 384–385
 acquired neurogenic dysfluency differentiated from, 248–253
 acquired neurological disorders associated with, 240
 acquired stuttering, 240
 aerodynamic disruptions and, 384–385, 389, 395–398
 apraxia of speech and, 244–245
 biofeedback therapy for, 378
 core components of, 378–379
 cortical stuttering, 240
 as drug-induced, 65
 electroglottography (EGG) and, 383–384, 388–389, 392, 394, 400–404
 hard articulatory contact, 385
 instrumentational treatment of, 377–406
 interiorized stuttering, 239–240
 laryngeal system and, 379, 382–384, 392–395
 as learned avoidance, 266
 lesions and, 241
 limbic system and, 339
 neurogenic stuttering, 240
 neuroimaging techniques and, 247–248

occult stuttering, 239–240
overview of, 67
Parkinson's disease and, 69
pharmacology for, 28, 67–70
physiological causes of, 390–404
prolonged silent blocks and, 384–385
respiratory system and, 379, 380–382, 388, 390–392
secondary components of, 378–379
stress and, 67, 251
treatment for, 265, 377–406
vascular lesions and, 254–255
vocal folds and, 382, 383, 386, 388, 392, 395
voice offset and, 382
voice onset and, 382, 384, 386
Successive approximation, 436
Sucking reflexes, 334
Supranuclear palsy, 334
Surgery, 261–262, 322, 325
Sydenham's chorea, 49
Symptomotology approach, 120
Syntactic forms, 125–126

Tardive dyskinesia, 54–55
Templin–Darley Screening Test of Articulation, 416, 431, 446, 450, 454
Tenuous fluency, 378
Test of Auditory Comprehension of Language, 450
Test of Oral and Limb Apraxia, 433
Thyroid disease, 10
Thyroplasty, 101
Tics, 44, 51–52
Timing of voicing, 100–101
Tonal languages, 287–288
Tone, 290
Tongue, 85, 96, 104
Top-down treatment of dysarthria
 case study on, 145–147
 deductive thinking and, 121
 definition of, 121
 of dysarthric speech, 119–150
 metacommunicative functions and, 121
 overview of, 121
 primary level of language processing and, 124–133
 secondary level of language processing and, 133–145

Torsion dystonia, 331
Touch-cue method, 443
Tourette's syndrome, 10, 51–52, 68, 331–332
Traditional articulation therapy, 435
Training for speech–language pathologists, 3–5
Transcortical motor aphasia, 19
Transcortical sensory aphasia, 19, 198
Traumatic brain injury, 10, 96, 100, 106–108
Traumatic midbrain dysphonia, 338–339
Treatment. *See also* Pharmacology; Speech therapy
 for acquired neurogenic dysfluency, 261–268
 for apraxia of speech, 218–223, 434–437
 behavior therapy, 102
 biofeedback therapies, 98, 266–267
 contextual facilitation, 436
 continuous positive airway pressure (CPAP) and, 98, 102–103
 contrast therapy, 436
 for developmental apraxia of speech, 434–446
 for disordered speech motor control, 13–15, 17–20
 for dysarthria, 97–150
 expense of, 387
 fluency-modification therapies, 265–267, 268
 imitation and, 218–219, 225
 instrumentational treatment of stuttering, 377–406
 integral stimulation, 436
 moto-kinesthetic speech training, 435
 multiple phoneme approach therapy, 435
 paired stimuli, 436
 palatal lift and, 98, 103
 for paraphasias, 224–226
 phoneme placement, 435
 of physiological causes of dysfluency, 398–404
 of prosodic disorders, 298–301
 sensory-motor approach therapy, 435
 for spasmodic dysphonia (SD), 354–356, 404

speech pattern remediation, 436
for stuttering, 377–406
successive approximation, 436
syllable-timed speech and, 267
traditional articulation therapy, 435
velopharyngeal system and, 98, 102–103
Tremors
  description of, 43–44
  essential tremor, 332, 333
  laryngeal tremor, 333
  Parkinson's disease and, 43, 83
  pharmacology for, 53
  phonatory tremors, 71, 72
  postural tremor, 331, 333
Tumors, 10

Upper motor neuron disease, 258–259

Vascular lesions, 254–257
Velar postural abnormalities, 355
Velopharyngeal system, 89, 98, 102–103
Verbal dyspraxia, 414
Verbal paraphasia, 203, 204, 205
Veteran's Administration, 79
Videonasoendoscopy, 355
Videostroboscopy, 93
Visi-Pitch, 101, 295, 299
Visual inputs, 198

Vocal folds, 382–388, 392, 395, 404
Vocal stress, 279, 288–289, 293, 295, 300–301
Voice onset time (VOT), 297, 382, 384, 386
VOT. *See* Voice onset time (VOT)

Wada Test (WT), 281
WA. *See* Wernicke's aphasia (WA)
Wearing-off effect, 61
Wechsler Adult Intelligence Scale, 261
Wechsler Intelligence Scales for Children–Revised, 432
Wernicke's aphasia (WA). *See also* Aphasia; Broca's aphasia
  activation decay rate and, 204
  combination errors and, 208
  conduction aphasia distinguished from, 209
  fundamental frequency (F0) and, 285
  intonation processing problems with, 286
  lesions and, 210
  paraphasia and, 203, 225
Wernicke's aphasia (WA) symptoms of, 19
Wilson's disease, 10, 12
Word specificity, 125
Word substitution, 125
WT. *See* Wada Test (WT)